NEW WEBSTER'S

MEDICAL
DICTIONARY

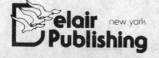
new york
Publishing

ISBN: 0-8326-0048-2

abdomen, that part of the human body which lies between the thorax and the pelvis, containing the stomach, liver, spleen, pancreas, kidneys, bladder, and intestines.

abdominoscopy, examination, especially by means of an instrument, of the abdomen or its contents.

abducens, the sixth cranial nerve, which supplies the external rectus muscle of the eye.

abducent muscles, muscles that pull back certain parts of the body from the mesial line.

abduct, to draw away from the main axis of the body or from a part of the body.

abductor, a muscle that moves certain parts from the axis of the body.

aberrant, 1. straying from the usual or normal method or course of action. 2. an aberrant structure, esp. in regard to variable chromosome numbers.

aberration, 1. deviation from the right course. 2. deviation of refracted light rays. 3. mental disorder.

ablate, to remove surgically.

ablation, the act of removal of a bodily part by surgery.

abnormal, deviating from normal.

abnormality, the state or quality of being abnormal.

abort, to miscarry in giving birth.

abortion, the act of spontaneous or induced expulsion of a fetus before it is at a viable stage. See also **miscarriage.**

abortionist, one who induces abortions, esp. illegal or unauthorized abortions.

abortus fever, see **brucellosis.**

abrade, to rub or wear down skin, primarily through friction.

abrasion. 1. the act of abrading. 2. an injury of the skin by abrading of the outer layer. 3. any scraped area.

abscess, a collection of purulent matter in the tissue of a body organ or part, with pain, heat, and swelling.

absolute, perfect or pure, as, absolute alcohol (ethyl alcohol containing not more than one percent by weight of water).

absorb, to soak up; suck up; incorporate; take in by capillarity.

absorbent, anything that absorbs; a substance applied to a wound to stanch or arrest the flow of blood.

absorption, the act or process of absorbing.

acantha, 1. the spine. 2. one of the acute processes of the vertebrae.

acariasis, a skin disease caused by mites. See also **scabies.**

accommodation, the adjustment of the eye lens whereby it is able to focus a clear image onto the retina.

accouchement, confinement; childbirth.

accoucheur, a surgeon who attends women in childbirth; obstetrician.

accoucheuse, midwife.

acetabulum, the cavity that receives the head of the thigh bone.

acetic, having the properties of vinegar.

acetic acid, an acid, often prepared by the oxidation of alcohol, and with water forming the chief ingredient of vinegar. Acetic acid is used as a reagent, caustic; sometimes taken internally.

acetone, a colorless liquid found in minute amounts in the body and in larger amounts in the blood and urine in diabetes, faulty metabolism, and after lengthy fasting. It can be produced synthetically.

acetylsalicylic acid, see **aspirin.**

achalasia, failure of the sphincter or other muscular valves to relax normally and allow the gastrointestinal contents to pass on.

ache, a dull pain.

ache, to suffer from an ache or pain; to be distressed.

Achilles heel, the point of weakness that is most vulnerable or suscepti-

ble.

Achilles tendon, the tendon that joins the heelbone and the muscles of the calf.

achondroplasia, defective development of cartilage causing dwarfism.

achromatin, that portion of the nucleus of a cell which is unstainable.

achromatopsia, see **color blindness.**

achromatous, having no color; of a lighter color than is usual or normal.

acid, 1. a compound that contains hydrogen as an essential constituent and has a sour taste, changes blue vegetable colors to red, neutralizes alkalis, and combines with bases to form salts. 2. informally, the hallucinogenic drug LSD-25.

acid-fast, not easily decolorized by acids when stained, as the tubercle bacillus.

acidity, the quality of being acid or sour.

acidophile, a tissue, organism, cell, or substance that shows an affinity toward an acidic environment.

acidophilic, 1. having the quality of being easy to stain with acid. 2. thriving or flourishing in an acid environment.

acidosis, abnormally high concentration of acid in the blood and body tissues.

acne, 1. an eruption of hard, inflamed tubercles or pimples on the face, esp. during adolescence. 2.

an inflammatory disease of the skin, arising from the obstruction of the sebaceous glands.

acoustic, pertaining to the sense or organs of hearing, or to the science of sound.

acoustics, 1. the science of sound. 2. the cause, nature, and phenomena of the vibrations of elastic bodies that affect the organ of hearing. 3. the properties determining audibility or fidelity of sound in an auditorium.

acquired character, a biological change that results from use or environment rather than from heredity.

acrid, sharp or biting to the taste or smell.

acriflavine, an acridine derivative used chiefly in medicine as an antiseptic.

acromegaly, a rare glandular disease, associated with overgrowth of bone, esp. in the jaws, hands, and feet.

acromial, pertaining to the acromion.

acromion, the outward end of the spine of the scapula or shoulder blade.

acrophobia, a pathological dread of high places.

ACTH, acronym for adrenocorticotropic hormone, a pituitary hormone that stimulates the cortex of the adrenal glands.

actin, a protein important in contraction of muscles.

actinodermatitis, see sunburn.

actinomycete, a member of the order Antinomycetales, which contains rod-shaped or filamentous bacteria.

actinomycin, one of the yellow-red or red polypeptide antibiotics separated from soil bacteria.

actinomycosis, a fungous disease in animals that is sometimes communicated to man; it most often invades the jaw.

actinotherapy, treatment of disease by rays of light, esp. ultraviolet or infrared radiation.

acuity, sharpness; acuteness; keen sense of perception.

acupuncture, an ancient Chinese technique of puncturing certain points in the body with long thin needles to treat painful conditions and to produce local anesthesia.

acute, a term applied to a disease that is attended by more or less violent symptoms and comes speedily to a crisis.

adactylia, absence of fingers or toes or both from birth.

adactylous, without fingers or toes.

Adam's apple, the prominence of the thyroid cartilage on the fore part of the throat, predominantly in men.

adaptation, a change, as of an organism's structure, to conform to environment.

addict, one who is addicted to a practice or a habit, esp. to narcotics.

addiction, 1. the state of being addicted. 2. habitual, compulsive use of narcotics.

addictive, 1. causing addiction. 2. one of a class of drugs that are habit-forming in nature.

Addison's disease, a disease characterized by asthenia, digestive disturbances, and usually a brownish coloration of the skin caused by disturbance of function of the suprarenal glands.

additive, a substance added in small amounts to another for improvement, as a drug added to medicine.

adduct, to draw (one's limb) toward the body's main axis.

adduction, the action by which a part of the body is drawn toward the bodily axis.

adductor, the muscle that draws toward the mesial line of the body.

adenalgia, a glandular pain.

adenectomy, the surgical removal of a gland.

Aden fever, see **dengue.**

adenine, a white, crystalline alkaloid, obtained from tea, glandular organs, or uric acid; used chiefly in medicine.

adenitis, inflammation of gland or lymph nodes.

adenocarcinoma, a malignant tumor that appears in glandular epithelium.

adenofibroma, a benign tumor of connective tissue frequently found in the uterus.

adenoid, an enlarged mass of lymphoid tissue in the upper pharynx that hinders nasal breathing.

adenoidectomy, surgical removal of the adenoids.

adenoma, a benign tumor originating in a gland.

adenomatosis, the condition of multiple glandular enlargement.

adenomatous, pertaining to adenoma.

adenopathy, disease of glands.

adenosarcoma, a malignant growth with characteristics of adenoma and sarcoma.

adenosine, a crystalline nucleoside, derived from the nucleic acid of yeast, which upon undergoing hydrolysis yields adenine and ribose.

adenosine diphosphate, a coenzyme, found in all living cells, important to the transfer of energy through the cell during glycolysis.

adenosine triphosphate, a nucleotide that occurs in all cells. It represents the reserve energy of muscle and is important to many biochemical processes that produce or require energy.

adenosis, see **adenopathy.**

adhesion, 1. a growth of scar tissue resulting from an incision. 2. the abnormal union of adjacent tissues resulting from inflammation.

adhesive tape, tape with a gummy substance on one side and having various uses, such as holding a bandage in place.

adipose, fat stored in the cells of adipose tissue.

adiposis, see **obesity.**

adiposis dolorosa, scattered areas of fat accumulations under the skin. The condition usually affects menopausal women.

adjuvant, a substance added to a prescription to aid the operation of the principal ingredient or basis.

Adler's theory, an approach to psychology based on the hypothesis that behavior is governed by an effort to compensate for inferiority or deficiency.

ad nauseam, to the point of being sickening.

adnexa, adjoining parts; accessory parts of a structure, as for instance ovaries and fallopian tubes.

adolescence, youth; the period of life between childhood and the full development of the body, or from puberty to full maturity.

adolescent, one who is in the teens and is in adolescence.

adrenal, pertaining to the adrenal gland or its secretions.

adrenal gland, a small endocrine gland consisting of a cortex and a medulla, attached to the kidney.

Adrenalin, a drug used as a heart stimulant, muscle relaxant, etc. (trademark).

adrenaline, epinephrine, a hormone secreted by the medulla of the adrenal gland.

adrenergic, liberated or activated by adrenaline or a similar substance.

adrenocorticotropic, affecting the adrenal cortex.

adrenocorticotropic hormone, see **ACTH.**

adsorbent, having the ability or tendency to adsorb.

adsorption, adhesion of a thin layer of liquid or gas to the surface of a solid body or liquid; the adhesion of molecules to a surface, as distinguished from absorption, the soaking up of a substance into the texture of a material.

adventitia, an external connective tissue that covers an organ.

aeremia, the presence of air in the blood.

aerobe, a microorganism whose existence requires the presence of air or free oxygen, as opposed to anaerobe.

aeromedicine, that branch of medicine concerned with disorders that result from or occur during flying.

aeroneurosis, a psychoneurotic condition occurring in airmen and aviators resulting from nervous tension, worry, or fatigue, characterized by mild depression, abdominal pain, insomnia, and nervous irritability.

aerophagia, the swallowing of air.

aerosol, 1. atomized particles ejected into the air from a pressurized can. 2. a solution of bactericidal substances that are atomized to sterilize the air of a room.

Aesculapian, 1. of or pertaining to Aesculapius, the Greco-Roman god of healing. 2. referring to the art of healing.

afebrile, without fever.

affection, 1. love, feeling. 2. an abnormal or morbid condition of body or mind.

affect, 1. emotion or feeling, as distinguished from cognition and volition. 2. an emotion with accompanying physical movements.

afferent, leading or conducting inward toward a center point, as certain nerves and veins; opposed to efferent.

afflict, to give, as pain that is continued or of some permanence, to the body or mind.

affliction, the state of being afflicted; a state of acute pain or distress of body or mind; the cause of this.

afflux, a flowing to, or that which flows to, as a stream of blood or other fluid to any part of the body.

afterbirth, the placenta and fetal membranes, which are expelled from the uterus after the birth of a child. Also called secundines.

afterbrain, the myelencephalon.

aftercare, the treatment and care required by a convalescent patient.

afterhearing, hearing sounds after the stimulus causing the sound has stopped.

afterimage, the image or sense impression that remains after the stimulus has disappeared.

afterpains, cramplike pains caused by contraction of the uterus after birth has occurred.

aftertaste, a taste that succeeds eating or drinking.

agar-agar, a gelatinous product derived from certain Asiatic seaweeds, used as a medium in bacteria culture, as a purgative, or as a stabilizer in certain foods.

agenesis, 1. a lack of or an imperfect development, as of a body part. 2. sterility.

agglutination, the clumping together of bacteria or other cells because of the introduction of an antibody.

agglutinin, an antibody that causes agglutination.

agglutinogen, any substance that stimulates the development of a specific agglutinin.

aglaucipsia, see **color blindness.**

agnosia, inability to comprehend a sensory perception, although the sensory sphere is intact. Agnosia results from disorders of the brain or nervous system.

agonad, one without sex glands.

agonal, relating to or

characteristic of agony.

agonist, a contracting muscle that is controlled by another opposing muscle.

agony, 1. extreme bodily or mental pain. 2. death struggle.

agoraphobia, pathological fear of open spaces.

agranulocyte, a leukocyte that does not have cytoplasmic granules.

agranulocytosis, a serious, destructive blood disease distinguished by a decrease of the leukocytes.

agraphia, a form of aphasia; a cerebral disorder, in which the patient is unable to express ideas by written signs.

agromania, pathological desire for solitude.

agrypnia, see **insomnia.**

ague, 1. an intermittent malarial fever with periodic chills. 2. a fit or attack of shivering. 3. a chill.

aguish, of or like ague.

air embolus, see **embolus.**

airsickness, a form of motion sickness affecting persons aboard an aircraft in flight. See **motion sickness.**

akinesia, complete or partial absence of muscle movement.

ala, an anatomical appendage resembling a wing.

alalia, the inability to speak because of defect or paralysis of the vocal organs.

alar, pertaining to or like a wing.

alba, 1. white. 2. the white

matter of the brain.

albedo, whiteness.

albinic, of or pertaining to albinism.

albinism, lack of pigment; inability to produce pigment.

albino, a person of abnormally pale, milky complexion, with light hair and pink eyes, resulting from a deficiency in pigmentation.

albumen, see **albumin.**

albumin, a member of a class of water-soluble proteins that are found in the juices and tissues of animals, in the white or clear viscous part of eggs, and in vegetables, and that contain sulfur, oxygen, hydrogen, carbon, and nitrogen.

albuminoid, having the characteristics of albumin.

albuminous, pertaining to or having the properties of albumin.

albuminuria, a condition in which the urine contains albumin, often indicating kidney disease.

alcohol, 1. any of a class of chemical compounds derived from hydrocarbons by replacing one or more of the hydrogen atoms with an equal number of hydroxyl radicals. 2. term for ethyl alcohol, the alcohol of commerce and medicine.

alcoholic, 1. pertaining to alcohol. 2. a habitual drunkard.

alcoholism, the condition of habitual drunkards who are poisoned by alcohol.

alcoholize, 1. to convert into alcohol. 2. to rectify (spirit) until it is wholly purified. 3. to make drunk or put under the influence of alcohol.

alcoholophilia, pathological craving for alcohol.

alcoholuria, alcohol in the urine.

aldehyde, a transparent colorless liquid produced by the oxidation of pure alcohol.

alethia, inability to forget.

aleukaemia, see **aleukemia.**

aleukemia, deficiency of white blood cells.

aleukocytosis, insufficient production of white blood cells.

alexia, a cerebral disorder marked by inability to read, or to read aloud.

algesia, supersensitiveness or increased sensitivity to pain.

algesic, painful.

alginuresis, ache on passing urine.

algolagnia, abnormal sexual pleasure derived from inflicting or enduring pain; sadism or masochism.

algophobia, an extreme dread or fear of pain.

alienation, 1. legal insanity. 2. mental sickness.

alienism, the scientific study and treatment of mental alienation or insanity.

alienist, one who studies or practices the psychiatric treatment of mental diseases.

aliment, food; nutriment.

alimental, of or pertaining to aliment.

alimentary, pertaining to aliment or food.

alimentary canal, the canal from the mouth to the anus through which food passes; digestive tract.

alimentation, the act or power of affording nutriment; the state of being nourished.

alimentology, the science of nutrition.

alinasal, pertaining to the wings of the nose.

alkali, any of various alkali metals that neutralize acids to form salts and turn red litmus paper blue; any of various other more or less active bases, as calcium hydroxide.

alkaline, the quality that constitutes an alkali.

alkalinity, 1. the state of being alkaline. 2. an excess of alkali.

alkalinuria, presence of alkali in the urine.

alkaloid, relating to or containing alkali.

alkalosis, a condition wherein the concentration of alkali in the body is higher than normal.

allele, in genetics, either a dominant or a recessive member of any pair of alternative characters, as tallness and shortness, which are present as genes and segregate at the time of sex cell production.

allelomorph, see **allele.**

allergen, any substance that induces allergy.

allergic, pertaining to or affected with allergy.

allergist, a medical specialist in the field of treating allergies.

allergy, excessive sensitivity producing a bodily reaction to certain substances, as food, pollen, drugs, or heat or cold, which are harmless to most persons; common allergies are hay fever, hives, and asthma.

allopath, a person who practices allopathy.

allopathy, method of treating disease by the use of agents producing effects different from those of the disease treated; opposed to **homeopathy.**

all-or-none, denoting either a complete response to a stimulus by a nerve or muscle, or none at all.

allotopia, displacement or malposition of an organ.

allotropism, a condition in which an element is present in two or more distinct forms with unlike properties.

almoner, a social worker who helps hospital patients with financial and social problems.

aloe, medicinal plant that yields a purgative drug, aloin.

alopecia, partial or total loss of hair from natural or abnormal causes.

altitude sickness, a condition caused by lack of oxygen at high altitudes.

alum, common or potash alum is used as an astringent and a styptic.

aluminosis, inflammation

of the lungs caused by inhaling aluminum dust, an occupational disease of alum workers.

alveolar, pertaining to the sockets of the teeth.

alveolar abscess, an abscess at the root of a tooth.

alveolus, 1. the socket of a tooth. 2. a terminal air sac deep within the lungs.

A.M.A., American Medical Association.

amalgam, an alloy of mercury with another metal or metals.

amaranth, a purplish-red nitrogen dye used to color medicines, cosmetics, and food.

amastia, absence of breast development.

amaurosis, partial or complete loss of sight from loss of power in the optic nerve or retina, without any visible defect in the eye except an immovable pupil.

amaurotic, pertaining to or affected with amaurosis.

ambidextrous, having the faculty of using both hands with equal ease and facility.

ambivalence, coexistence of contradictory feelings about a particular person, object, or action.

ambiversion, the state of being an ambivert.

ambivert, a person possessing characteristics of both the introvert and the extrovert.

amblyopia, dullness or dimness of eyesight without any apparent defect in the organs; the first stage of amaurosis.

ambulant, able to move from place to place; not confined to bed.

ambulance, vehicle fitted with suitable appliances for moving the injured and sick.

ambulate, to walk; travel; move about.

ambulatory, pertaining to an illness or condition that can be treated while the patient is able to walk about and is not confined to bed.

ameba, see amoeba.

amebiasis, see amoebic dysentery.

amelioration, improvement; moderation of a patient's condition.

amenorrhea, a morbid or unnatural suppression of menstruation.

amentia, imbecility; idiocy or dotage; deficiency of mental capacity.

ametropia, an abnormal condition of the eye with respect to refraction of light, as in myopia, etc.

amino acid, an organic compound forming the basic constituent of proteins.

aminopyrine, a drug used as a fever preventive and pain reliever.

amitosis, the direct method of cell division, characterized by simple cleavage of the nucleus, without formation of chromosomes.

amnesia, partial or complete loss of memory.

amnion, the innermost membrane surrounding the fetus.

amniotic fluid, the liquid or albuminous fluid contained in the amnion in which the embryo floats and which protects the fetus from injury.

amniotitis, inflammation of the amnion.

amoeba, a member of a genus of protozoa, a one-celled semifluid animal. Some species are parasitic in the human body and cause disease.

amoebic, 1. of or pertaining to amoebae. 2. characterized by or caused by the presence of amoebae, as certain diseases.

amoebic dysentery, a form of dysentery characterized by ulceration of the intestinal tract, caused by the amoeba.

amok, see amuck.

amorphous, having no determinate form.

amphetamine, a compound used as a drug to stimulate the central nervous system; prolonged use may cause drug dependence.

amphoteric, able to react as an acid or base, depending on environmental circumstances; having or showing the characteristics of both a base and an acid.

ampoule, see ampul.

ampul, a small, hermetically sealed vessel that holds a solution for hypodermic injection.

ampule, see ampul.

ampulla, a dilated section of a duct or canal.

ampullaceous, of, pertaining to, or like an ampulla.

amputate, to cut off, as a limb or other member, by a surgical operation; to remove all or part of by cutting.

amputation, the act of amputating.

amputee, one who has had one or more limbs, or parts of limbs, amputated.

amuck, a furious, reckless state, comparable to a psychotic disturbance, in which the afflicted runs about frantically, attacking at large.

amusia, music deafness; inability to produce or comprehend musical sounds.

amyelia, underdevelopment or congenital absence of spinal cord.

amyelineuria, partial paralysis or impaired functioning of the spinal cord.

amygdalin, a white glycosidic powder, obtained from bitter almonds, chiefly used medically as an expectorant.

amylase, any of the enzymes that convert starch into sugar, as in saliva.

amyloid, 1. starchlike; resembling starch. 2. a protein complex of starchlike characteristics forming a hard substance in tissues during diseases.

amylolysis, the conversion of starch into sugar, esp. by enzymes.

amylopsin, an enzyme of the pancreatic juice, capable of converting starch into sugar.

amylum, starch.

amyocardia, weakness of the heart muscle.

amyosthenia, lack of muscle tone; muscular weakness.

amyotonia, extreme flaccidity and smallness of the muscles, occurring mostly in early childhood.

amyotrophic lateral sclerosis, a chronic disease marked by muscular weakness and atrophy resulting from degeneration of the nerve tracts that supply the muscles, causing virtual paralysis.

amyotrophy, painful muscle wasting, usually of the deltoid muscle.

ana, in equal quantities; of each: used in medical prescriptions with reference to ingredients.

anabiosis, a return to life from a state resembling death.

anabolism, constructive metabolism: opposed to catabolism.

anabolite, a complex substance synthesized from a simpler form by constructive metabolism.

anadipsia, intense thirst.

anaemia, see **anemia.**

anaerobe, a microorganism that lives without air or free oxygen.

anaesthesia, see **anesthesia.**

anaesthetic, see **anesthetic.**

anaesthetist, see **anesthetist.**

anakusis, complete deafness.

anal, pertaining to or situated near the anus.

analeptic, invigorating; giving strength after disease; awakening, especially from drug stupor.

analgesia, absence of sensibility to pain while retaining consciousness.

analgetic, 1. pertaining to or causing analgesia. 2. a remedy that relieves pain.

analysand, one who undergoes psychoanalysis.

analysis, 1. the resolution of a compound substance into its constituent elements or component parts. 2. see **psychoanalysis.**

analyst, 1. one who analyzes. 2. see **psychoanalyst.**

analytic, pertaining to analysis.

anamnesis, the original case history of a psychiatric or medical patient.

anaphase, the stage in mitosis in which the chromosome halves move away from each other toward opposite ends of the cell.

anaphia, lack of or diminished sense of touch.

anaphoresis, insufficient or defective activity of the sweat glands.

anaphoretic, a substance that prevents sweating.

anaphrodisia, diminished sexual desire or sexual impotence.

anaphrodisiac, a substance capable of dulling or reducing sexual appetite.

anaphylaxis, increased susceptibility to the action of a foreign protein, such as penicillin, as the result of a first injection of

the substance. A special form of severe shock can follow a second injection.

anaplastic, of or pertaining to anaplasty.

anaplasty, plastic surgery.

anarthria, loss of the ability to articulate words.

anasarca, dropsy, of considerable extent, in the subcutaneous connective tissue.

anastigmat, a system of lenses in which astigmatic defects are overcome.

anastigmatic, not astigmatic: applied esp. to a lens, or a system of lenses, in which astigmatic defects are overcome.

anastomose, to unite or run into each other; to communicate with each other by minute branches or ramifications, as the arteries and veins.

anastomosis, union of vessels such as arteries and veins.

anastomotic, pertaining to anastomosis.

anatomist, one who is skilled in dissection or in the principles of anatomy.

anatomy, 1. the structure or study of the body. 2. dissection or cutting apart of an organized body.

ancon, the upper end of the ulna or elbow.

ancylostomiasis, hookworm disease, caused by any of certain bloodsucking nematode worms equipped with mouth hooks, which feed off the lining of the intestine of men and animals. The disease is characterized by severe anemia.

androgen, a substance, as androsterone, which promotes the development of secondary male sex characteristics.

androgynous, 1. having two sexes; being male and female; hermaphroditical. 2. having or partaking of the mental and physical characteristics of both sexes.

androsterone, a male sex hormone found in urine.

anemia, a deficiency of hemoglobin, resulting in a lack of energy and vitality; a state of the system marked by a deficiency in certain constituents of the blood.

anemic, pertaining to or affected with anemia.

anencephaly, impaired development of the brain and spinal cord.

anesthesia, 1. diminished or lost sense of feeling because of disease. 2. an artificially produced state of insensitivity, esp. to pain.

anesthesiologist, a physician specializing in anesthesiology.

anesthesiology, the science of the administration of anesthetics.

anesthetic, 1. of or belonging to anesthesia. 2. a substance having the power to deaden feeling or sensation.

anesthetist, one who administers anesthetics.

anesthetize, 1. to bring under the influence of an anesthetic agent. 2. to render insensible to pain.

aneurin, vitamin B_1.

aneurysm, a localized dilation of an artery, caused by the pressure of the blood acting on a part weakened by disease or injury.

angel's wing, abnormal prominence of the shoulder blades; also called winged scapulae.

anglitis, inflammation of a blood or lymphatic vessel.

angina, 1. any inflammatory affection of the throat or fauces. 2. a disease accompanied by spasms and a sense of suffocation.

angina pectoris, a disease characterized by paroxysms of acute pain in the chest, with a sense of suffocation, associated usually with morbid conditions of the heart or arteries caused by ischemia of the heart muscle.

angiocardiogram, an X ray of the heart and great blood vessels after the intravenous injection of a solution that makes the shape of these organs visible.

angiocarditis, inflammation of the heart and larger blood vessels.

angiology, the branch of anatomy that deals with the blood vessels and lymphatics.

angioma, a tumor consisting chiefly of dilated or newly formed blood or lymph vessels.

angioneurectomy, surgical removal of nerves and blood vessels.

angioplasty, repair of blood

vessels by plastic surgery.

angiospasm, spasmodic contractions of blood vessels.

angostura bark, the bitter aromatic bark of a South American rutaceous tree from which a stimulant and a medicine to reduce fever is extracted.

angst, anguish; feeling of dread.

anguish, 1. extreme pain or distress of either body or mind. 2. any keen affection of the emotions or feelings.

anhydrosis, diminution or complete absence of sweat.

anhydremia, lowering or lessening of the normal fluid content of the blood.

anhydrous, free of water.

animalcule, a minute animal, esp. one that is microscopic or invisible to the naked eye.

animal heat, heat formed in the body by metabolic acitvity.

animal magnetism, 1. any force or power in certain individuals said to give them the ability to induce hypnosis. 2. allure for persons of the opposite sex because of one's physical characteristics.

animal spirits, vigor, exuberance resulting from physical well-being and energy.

aniridia, complete or partial absence of the iris of the eye.

anisocytosis, inequality in size of cells, esp. red blood cells.

ankle, the joint connectng the foot and the leg.

anklebone, see talus.

ankylocolpos, partial closure of the vagina from adhesions.

ankylosis, 1. stiffness and immovability of a joint, as a result of disease or surgery. 2. morbid adhesion of the articular ends of contiguous bones.

ankylose, to affect with ankylosis; to grow together.

anlage, 1. the initial accumulation of cells in a growing organ or part. 2. the initial step in any development.

annular, having the form of a ring; pertaining to a ring.

annular ligament, a ring-shaped ligament.

anodmia, see anosmia.

anodyne, 1. any medicine that allays pain. 2. anything that diminishes stress.

anomalistic, pertaining to an anomaly.

anomalous, pertaining to an anomaly; irregular; peculiar; abnormal.

anomaly, 1. deviation from the common rule. 2. a malformation. 3. something abnormal.

anomia, loss of ability to remember names of persons and objects.

anonychia, absence of nails.

anopheles, a mosquito which, when infected with the organisms causing malaria, may transmit the disease to human beings by biting.

anorexia, pathological loss of appetite.

anorexia nervosa, loss of appetite accompanied by psychotic symptoms.

anosmia, deficiency or loss of the sense of smell.

anovulation, cessation of productin or discharge of ova.

anoxemia, a condition characterized by an abnormally low amount of oxygen in arterial blood.

anoxia, insufficient oxygen supply in body tissues.

antacid, an alkali, or a remedy for acidity in the stomach.

antagonism, opposition to the action of a substance on living tissues or cells.

antagonist, 1. a drug that counteracts the action of another drug. 2. a muscle that counteracts another muscle.

antalkali, a substance that neutralizes an alkali.

ante cibum, indicated on a prescription as a.c., meaning before a meal.

anteflexion, a bending forward, esp. of the body of the uterus.

antemortem, before death.

antenatal, before birth.

antepartum, before the onset of labor.

anterior, in front, as opposed to posterior.

anteversion, turning forward; displacement, as by tipping forward of an organ.

anthelmintic, a medicine that destroys parasitic intestinal worms.

anthracosis, black lung disease, a pneumoconiosis caused by breathing coal dust and silica, occurring mainly in those who work in coal mines.

anthrax, 1. a carbuncle. 2. a malignant ulcer. 3. a malignant infectious disease of certain warmblooded animals, which may be transmitted to man.

anthropophobia, a pathological fear of human companionship or of society in general.

anthropoid, 1. resembling man. 2. any of the larger apes.

anthropologic, pertaining to anthropology.

anthropologist, one who specializes in anthropology.

anthropology, the science of man and mankind, including the study of the physical and mental constitution of man, his cultural development and social conditions, as exhibited both in the present and in the past.

anthropometric, about or referring to anthropometry.

anthropometry, the comparative measurement and study of the human body.

antibacterial, an agent destroying or stopping the growth of bacteria.

antibiosis, a relationship between two organisms that is harmful to one, as parasitism.

antibiotic, any of a variety of substances produced by fungi or synthetically which, in diluted solution, inhibit or destroy bacteria; included are penicillin and the "mycin" drugs.

antibody, any of various substances existing in the blood or developed in immunization that counteract toxins or bacterial poisons in the system.

anticoagulant, any agent that prevents coagulation, esp. of the blood.

antidiuretic, an agent that acts to reduce excretion of urine.

antidotal, having the quality of an antidote.

antidote, a medicine that neutralizes the effects of poison.

antienzyme, 1. a substance that retards, inhibits, or prevents enzymatic action. **2.** a chemical substance (an antibody) produced by an organism to inhibit or counteract the effect of a foreign enzyme.

antifebrile, having the quality of abating fever.

antigalactic, an agent that diminishes or prevents the secretion of milk.

antigen, a substance that gives rise to an antibody when introduced into blood or tissue.

antihistamine, any of a number of compounds that inactivate histamine in the body, used mainly for the treatment of allergies and colds.

antimalarial, 1. preventing malaria or its growth. **2.** any such agent.

antimicrobial, destroying or retarding the growth of microbes.

antimonic, of or containing antimony.

antimony, a metallic element used chiefly in alloys and in medicine.

antimycotic, an agent inhibiting the growth of or destroying fungi.

antipathy, natural aversion.

antiperiodic, efficacious against periodic diseases, as intermittent fever.

antiperistalsis, peristalsis moving toward the oral end (reverse of the usual direction).

antiphlogistic, 1. counteracting inflammation or an excited state of the system. **2.** a medicine that checks inflammation.

antipyretic, a remedy efficacious against fever.

antipyrine, a white, crystalline powder used to reduce fever or relieve pain.

antiscorbutic, 1. counteracting scurvy or a scorbutic tendency. **2.** a remedy for or a preventive of scurvy.

antisepsis, 1. the inhibition or destruction of microorganisms. **2.** prevention of sepsis.

antiseptic, 1. pertaining to or effecting antisepsis. **2.** devoid of germs. **3.** an agent that inhibits the growth of microorganisms.

antiserum, a serum containing antibodies for a specific antigen.

antisocial, opposed or averse to social intercourse or relations.

antispasmodic, 1. something that relieves spasms. **2.** relieving or preventing spasms.

antitetanus, a substance used to destroy the germ of tetanus or lockjaw.

antithyroid, capable of preventing overactivity of the thyroid gland.

antitoxic, counteracting poisons or toxic influences.

antitoxin, a substance formed in the body, capable of counteracting a specific toxin or infective agency.

antitussive, apt to control or capable of controlling or counteracting a cough.

antivene, see **antivenin.**

antivenin, 1. an antitoxin produced in the blood by repeated injections of venom, as of snakes. 2. the antitoxic serum obtained from such blood.

antiviral, something that is effective in inhibiting a virus.

antivitamin, a substance that makes a vitamin powerless.

antivivisectionist, one who is opposed to scientific experimentation on living animals.

antrum, any nearly closed chamber or cavity in a hollow organ, esp. the cavity in bones.

anuresis, inability to bring about the act of urination.

anuria, 1. total suppression of urine. 2. failure to urinate because of lack of urine.

anus, the lower orifice of the alimentary canal.

anvil, the incus, one of the three small bones in the ear.

anxiety, pain or uneasiness

of mind in respect to some future or uncertain event.

aorta, the great artery or trunk of the arterial system, proceeding from the left ventricle of the heart, and giving origin to all the arteries except the pulmonary.

aortic stenosis, narrowing of the aorta resulting from lesions of the wall caused by scar tissue or infection as rheumatic fever; hypertrophy of the heart is a usual result.

aortitis, inflammation of the aorta.

apareunia, inability to have sexual intercourse.

apathetic, 1. affected with or proceeding from apathy. 2. devoid of feeling; insensible. 3. displaying no emotion; indifferent.

apathy, 1. want of feeling. 2. privation of passion, emotion, or excitement. 3. insensibility; indifference.

aperient, 1. gently purgative. 2. a medicine that gently opens the bowels; a laxative.

aperiodic, 1. not periodic, as a fever. 2. of irregular occurrence.

aperitif, see **aperitive.**

aperitive, a stimulant for the appetite.

aphagia, inability to swallow.

aphakia, absence of the crystalline lens of the eye.

aphasia, loss of the faculty of speech, or of connecting words and ideas.

aphemia, motor aphasia, esp. a form marked by inability to express ideas in spoken words.

aphonia, loss of voice.

aphonogelia, the inability to laugh out loud.

aphrasia, a nervous disorder that causes inability to use connected phrases when speaking.

aphrodisia, sexual passion.

aphrodisiac, 1. exciting sexual desire. 2. food or medicine exciting sexual desire.

aphtha, a small ulcer occurring usually in the mouth.

aphthous fever, see **foot-and-mouth disease.**

aplasia, congenital absence or defective development of a tissue or organ.

apnea, temporary cessation of breathing.

apocrine, pertaining to cells that lose part of their cytoplasm while functioning, esp. gland cells, such as the cells of the mammary glands and of certain sweat glands.

apodal, having no feet.

apomorphine, a drug used as an emetic and expectorant.

aponeurosis, a white, shining, and very resistant membrane surrounding the voluntary muscles and large arteries.

apoplectic, pertaining to apoplexy; predisposed to apoplexy.

apoplexy, abolition or sudden diminution of sensation and voluntary motion, resulting from congestion or rupture of a blood vessel of the brain (stroke).

appendectomy, surgical excision of the vermiform appendix.

appendicitis, inflammation of the appendix.

appendicular, relating to an appendage or limb.

appendix, something appended or added; medically the term usually refers to the vermiform appendix, a small hollow blind process attached to the cecum.

appestat, an area of the brain supposed to control appetite for food and satiety.

appetite, the natural desire for food, not necessarily hunger.

apyrexia, absence of or intermission of fever.

aqua, 1. water. 2. a solution, esp. used in pharmacy.

aqueous, of, like, or containing water; watery.

aqueous humor, the watery fluid that fills the anterior and posterior chambers of the eye between the crystalline lens and the cornea.

arachnoid, weblike.

arachnoid membrane, the semitransparent, thin center membrane that covers the brain and spinal cord.

arcuate, bent or curved in the form of a bow or an arc.

arcus, an arc or arch.

arcus senilis, the opaque white ring that appears in old age around the corneal periphery because of cholesterol deposits.

areola, 1. a small area or space. 2. a space between two tissues. 3. the colored circle or halo surrounding the nipple or surrounding a pustule. 4. the part of the iris surrounding the pupil of the eye.

areole, see **areola.**

ariboflavinosis, a disease caused by a deficiency of riboflavin (vitamin B_2 or G) in the diet.

arnica, a composite plant, also called mountain tobacco. A tincture of its dried flower heads is used as an application to wounds and bruises.

aromatic, a plant, drug, or medicine that yields a fragrant odor and often a warm, pungent taste.

arrector pili, the minute muscles arising in the skin connected with the hair follicles that contract when stimulated by cold or fright, causing the hair to "stand on end" and the condition called "gooseflesh."

arrhythmia, absence or disturbance of rhythm, as in heartbeat.

arrhythmic, without regularity or rhythm.

arsenic, an element of grayish-white substance with a metallic luster, forming poisonous compounds used in medicine and industry.

arterial, pertaining to an artery or to the oxygenated blood contained in the arteries.

arterialize, to change venous blood to arterial blood by oxygenation.

arteriectomy, removal of an artery or part of an artery by surgery.

arteriography, the visualization of an artery or arterial system by X ray after the injection of a radiopaque medium.

arteriola, see **arteriole.**

arteriolar, pertaining to arterioles.

arteriole, 1. a small muscle-walled artery. 2. a terminal (end) artery feeding the capillaries.

arterioplasty, an operation to repair or reconstruct an artery.

arteriosclerosis, a disease in which thickening of the walls of arteries impedes circulation of the blood.

arteriospasm, spasm of an artery.

arteriostenosis, temporary or permanent narrowing of the duct of an artery.

arteriovenous, relating to the veins and arteries.

arteritis, inflammation of an artery.

artery, one of a system of cylindrical vessels or tubes that convey the blood from the heart to all parts of the body, to be brought back again by the veins.

arthralgia, pain, esp. neuralgic pain, in a joint.

arthritic, pertaining to or affected by arthritis.

arthritis, any inflammation of the joints.

arthrography, the inside of a joint shown by X rays. It is usually necessary to inject the joint with a substance opaque to X rays.

arthropathy, any disease of a joint.

arthroplasty, 1. surgical repair of a joint. 2. the making of an artificial joint.

arthrosclerosis, stiffening or hardening of a joint or joints, occurring esp. in the aged.

arthrosis, 1. a joint. 2. any disease causing trophic degeneration of a joint. 3. an articulation or suture of two bones or cartilages.

arthrosynovitis, inflammation of the membrane lining of a joint.

articular, pertaining to the joints.

articulate, 1. to unite by means of a joint. 2. pertaining to one who speaks with ease or facility of vocabulary.

articulation, 1. a joining or juncture, as of the bones. 2. the part between two joints. 3. a joint. 4. distinct and clear speech.

articulatory, of or concerned with articulation.

artifact, any unnatural change in structure or tissue.

artificial insemination, mechanical injection of spermatozoa into the uterus.

artificial respiration, a method by which air is rhythmically forced into and out of the lungs of a person whose respiration has ceased.

arytenoid, ladle-shaped; usually referring to the two cartilages of the larynx to which the vocal cords are attached.

asbestosis, a lung disease caused by the inhalation of asbestos particles.

ascaris, an intestinal worm.

ascites, the presence of excessive fluid in the abdominal cavity.

ascorbic acid, the antiscorbutic vitamin C, abundant in citrus fruits, tomatoes, and green vegetables; also produced synthetically.

asepsis, absence of microorganisms; prevention of sepsis; sterile.

aseptic, free from disease-causing germs.

asexual, not sexual.

Asian cholera, an acute, infectious, epidemic disease. See **cholera.**

Asian influenza, a variant epidemic form of influenza, probably originating in China. Also called Asian flu.

aspergillosis, condition characterized by the presence of a fungus of the genus *Aspergillus* in tissues or on a mucous surface.

aspermia, failure to produce or ejaculate sperm.

asperity, roughness or harshness to the touch, taste, hearing, or feelings.

asphyxia, lack of oxygen or an excess of carbon dioxide in the system as a result of some interference with respiration; suffocation.

asphyxiate, to bring to a state of asphyxia.

aspirate, 1. to remove fluid

from a body. 2. to inhale fluid into the lungs.

aspiration, 1. the removal of fluid from the body using an aspirator. 2. drawing in or out as by suction.

aspirator, a device that uses suction to remove air, liquids, or granular substances from a cavity of the body.

aspirin, 1. a white crystalline derivative of salicylic acid used to relieve pain and reduce fever. 2. a tablet made of this.

astasia, the inability to stand or sit erect resulting from loss of motor coordination.

asteatosis, any disease in which there is a loss of activity of the sebaceous glands or scantiness of their secretions.

asternal, not connected to the sternum or breastbone.

astereognosis, inability to recognize forms or objects by touch.

asthenia, debility; want of strength.

asthenic, characterized by asthenia; weak; frail; slight in build.

asthenopia, weakness of the eye muscles or visual power because of fatigue.

asthma, a chronic, paroxysmal disorder of respiration, characterized by difficulty in breathing.

asthmatic, 1. pertaining to asthma; affected by asthma. 2. a person suffering from asthma.

astigmatic, pertaining to or

exhibiting astigmatism.

astigmatism, a defect of the eye or of a lens whereby rays of light from an external point fail to converge to a focus, thus giving rise to imperfect vision or images.

astragalus, the talus, or anklebone.

astraphobia, pathological fear of lightning and thunderstorms.

astringent, 1. contracting; styptic. 2. an agent that contracts the organic tissues and canals of the body, thereby checking or diminishing bleeding or excessive discharges. 3. an astringent substance, as alum, catechu, etc.

astrocyte, a star-shaped neurological cell.

astrocytoma, a tumor formed by astrocytes.

asystole, faulty contraction of the ventricles of the heart, preventing it from performing a complete systole.

Atabrine, quinacrine, used in the treatment of malaria (trademark).

atactilia, failure of the sense of touch.

ataractic, a drug that decreases anxiety or tension; a tranquilizer.

atavism, the recurrence of any peculiarity or disease of an ancestor.

ataxia, irregularity in the functions of the muscles.

atelocheilia, see **harelip.**

atelectasis, 1. partial collapse of the lung. 2. failure of the lung to expand completely, esp. at birth.

atheroma, a condition in

which there is a deposit of lipids (fats) within the inner walls of an artery, often causing arteriosclerosis.

atherosclerosis, a disease in which an artery is dangerously narrowed by lipid deposits in the inner walls; one of the three types of arteriosclerosis.

athetosis, a condition in which the hands and feet continually perform involuntary, slow, irregular movements.

athlete's foot, ringworm of the feet, a contagious disease caused by a fungus that grows in wet or damp areas.

athrombia, defective clotting of the blood.

atlas, the first vertebra of the neck.

atomizer, an apparatus for reducing a liquid to a spray for disinfecting, cooling, perfuming, etc.

atonic, characterized by atony.

atony, 1. a want of tone; flaccidity. 2. defect of muscular power; debility.

atopy, an allergic disorder, as acquired or inherited hypersensitivity of the skin to a drug or other agent.

atresia, closure of a normal body orifice, such as anus or vagina, caused by failure of development or disease.

atrioventricular, relating or referring to both the ventricles and atria (auricles) of the heart.

atrium, either of the two receiving chambers of the heart; the auricles.

atrophic, pertaining to or characterized by atrophy.

atrophy, a wasting away of the body or of an organ or part, as from defective nutrition or other causes; degeneration.

atropine, a highly poisonous alkaloid obtained from the deadly nightshade, used esp. to dilate the pupil of the eye and alleviate spasms.

attenuate, to make thin; to make slender or fine; to reduce in density; to dilute; to weaken; to lower; to reduce.

attic, that portion of the ear lying above the tympanic cavity.

audiogram, a record of the audiometer.

audiometer, an instrument for testing the power of hearing.

auditory, relating to hearing or to the sense or organs of hearing.

auditory nerve, the nerve of hearing, going from the organs of hearing and the semicircular canals to the brain; the eighth cranial nerve.

aura, a feeling or sensation that precedes an attack of some kind, such as hysteria or epilepsy.

aural, relating to the ear.

Aureomycin, an antibiotic isolated from a fungus (trademark).

auricle, 1. the external ear. 2. either of the two cavities in the heart, situated above the two ventricles and resembling in shape the external ear.

auricular, 1. pertaining to the ear or the sense of hearing. 2. pertaining to one of the auricles of the heart.

auriscope, an instrument for examining the eardrum.

aurotherapy, the use of gold salts in the treatment of disease.

auscultate, to examine by listening to the sounds of the viscera by auscultation.

auscultation, a method of distinguishing the state of the internal parts of the body, particularly of the chest, by observing the sounds arising there through the application of the ear or the stethoscope.

autism, the tendency to escape reality through daydreams or fantasy.

autoclave, airtight vessel for sterilizing objects by means of high-pressure steam.

autodigestion, digestion of tissues or destruction of cells by their own secretions.

autogenous, self-produced; generated within the body.

autograft, a graft made by taking tissue from one part of the body and using it at another part of the same body.

autohypnosis, self-induced hypnosis.

autoinfection, infection of the body from within.

autoinoculation, inoculation or vaccination of a healthy part with virus from a diseased part of the same body.

autointoxication, poisoning by toxic substances formed within the body.

autologous, grafted, transplanted, or relocated within the same body.

autolysin, any agent or substance that produces autolysis.

autolysis, digestion or disintegration of tissue by ferments generated in the cells.

automatism, performance of actions without conscious volition, as sleepwalking.

autonomic nervous system, that part of the nervous system which innervates the blood vessels, heart, viscera, smooth muscles, and glands and regulates involuntary actions.

autoplasty, the repairing of lesions with tissue from another part of the same body.

autopsy, dissection and inspection of a body after death to determine the cause of death; a postmortem examination.

autosome, any chromosome that is not a sex chromosome.

autosuggestion, suggestion by the mind to itself of ideas that operate to produce actual or physical effects.

autotherapy, 1. spontaneous cure. 2. the treatment of disease using the patient's own body secretions.

autotoxemia, self-poisoning by absorption of a poisonous substance produced in the body.

autotoxin, a poisonous principle formed within the body and acting against it.

avitaminosis, a disease caused by vitaminic deficiency.

avulse, to separate or detach forcibly, as the flesh of a wound.

avulsion, a pulling or tearing apart or off, as by surgery.

axanthopia, the inability to see the color yellow.

axilla, armpit.

axis, the pivotal vertebra of the neck on which the head turns.

axon, a long, single nerve cell process that carries transmitted nerve impulses away from the body of the cell.

azoospermia, absence of spermatozoa from the seminal fluid.

azote, nitrogen.

azotemia, a large accumulation of nitrogenous waste in the blood resulting from a kidney malfunction.

azotic, of or pertaining to azote; nitric.

azoturia, 1. an overabundance of urea in the urine. 2. an excess of other nitrogenous substances in the urine.

azygous, not one of a pair; single. Applied to certain muscles, etc.

Babinski reflex, a normal reflex action in children up to one year of age in which the large toe extends upward when the sole of the foot is stroked. In adults the reflex is a sign of certain diseases of the brain or spinal cord.

baby, a very young child; an infant.

bacillary, relating to or caused by bacilli.

bacillemia, the presence of bacilli in the blood.

bacilluria, the presence of bacilli in the urine.

bacillus, any rod-shaped bacterium that produces spores in the presence of free oxygen.

bacitracin, an antibiotic effective against bacterial infections.

back, 1. the posterior part of the trunk. 2. the region of the spine.

backache, pain or discomfort generally located in the small of the back and often caused by muscle stress.

backbone, the bone of the back; the spine; the vertebral column.

bacteria, see **bacterium**.

bacterial, of, pertaining to, or caused by bacteria.

bactericidal, capable of killing bacteria.

bactericide, anything capable of destroying bacteria.

bacteriologic, pertaining to or concerned with bacteriology.

bacteriology, the study of bacteria and the part they

play in medicine, agriculture, and industry.

bacteriolysis, the process of dissolving or destruction of bacteria.

bacteriophage, any of a group of viruses that effect bacteriolysis on specific viruses found in sewage or body products.

bacteriophobia, pathological fear of bacteria.

bacterioscopy, microscopic investigation of bacteria.

bacteriostasis, 1. prevention of the growth of bacteria. 2. a substance used for bacteriostasis.

bacterium, (singular of bacteria) any of the microscopic organisms of the class Schizomycetes, having round, spiral, or rod-shaped bodies, which occur in soil, water, organic matter such as sewage, and animal tissues. Typhoid or pneumonia bacteria are disease-producing, whereas others are useful in bringing about fermentation in many industrial processes.

bacterization, 1. the condition of being bacterized. 2. the process of bacterizing.

bacterize, to expose to the decomposing effects of bacteria.

bag of waters, see **amnion.**

baker's itch, eczema caused by handling yeast and dough.

baker's leg, see **knock-knee.**

balanitis, inflammation of the glans penis.

balanus, the glans of the penis or the glans of the clitoris.
discharge.

basal metabolism, the amount of energy required by a person to maintain minimum vital functions.

basement membrane, a thin layer of connective tissue cells underlying the epithelium.

basiphobia, pathological fear of walking.

basophil, cell or tissue easily stained with basic dyes.

bathophobia, pathological fear of looking down from high places; fear of depth.

bathycardia, a condition in which the heart is positioned abnormally low in the thorax.

battle fatigue, a neurosis suffered by soldiers after prolonged combat duty and exposure to danger, rendering them incapable of further fighting.

B complex, see **vitamin B complex.**

bedpan, a utensil for urination or defecation by bed-ridden persons.

bedside manner, the attitude and approach of the physician toward his patient.

bedsore, 1. a sore liable to affect bedridden persons on the parts of the body subjected to the most pressure. 2. afflicted with skin irritation caused by prolonged illness in bed.

bed-wetting, see **enur-**

esis.

behavior, the aggregate of observable actions or activities of the individual as matter for psychological study.

behaviorism, a theory or method of psychological procedure that regards objective facts of behavior or activity, in the broadest sense, of both men and animals as the proper matter for study.

behaviorist, 1. an advocate of behaviorism. 2. one who follows the methods of behaviorism.

behavioristic, pertaining to behaviorism or behaviorists.

belch, to involuntarily expel wind from the stomach in a noisy manner.

belladonna, a poisonous plant from the leaves and root of which atropine is derived.

Bell's palsy, facial paralysis caused by an acute inflammatory reaction in or around the seventh, or facial, nerve.

belly, that part of the human body which extends from the breast to the thighs, containing the bowels; the abdomen.

bellyache, pain in the abdomen.

bellybutton, colloquial: navel.

belonephobia, pathological fear of sharp-pointed objects.

Benadryl, one of the antihistaminic drugs (trademark).

bends, see **caisson disease.**

benign, 1. mild. 2. not malignant. 3. not severe or violent.

Benzedrine, a drug used to stimulate the central nervous system (trademark).

benzoate of soda, a water-soluble powder used in medicine and as a food preservative.

benzocaine, a crystalline ester, employed, usually in an ointment, as a local anesthetic.

beriberi, a form of multiple neuritis caused by a lack of vitamin B_1, characterized by loss of muscular power, emaciation, and exhaustion.

betweenbrain, see **diencephalon.**

bhang, see **hashish.**

bicarbonate of soda, see **sodium bicarbonate.**

biceps, 1. a muscle having two heads or origins. 2. the name of two muscles, one of the upper arm, the other of the thigh.

bicipital, pertaining to the biceps.

bicuspid, 1. having two cusps or projections. 2. one of eight human bicuspid teeth, located in pairs behind the canine teeth in the upper and lower jaws. 3. a premolar.

bifid, cleft or divided into two parts; forked.

bifocal lens, a lens with two parts; one for near and one for distant vision.

bifocals, eyeglasses with bifocal lenses.

bifurcation, a forking or division into two branches.

bile, a bitter, viscid, yellow

or greenish alkaline liquid secreted by the liver and aiding in digestion.

bile acid, an acid found in bile that promotes the digestion of fats and aids in the absorption of many water-insoluble, organic substances.

bile duct, the tube through which the liver secretion passes as it leaves the gall bladder.

bilharziasis, see **schistosomiasis.**

biliary, pertaining to the bile or gallbladder or to the bile-conveying passages.

bilious, suffering from, caused by, or attended with disorder of the liver or bile.

bilirubin, a reddish-yellow pigment of urine, blood, or bile.

biliverdin, a greenish pigment found in bile.

bilobed, divided into two lobes.

bilocular, divided into two cells or small compartments.

bimanual, involving the use of both hands.

binocular, pertaining to or employing both eyes.

binovular, derived from two eggs; as binovular twins, where each baby comes from a separate egg.

bioassay, quantitative determination or estimate of the biological activity or potency of a substance, such as a hormone, by observation of its action on a test organism.

bioastronautics, the study of the biological, be-

havioral, and medical effects of flight and space travel; space medicine.

biocatalyst, a substance that accelerates or modifies a physiological process, such as a hormone.

biochemistry, the science of the chemical processes of living things.

biocide, destruction of living organisms by such unphysiologic effects of civilization as pollution, nuclear fallout, and pesticides.

bioclimatology, the study of the relations of climate and life, particularly the effects of climate on the health and activity of living things.

biogravics, a branch of science, developed since the start of space flight, that studies the effects of weightlessness and excessive gravitational force on living organisms.

bioinstrument, an apparatus fastened to the body to record physiological information.

biological clock, an internal mechanism in living organisms that commands the rhythmic cycles of diverse involuntary activities.

biological electricity, the electricity created by living beings and cells.

biologist, one skilled in or one who studies biology.

biology, the science of life and living things.

biomedicine, a field of medical science concerned with the ability of a human being to live and function in abnormal environments.

biometry, 1. the measurement of life; the calculation of the probable duration of human life. 2. the branch of biological science concerned with the quantitative statistics of the properties and phenomena of living things.

biophysics, the study of living things using the method and principles of physics.

biopolymer, a polymeric material, such as protein, produced in a living system.

biopsy, the examination of tissue from a living subject for diagnostic purposes.

biosynthesis, the synthesis of a chemical within and by a living organism.

biotelemetry, the remote measuring and evaluation of life functions, as in spacecraft and artificial satellites.

biotin, a crystalline growth vitamin of the vitamin B complex, vital in the prevention of animal death from an excess of egg white in the diet; presumably also important for man.

biotype, a group of organisms or individuals having many of the same or similar genetic traits and physiological characteristics.

biovular, originating from two ova, such as fraternal twins.

biparous, giving birth to twins.

bipartite, composed of two parts.

biped, an animal having two feet, as man.

bipedal, having two feet.

birth, the act or process of being born.

birth control, the prevention or regulation of conception by the use of drugs, by devices used by either male or female, by restriction of sexual intercourse to the so-called safe period, or by surgical sterilization.

birthmark, a congenital mark on the body. See also **nevus.**

birthrate, the ratio of the number of births in a given time and population to the total population (usually expressed in terms of the number of births per one thousand of population).

birth trauma, severe emotional stress experienced by a child at birth, considered in psychoanalytic theory a likely source of neurosis in later years.

bisexual, 1. having the organs of both sexes in one individual. 2. of two sexes.

bisexuality, 1. hermaphroditism. 2. sexual attraction to individuals of both sexes.

bisferious, see **dicrotic.**

bismuth, a brittle metallic element, having compounds used in medicine.

bitemporal, pertaining to both temporal bones.

bistoury, a small, narrow surgical knife, used for minor incisions.

Black Death, the bubonic plague, which first occurred in Europe in epidemic form during the fourteenth century; characterized by black spots on the skin. See also **plague.**

black eye, 1. an eye with a black or blackish-brown iris. 2. an eye with the surrounding flesh or skin discolored by a blow or bruise.

blackhead, a comedo or skin blemish consisting of a blackish fatty secretion in a follicle.

black lung, see **pneumoconiosis.**

blackout, temporary loss of vision or consciousness; loss of memory.

black out, to suffer a transient loss of vision, memory, or consciousness.

black vomit, 1. a dark-colored substance, consisting chiefly of altered blood, vomited in some cases of yellow fever. 2. yellow fever.

blackwater fever, an acute form of malaria occurring in tropical and semitropical regions, characterized by febrile paroxysms and bloody urine.

bladder, 1. a distensible sac with muscular and membranous walls, serving as a receptacle for the urine secreted by the kidneys. 2. any similar sac or receptacle, as the gallbladder. 3. a vesicle, blister, etc. filled with fluid or air.

bland, soothing, mild.

blastema, the mass of undifferentiated cells from which an organ or a body part is evolved during embryonic development.

blastocyst, the blastula, having a knob of cells at one side that develops into the embryo, the remainder developing into the placenta.

blastogenesis, the theory of the transmission of hereditary characteristics by genes.

blastoma, a tumor originating in immature cells.

blastomere, any of the cells into which the ovum segments after fertilization.

blastomycete, a yeastlike fungus capable of causing disease.

blastula, the stage in embryonic development at the end of or immediately following the stage of cleavage of the ovum, consisting of a ball made up of a single layer of cells enclosing a fluid-filled cavity.

bleb, a blister or pustule; a small vesicular body.

bleeder, see **hemophilia.**

blemish, a noticeable defect, flaw, or imperfection, usually of the skin.

blennorrhagia, 1. a profuse mucous discharge, esp. a gonorrheal discharge from the penis or vagina. 2. gonorrhea.

blennuria, an excess of mucus in the urine.

blepharitis, inflammation of the edges of the eyelids.

blepharon, the eyelid.

blind, devoid of the sense

of sight; not having sight.

blindness, see **amaurosis.**

blind spot, the point in the retina that is insensitive to light; situated where the optic nerve enters the eye.

blister, a thin vesicle on the skin containing watery matter or serum, as from an injury; a pustule.

blood, the fluid that circulates in the arteries and veins or principal vascular system, being of a red color and consisting of a pale yellow plasma containing semisolid corpuscles, some red and some white.

blood bank, an institution for storing and processing blood or blood plasma.

blood cell, a basic structural unit of the blood. See also **blood corpuscle.**

blood clot, the jellylike mass formed as liquid blood congeals when blood vessels are injured.

blood corpuscle, 1. a cell circulating in the blood. 2. a red cell or corpuscle; see also **erythrocyte.** 3. a white cell or corpuscle; see also **leukocyte.**

blood count, determination of the number and proportion of red and white cells in a specific volume of blood.

blood group, one of several classifications into which human blood can be divided, based on the proportion of specific antigens.

blood heat, the normal temperature, about 98.6°F, of human blood.

bloodless, 1. without blood; 2. drained of blood. 3. dead.

bloodletting, the act of letting blood or bleeding, as by opening a vein, as a remedial measure. See also **phlebotomy.**

bloodmobile, a motor vehicle equipped to receive donations of human blood.

blood plasma, the clear, almost colorless fluid of the blood when separated from blood corpuscles by centrifuging: used in blood transfusions, since it clots as easily as whole blood.

blood platelet, a minute circular or oval body found in blood, necessary for blood clotting.

blood poisoning, a diseased condition of the blood caused by the presence of toxic matter or microorganisms; toxemia; septicemia; pyemia.

blood pressure, the pressure exerted by the blood against the inner walls of the blood vessels, varying in different parts of the body, with exertion, excitement, strength of the heart, age, or health.

blood serum, the yellowish, clear liquid remaining after all solid constituents of the blood have been removed.

bloodshot, red and inflamed because of excessively dilated capillaries: said of the eye.

bloodstream, the blood flowing through the circulatory system.

blood sugar, glucose, supplied by the liver, circulating in the blood.

blood test, the test of a blood sample to determine such qualities as blood type, or such quantities as sugar content.

blood vessel, any of the vessels of the body, arteries, veins, capillaries, through which the blood circulates.

blotch, an inflamed eruption or discolored patch on the skin.

blue baby, an infant with a bluish color caused by congenital heart disease or defective lungs.

blue-yellow blindness, a rare form of color blindness in which the individual cannot differentiate between blue and yellow.

boil, a painful, suppurating, inflammatory sore forming a central core, caused by microbic infection; a furuncle.

bolus, a soft round mass of anything medicinal to be swallowed at once, larger and less solid than an ordinary pill.

bone, the hard, porous material that forms the skeleton.

borborygmus, the rumbling sound caused by the movement of gas or fluid in the large intestine.

boric acid, an acid derived from boron trioxide, esp. a white crystalline acid

occurring in nature or prepared from borax and used as a weak antiseptic.

botulin, a neurotoxin sometimes found in improperly canned meats and vegetables.

botulinus, the bacterium **Clostridium botulinum,** which forms the toxin causing botulism.

botulism, a severe form of poisoning caused by eating spoiled food containing the toxin botulin.

bougie, 1. a slender, flexible instrument for dilating or opening passages of the body. 2. a pencil of medicated paraffin or other readily melting substance for introduction into the body. 3. a suppository.

bowels, see **intestines.**

bowleg, an outward curvature of the legs, causing a separation of the knees when the ankles are in contact.

brachial, pertaining to the arm, esp. the upper arm or brachium.

brachialgia, pain in the arm.

brachium, the upper arm, from the shoulder to the elbow.

brachycephalic, short-headed; having a breadth of skull at least four-fifths as great as the length from front to back: opposed to **dolichocephalic.**

brachycranial, short-skulled or broad-skulled.

brachydactylous, having fingers and toes shorter

than normal.

bradycardia, abnormally slow heart action.

bradyuria, extremely slow passing of urine.

bradykinesia, exaggerated slowness of movement.

bradypnoea, slow or labored breathing.

brain, the soft, convoluted mass of grayish and whitish nerve substance filling the cranium of man and other vertebrates, which governs or coordinates mental and physical motions.

brain case, the bony cranium or skull that surrounds the brain.

brain fever, see **cerebrospinal meningitis.**

brain stem, all of the brain except the cerebellum and cerebrum.

brainpan, the skull; the cranium.

brain wave, an electric impulse given off by tissues of the brain.

breakbone fever, see **dengue.**

breast, 1. either of the two soft protuberances on the thorax in females, containing the milk-excreting organs. 2. the analogous rudimentary organ in males.

breastbone, see **sternum.**

breath, the air inhaled and exhaled in respiration; respiration, esp. as necessary to life.

breathe, to inhale and exhale air, or respire.

breathing, the act of one who or that breathes; respiration.

breech, 1. the lower part of the body behind. 2. the posterior or buttocks.

breech birth, see **breech delivery.**

breech delivery, delivery of a fetus when the breech or buttocks or the feet appear first in the birth canal.

bregma, the point of junction of the sagittal and coronal sutures of the skull.

Bright's disease, kidney degeneration accompanied by imperfect uric acid elimination and high blood pressure. See **nephritis.**

Brill's disease, an infectious disease considered to be a relatively mild form of typhus.

broad-spectrum, pertaining to antibiotics that effectively combat a large variety of organisms.

Brocca's area, the speech center, situated on the left side of the brain.

bromic acid, an unstable, strongly oxidizing acid, occurring only in solution or in a salt: used as an oxidizing agent in the manufacture of medicines and dyes.

bromide, a salt of hydrobromic acid, esp. potassium bromide, strontium bromide, etc., that acts as a cerebral and cardiac depressant and is used in medicine as a sedative and a hypnotic.

brominism, a morbid condition caused by excessive use of bromides.

bronchadenitis, inflammation of the bronchial lymph glands.

bronchi, plural of **bronchus.**

bronchia, the ramifications of the bronchi or two main branches of the trachea through which air reaches the lungs.

bronchial, pertaining to the bronchia or the bronchi.

bronchial asthma, a respiratory disorder characterized by inflammation of the bronchi and causing difficulty in breathing.

bronchial tubes, the bronchi, or the bronchi and their ramifications.

bronchiectasis, an inflamed condition of the bronchial tubes, producing paroxysms of coughing and difficult breathing.

bronchiole, a tiny branch of a bronchus.

bronchiolitis, an inflammation of the bronchioles.

bronchitic, a person suffering from bronchitis.

bronchitis, an inflammation of the lining membrane of the bronchi or bronchia.

bronchodilatation, dilation of a bronchus with a bronchodilator, a drug that dilates the bronchus and the bronchial tubes.

bronchopneumonia, inflammation of the bronchia and lungs: a form of pneumonia.

bronchoscope, an instrument used to examine the trachea.

bronchoscopy, examination of the interior of the bronchus with a bronchoscope.

bronchus, either of the two main branches of the trachea, or any of their ramifications.

brontophobia, pathological fear of thunder.

brow, 1. the ridge or prominence over the eye. 2. the forehead.

brucellosis, any of a variety of infectious diseases caused by a parasitic bacterium (genus **Brucella**).

bruise, 1. an injury caused by bruising; a contusion; a discoloration of the skin from bruising. 2. to injure by a blow or by pressure without laceration.

bruit, any sound heard within the body, as by means of a stethoscope.

bubo, an inflammatory swelling of the lymphatic gland, esp. in the groin or armpit.

bubonic plague, an epidemic disease caused by infection from rodents and fleas and characterized by the formation of buboes.

buccal, 1. of or pertaining to the cheek. 2. pertaining to the sides of the mouth or to the mouth. 3. oral.

Buerger's disease, a disease affecting both arteries and veins, principally in the lower leg; the cause is unknown.

bucktooth, a projecting front tooth.

bulla, 1. a vesicle or elevation of the epidermis containing a watery fluid. 2. an inflated portion of the bony external meatus of the ear.

bunion, a knob on the side of the ball of the great toe resulting from chronic inflammation of the bursa.

burn, an injury or wound caused by burning; a mark made by burning.

bursa, a pouch, sac, or vesicle, esp. a sac containing synovia, called synovial bursa, to facilitate motion, as between a tendon and a bone.

bursectomy, removal of a bursa by surgery.

bursitis, inflammation of a bursa.

bypass, installation of an alternate route for the blood to bypass an obstructed vital artery.

byssinosis, a lung disease caused by inhaling cotton dust over a long period, occurring in flax and hemp workers.

cachet, a hollow wafer or capsule for enclosing an ill-tasting medicine.

cachexia, a state of extreme wasting occurring in persons with chronic diseases, as certain malignancies.

cachinnation, hysterical laughter.

cachou, a pill or pastille for sweetening the breath.

cacidrosis, excessive, offensive sweating.

cacoëthes, 1. a strong compulsion; mania. 2. a bad habit, as of incessant talking.

cadaver, a dead body, esp. of a human being used for dissection; a corpse.

cadaverous, pertaining to a dead body; esp. having the appearance or color of a dead human body.

caduceus, the emblem of the medical profession.

caducity, tendency to fall; frailty; the infirmity of old age; senility.

caecal, see **cecal.**

caecostomy, see **cecostomy.**

caecum, see **cecum.**

caesarean operation, the operation by which a fetus is taken from the uterus by cutting through the walls of the abdomen and uterus.

caffeine, a slightly bitter alkaloid used as a stimulant and diuretic and found in coffee, tea, etc.; poisonous when taken in large doses.

caisson disease, a painfully paralyzing, sometimes fatal sickness resulting from a too rapid lowering of air pressure, as in the change from the compressed air of a caisson to surface air pressure, which causes dissolved nitrogen to be released as bubbles in the blood and tissues; the bends.

calamine, a pink, water-insoluble powder consisting of zinc oxide and a small amount of ferric oxide, used in lotions and ointments to treat skin disorders.

calcaneus, the largest bone of the tarsus; the bone that forms the heel.

calcar, a spurlike projection.

calcareous, partaking of the nature of, having the qualities of, or containing calcium carbonate.

calcic, of or pertaining to lime; containing calcium.

calciferol, vitamin D_2, a crystalline, fat-soluble compound, occurring naturally in milk and fish-liver oils.

calcification, the process of changing a substance through the deposition of lime.

calcination, the drying of a substance by roasting to make a powder.

calcine, to reduce to a powder or to a friable state by the action of heat.

calcinosis, a state characterized by abnormal deposits of lime salts in tissues.

calcipenia, calcium deficiency in the body.

calcium, the basic element of lime, an essential ingredient of bones and teeth.

calcium carbonate, a colorless crystal or gray powder used as an antacid.

calculous, pertaining to, caused by, or affected with a calculus or calculi.

calculus, a stonelike mass sometimes formed in the gallbladder, kidneys, or other organs or ducts of the body.

calf, the fleshy back part of the human leg below the knee.

calisthenics, the art or practice of exercising for health, strength, or grace of movement.

callosity, abnormal hardness and thickness of skin and other tissues.

callous, 1. hard, as skin. 2. indurated, as portions of the skin exposed to friction.

callus, 1. a hardened or thickened portion of the skin; a callosity. 2. a new growth of osseous matter at the ends of a fractured bone, serving to unite them.

caloric, of or pertaining to heat or calories.

calorie, 1. the quantity of heat necessary, at normal atmospheric pressure, to raise the temperature of one gram of water one degree centigrade. 2. a unit of food measurement, having an energy-producing value of one large calorie.

calorific, capable of producing heat; causing heat; heating.

calorimeter, any of several apparatuses for measuring quantities of heat absorbed or produced by the body.

calory, see **calorie.**

calvaria, the cranium; skull.

calyx, a cuplike part, as one of the funnel-shaped structures that enclose the tips of the renal pyramids.

camp fever, see **typhus.**

camphor, a whitish, translucent, volatile, and aromatic crystalline substance, obtained chiefly from the camphor tree, used in medicine and as an irritant and stimulant.

camphor ice, an ointment composed chiefly of camphor, white wax, spermaceti, and castor oil, used for chapped or blemished skin.

canal, any cylindrical or tubular cavity in the body through which solids and liquids pass; a duct.

canaliculus, a tubular or canallike passage or channel, as in a bone.

cancellate, of spongy or porous structure.

cancellus, the spongy texture of bone.

cancer, a malignant growth or tumor, esp. originating in the epithelium, and characterized by abnormal cellular growth that spreads to other areas.

cancerate, to become cancerous.

cancerogenic, see **carcinogenic.**

cancerophobia, pathological fear of having cancer.

cancerous, pertaining to the nature of cancer.

cancroid, 1. resembling a cancer, as certain tumors. 2. a form of cancer of the skin.

canella, the cinnamonlike bark of a West Indian tree, used as a condiment and in medicine.

canine, pertaining to the four pointed teeth situated one on each side of each jaw, next to the incisors.

canker, 1. a kind of cancerous, gangrenous, or ulcerous sore or disease. 2. an eating, corroding, or other noxious agency producing ulceration, gangrene, rot, decay, and the like.

canker sore, an ulcerated sore of the lips or membranous lining of the mouth.

cannabis, the tops and leaves of Indian hemp used as a narcotic or intoxicant. See also **hashish, marijuana.**

cannula, a small tube of metal or the like that draws off fluid from or injects medicine into the body.

cannular, hollow or tubular; as a cannulated needle, a surgeon's hollow needle.

cantharidism, a morbid state caused by the use of cantharis.

cantharis, a substance obtained from dried and crushed blister beetles and used in medicine, esp. externally for raising blisters and formerly as a stimulant.

canthectomy, surgical excision of a canthus.

canthus, the angle or corner on each side of the eye formed by the junction of the upper and lower lids.

canula, see **cannula.**

capiat, an instrument for removing a foreign substance from the uterus or other body cavities.

capillarity, the state of being capillary.

capillary, one of the minute blood vessels between the terminations of the arteries and the beginnings of the veins.

capillary attraction, the apparent attraction between a liquid and a solid in capillarity.

capillary action, see **capillarity.**

capitate, having an enlarged or headlike end.

capitatum, one of the small bones, the capitate bone, in the hand.

capitellum, 1. the round eminence at the lower end of the uterus. 2. any small, rounded knob on a bone.

capsicum, the pod of the pepper plant which, when dried and prepared, is used in medicine as an irritant and a stimulant.

capsular, of, pertaining to, in, or of the nature of a capsule.

capsulate, enclosed in or formed into a capsule.

capsule, 1. a gelatinous case enclosing a dose of medicine. 2. a membranous sac or integument.

caput, 1. the upper part of an organ. 2. the head.

carbohydrate, a member of several groups of compounds including simple sugars such as glucose, double sugars such as sucrose, and polymers such as starch and cellulose; one of the major sources of food.

carbon 13, a rare carbon isotope used in cancer research and tracer studies.

carbon dioxide, a heavy, colorless, odorless, noncombustible gas, present in the atmosphere and formed during respiration.

carbon monoxide, a color-

less, odorless, very poisonous gas, which burns with a pale blue flame and is formed when carbon burns with an insufficient supply of air.

carbon monoxide poisoning, poisoning by inhalation of carbon monoxide. It causes dizziness, headache, and convulsions and can lead to paralysis and death.

carbuncle, a painful local inflammation of tissues, esp. of the back of the neck and trunk, characterized by hardness and having a tendency to spread like a boil.

carcinectomy, the surgical excision of a cancerous growth.

carcinogenic, pertaining to the development of cancer.

carcinoid, a benign tumor in the appendix or other intestinal tissue.

carcinoma, a malignant epithelial tumor that spreads and often recurs after excision; a cancer.

carcinomatophobia, pathological fear of cancer.

carcinomatosis, a state in which numerous carcinomas, disseminated from a primary source, grow in the body at the same time.

carcinomatous, pertaining to cancer; cancerlike.

carcinosarcoma, a malignant tumor having the elements of both carcinoma and sarcoma.

carcinosectomy, surgical excision of a cancer.

cardia, 1. the region of the

stomach connecting with the esophagus. 2. the heart.

cardiac, 1. pertaining to the heart. 2. exciting action in the heart through the medium of the stomach. 3. a person with a heart disease. 4. a medicine that excites action in the heart and animates the spirits.

cardiac cycle, the period from the beginning of one heartbeat to the next.

cardiac failure, the inability of the heart to pump sufficient blood to maintain the circulation and to meet the needs of the body.

cardiac hypertrophy, enlargement of the heart.

cardiac murmur, see **heart murmur.**

cardialgia, see **heartburn.**

cardiasthenia, neurasthenia with cardiac symptoms.

cardiectomy, surgical excision of the cardiac end of the stomach.

cardiogram, the record of heart action made by a cardiograph.

cardiograph, an instrument that traces and records the action of the heart.

cardiography, examination with a cardiograph.

cardiologist, a specialist in cardiology.

cardiology, the science of the heart, including the study of its diseases and functions.

cardioneurosis, neurosis with cardiac symptoms, as palpitations.

cardiopathy, any disease of the heart.

cardiophobia, pathological fear of heart disease.

cardiopulmonary, pertaining to both heart and lungs.

cardiosclerosis, hardening of the cardiac tissue and arteries.

cardiosphygmograph, an instrument for recording graphically the heartbeat and pulse.

cardiotomy, surgical incision of the heart.

cardiovalvulitis, inflammation of the valves of the heart.

cardiovascular, having reference to or involving the heart and blood vessels.

carditis, inflammation of the muscles of the heart.

caries, decay, as of bone or teeth.

carminative, 1. expelling wind from the body; relieving flatulence. 2. a carminative medicine.

carnophobia, pathological fear of eating meat.

carotene, the orange or red hydrocarbon pigment found in some vegetables and animal fats, capable of being converted into vitamin A.

carotid, of or pertaining to the two great arteries, one on either side of the neck, that convey the blood from the aorta to the head and brain.

carpal, relating to the joint of the carpus.

carpale, any bone of the carpus.

carpophalangeal, pertaining to the carpus and the phalanges or the finger bones.

carpus, 1. the part of the skeleton between the forearm and hand; the wrist. 2. the wrist bones collectively.

carrier, a person carrying bacteria that he can transmit to others although immune to their effects himself.

caron oil, an ointment composed of equal parts of limewater and olive oil, used as treatment for burns and scalds.

car sickness, nausea caused by motion, esp. when riding in a car.

cartilage, 1. an elastic tissue composing most of the skeleton in embryos, then largely being converted into bone. 2. the gristle or specialized connective tissue between bones.

cartilaginous, resembling cartilage; gristly; consisting of cartilage.

caruncle, a small, fleshy nodule.

cascara buckthorn, a buckthorn yielding cascara sagrada.

cascara sagrada, the dried bark of cascara buckthorn, used as a cathartic or laxative.

caseation, deterioration, as of tubercular tissue, into a soft, crumbly, cheeselike substance.

case history, a factual record of an individual's or family's personal history for use esp. in sociological, medical, or psychiat-

ric analyses.

casein, the principle protein in milk.

caseous, cheesy; as, caseous degeneration, pertaining to a morbid process in which tissues are converted into a thick, cheeselike mass.

caseous abscess, an abscess containing cheeselike matter.

case record, information gathered about an individual or group of individuals to serve as a psychological biography in social work, psychiatry, medicine, and sociology.

cassia, a tropical plant that yields senna, used as a purgative.

cast, 1. fibrous matter that takes the shape of the organ in which it is formed and is ejected from the body. 2. a mold made of plastic or plaster of paris, usually applied for immobilization, as in fractures, dislocations, and other injuries.

castor bean, the seed of the castor-oil plant.

castor oil, a viscid oil obtained from the castor bean, used as a cathartic or lubricant.

castrate, to remove the testicles or the ovaries.

castration, removal of the sex glands in either male or female.

catabolism, a breaking down of complex molecules into simpler ones, accompanied by an energy release; descending or destructive metabolism: opposed to **anabo-**

lism.

catalepsy, a nervous affection characterized by a temporary suspension of the senses and volition with rigidity of the muscles; trance.

cataleptic, 1. pertaining to catalepsy. 2. a person with catalepsy.

catalysis, the causing or accelerating of a chemical change by addition of a catalytic agent that is not permanently affected by the reaction.

catalyst, in catalysis, the substance that causes the chemical change.

catalyze, to act upon by catalysis.

catamenia, see **menses.**

catamnesis, a patient's medical history taken during, or after recovery from, an illness.

cataphasia, a speech disorder in which the afflicted involuntarily repeats the same words.

cataphora, a state of coma with short remissions.

cataphoria, a condition in which there is a tendency of the visual axis of each eye to incline below the horizontal plane.

cataplasia, a reversion of cells or tissues to an earlier or more primitive stage.

cataplasm, see **poultice.**

cataplexy, 1. a sudden, temporary loss of muscle power caused by emotional shock. 2. sudden prostration. 3. a form of hypnotic sleep.

cataract, a disease of the eye consisting of opacity of the crystalline lens or its capsule, which impairs or destroys vision.

catarrh, inflammation of a mucous membrane, esp. of the respiratory tract, accompanied by exaggerated secretions.

catatonia, 1. a state of suspended animation with loss of voluntary motion; catalepsy. 2. any of several schizophrenic syndromes in which the patient exhibits muscular rigidity and periods of stupor alternating with periods of agitation.

catatonic, pertaining to catatonia.

catechu, a strong, astringent substance prepared from the wood of various tropical Asiatic plants and used in medicine with prepared chalk to treat diarrhea.

catgut, a substance made from the intestine of sheep and other animals for use as an absorbable ligature.

catharsis, 1. purgation. 2. emotional release by recalling the memory of an event that was the cause of a psychoneurosis.

cathartic, pertaining to catharsis.

catheter, a hollow tube inserted into the body to allow the withdrawal or injection of fluids, usually inserted through the urethra into the bladder to draw off urine when natural discharge is arrested.

catheterization, use or passage of a catheter.

cauda, a tail or taillike termination.

caudad, toward the tail or posterior end of the body.

cauda equina, the terminal portion of the spinal cord that resembles a horse's tail.

caudal, relating to a cauda.

caudal anesthesia, insensibility to pain in the lower portion of the body, caused by injection of an anesthetic drug into the caudal or sacral part of the spinal canal.

caudate, having a tail or tail-like appendage.

caul, 1. a membrane investing some part of the intestines; the omentum. 2. a portion of the amnion or membrane enveloping the fetus, sometimes encompassing the head of a child at birth.

causalgia, burning pain.

caustic, a chemical capable of burning, corroding, or destroying tissue.

cauterization, the act or the effect of cauterizing.

cauterize, to burn or sear with fire, a hot iron, or caustics for beneficial purposes; to treat with cautery.

cautery, 1. a burning or searing, as of diseased tissue, by a hot iron or by caustic substances. 2. the instrument or chemical agent employed in cauterizing.

cava, 1. any body cavity. 2. see **vena cava.**

cavernous, 1. containing caverns. 2. of or like a cavern. 3. full of or containing small cavities or interstices; porous.

cavity, 1. a void or empty space in a body. 2. an opening. 3. a hollow part of the human body, the hollowness being pathological, as a dental cavity, or natural.

cecectomy, surgical removal of part of, or incision of, the cecum.

cecitis, inflammation of the cecum.

cecum, a sac or cavity with an opening only at one end, esp. the intestinal cecum, or "blind gut" in humans, at the beginning of the large intestine.

celiac, pertaining to the cavity of the abdomen.

celiac disease, 1. a disease common to the tropics, characterized by anemia, sore tongue, and gastrointestinal disturbance. 2. a dietary deficiency disease occurring in children.

cell, the basic unit of structure and function of all living things, made up of a small mass of protoplasm and containing a nucleus and cytoplasmic material.

cell membrane, the thin, semipermeable membrane enclosing the protoplasmic material of a cell.

cellular, pertaining to or characterized by having cells.

cellulase, an enzyme that hydrolyzes and depolymerizes cellulosic polysaccharides, including cellulose; obtained from a fungus and used in medicine.

cellulate, having cellular

structure.

cellule, a small cell.

cellulitis, inflammation of cellular tissue.

celluloneuritis, inflammation of nerve cells.

cellulose, the chief constituent of the cell walls of plants.

cell wall, the definite boundary or rigid permeable wall, formed by the protoplasm, which surrounds a biological cell.

cementum, the layer of bony tissue forming the outer surface of the root of the tooth within the gum.

cenogenesis, the introduction of new characters in the development of an individual, absent from early phylogeny of the species.

centigrade, divided into 100 degrees.

central nervous system, the part of the nervous system consisting of the brain and spinal cord, with their nerves and end-organs, which control and coordinate the entire voluntary nervous system.

cephalad, toward the head: opposed to **caudad.**

cephalalgia, see **headache.**

cephalic, 1. of or pertaining to the head. 2. situated or directed toward the head.

cephalic index, the ratio of the greatest breadth of the skull to the greatest length from front to back, multiplied by 100.

cephalometer, an instrument for measuring the head or skull; a craniometer.

cephalometry, the science of measuring the head or skull.

ceraceous, of the nature of wax; waxy.

cerate, a thick ointment composed of oils mixed with wax, resin, etc., and medicinal ingredients.

cerebellar, relating to the cerebellum.

cerebellitis, inflammation of the cerebellum.

cerebellum, a large section of the brain, the coordinating center for voluntary movements, equilibrium, and posture, composed of a central lobe and two lateral lobes, and located posterior to and underlying the cerebrum.

cerebral, 1. pertaining to the cerebrum or brain. 2. expressing an appeal to or use of the intellect.

cerebral accident, a sudden injury occurring inside the cerebrum, as a hemorrhage.

cerebral hemisphere, either of the two convoluted halves of the cerebrum.

cerebral palsy, paralysis caused by brain damage prior to birth or during delivery, and marked by a lack of muscular coordination, spasms, and difficulties in speech.

cerebral thrombosis, a clot in a blood vessel of the brain.

cerebrate, to have or exhibit brain action; to think.

cerebration, mental activity.

cerebrospinal, of or pertaining to the brain and spinal cord, or to these coupled with the spinal and cranial nerves.

cerebrospinal fever, see **cerebrospinal meningitis.**

cerebrospinal fluid, a serumlike liquid in the lateral ventricles of the brain.

cerebrospinal meningitis, an acute bacterial disease, involving inflammation of the membranes covering the brain and spinal cord, and manifested by fever and sometimes red spots on the skin.

cerebrum, the main, anterior part of the brain, divided into halves, or cerebral hemispheres, and considered the center of conscious and voluntary processes.

cerumen, see **earwax.**

cervical, 1. belonging to the neck. 2. pertaining to the narrow lower part of the uterus.

cervicitis, inflammation of the lower, necklike part of the uterus.

cervico-axillary, pertaining to the neck and armpit.

cervicobrachial, pertaining to the neck and arm.

cervicodorsal, pertaining to the neck and back.

cervicofacial, pertaining to the neck and face.

cervico-occipital, pertaining to the neck and the back of the head.

cervicoplasty, plastic surgery of the neck.

cervicovaginal, pertaining to the neck of the womb and the vagina.

cervix, 1. the neck, esp. the back of the neck. 2. any necklike part, esp. the narrow lower part of the uterus.

cervix vesicae, the neck of the bladder.

cesarean, see **caesarean.**

cestode, belonging to the Cestoda, a class or group of internally parasitic flatworms, including the tapeworms.

cestoid, ribbon-shaped, as tapeworms.

cetrimide, an antiseptic chemical.

cevitamic acid, ascorbic acid; vitamin C.

chalazion, a small tumor similar to a sebaceous cyst developing on the eyelid.

chancre, the initial lesion of syphilis.

chancroid, a soft, local venereal sore.

chancroidal, pertaining to chancroid.

chancrous, of or like a chancre.

change of life, see **climacteric** and **menopause.**

chap, 1. to split; crack; make rough, esp. the skin. 2. to become chapped, as the skin. 3. a crack in the skin.

chart, a sheet of any kind on which information is exhibited, esp. all relevant details about a patient, e.g., temperature, respiration, pulse.

cheek, 1. either side of the face below the eye and above the lower jawbone.

2. something resembling the cheeks, as for instance any rounded prominence, as the buttocks.

cheekbone, bone or bony prominence below the outer angle of the eye; the zygomatic bone.

cheilitis, inflammation of the lip.

cheilosis, a condition in which fissures and ulcers appear at the angles of the mouth, caused by vitamin B deficiency.

cheloid, see **keloid.**

chemoprophylaxis, the prevention of disease by chemical drugs or agents.

chemoreception, the physiological response of a sense organ to the reception of chemical stimuli.

chemotaxis, the movement of a cell or organism toward or away from a chemical stimulus.

chemotherapy, treatment of disease with chemicals.

cherophobia, pathological fear of and aversion to pleasure.

chest, the part of the body enclosed by the ribs and breastbone, extending from neck to abdomen; the thorax.

chested, pertaining to the chest of the body, as, broad-chested.

chiasma, a crossing as of two tendons or two nerves.

chicken pox, an acute, contagious, eruptive disease generally appearing in children.

chigger, see **chigoe.**

chigoe, an insect closely resembling the common flea, but of more minute size, which burrows beneath the skin and, becoming distended with eggs, produces a troublesome ulcer.

chilblain, 1. a blain or inflamed sore on the hands or feet, produced by cold. 2. to afflict with chilblains; to produce chilblains on.

childbearing, the act of producing or bringing forth children; parturition.

childbed, the state of a woman in childbirth or labor.

childbed fever, an infection of the mother occurring at childbirth; puerperal fever.

childbirth, see **childbearing.**

chill, cold; tending to cause shivering; depressingly affected by cold; shivering with cold.

chilly, producing the sensation of cold; so cold as to cause shivering.

chiropodist, one who treats ailments and irregularities of the feet; podiatrist.

chiropody, the science dealing with the treatment of foot ailments and irregularities; podiatry.

chiropractic, a system of therapeutics based upon the theory that disease is caused by interference with nerve function, the method being to restore normal condition by adjusting body structures, esp. the spinal column.

chiropractor, one who practices chiropractic.

chirospasm, see **writer's cramp.**

chloasma, a skin discoloration caused by deposits of pigment and occurring in patches or spots of yellowish-brown color.

chloral, 1. a colorless mobile liquid first prepared from chlorine and alcohol. 2. a white crystalline substance ("chloral hydrate") formed by combining liquid chloral with water, and used as a hypnotic and an anesthetic.

chloralose, a crystalline compound, made by combining chloral with dextrose: used in medicine as a hypnotic.

chloramphenicol, a synthetic antibiotic used to treat typhoid fever and other infections caused by Salmonellae.

chloride, a compound of chlorine with an element or radical; a salt of hydrochloric acid.

chloridize, to convert into a chloride; to treat with a chloride.

chlorinate, 1. to combine or treat with chlorine. 2. to disinfect, as water, by means of chlorine.

chlorination, the act of combining or treating with chlorine.

chlorine, a greenish-yellow gaseous element, highly irritating to the organs of respiration, occurring naturally combined in table salt.

chloroform, 1. a volatile, colorless liquid of an agreeable, fragrant taste and odor, prepared by distilling a mixture of alcohol, water, and chloride of lime, or as a byproduct of the chlorination of methane: used in refrigerants, propellants, and as an anesthetic. 2. to put under the influence of chloroform; to treat with chloroform.

chloroma, green cancer; a greenish tumor in certain bones, a condition mainly affecting young people.

chlorophyll, the green coloring matter of plants and leaves, used in the manufacture of carbohydrates.

chlorosis, loss of the normal green color in a plant, from lack of iron in the soil or other causes, exclusive of lack of sunlight.

chlorotic, relating to chlorosis.

chlorpropamide, a compound that lowers blood sugar, used to treat mild diabetes.

chlortetracycline, an antibiotic, having a wide antimicrobial spectrum, and also used as an animal feed supplement.

choke, to stop the breath of, by stricture of or obstruction in the windpipe; strangle; stifle; suffocate.

cholangitis, inflammation of the bile ducts.

cholecystectomy, surgical removal of the gallbladder.

cholecystitis, inflammation of the gallbladder.

cholecystolithiasis, the

presence of gallstones in the gallbladder.

cholecystopathy, any disease of the gallbladder.

cholecystotomy, removal of gallstones by surgical incision of the gallbladder.

choledochitis, inflammation of the bile duct.

choleic, pertaining to bile.

cholelithiasis, presence of bile stones in the gallbladder.

cholelithotomy, removal of gallstones by surgical incision of the gallbladder.

cholemia, presence of bile or bile pigments in the blood, causing jaundice.

cholera, any of several acute infectious diseases of humans and domestic animals, characterized by severe intestinal disturbances.

choleric, easily irritated; irascible; inclined to anger; quick-tempered.

cholerine, a mild form of Asiatic cholera.

cholesteatoma, a tumor occurring in the ear.

cholesterol, 1. a fat-soluble alcohol, present in body cells and animal fats and tissues. 2. a form of this compound used in making ointments and pharmaceuticals.

chololith, see **gallstone**.

chondralgia, pain in or around a cartilage.

chondritis, inflammation of a cartilage.

chondroma, a tumor in a cartilage.

chondromalacia, softening of cartilages.

chondropathy, any disease of cartilages.

chorda, any nerve filament, cord, or tendon.

chorditis, inflammation of the vocal chords.

chorea, St. Vitus's dance; convulsive motions of the limbs and strange and involuntary gesticulations.

choreiform, resembling chorea.

chorion, the vascular outer membrane enveloping a fetus, enclosing the amnion.

chorionic, relating to the chorion.

chorioretinitis, inflammation of the choroid and the retina.

choroid, 1. the middle coat of the eye. 2. pertaining to the choroid. 3. resembling the chorion and corium.

choroiditis, inflammation of the choroid membrane of the eye.

chromatid, one of a pair of chromosomal strands formed when a chromosome duplicates during cell reproduction.

chromatin, the constituent of a chromosome that is believed to carry the genes and that stains deeply with basic dyes.

chromatosis, abnormal skin pigmentation.

chromoprotein, a protein compound, as hemoglobin, made up of a protein combined with a pigment or a carotenoid.

chromoscope, an instrument for determining color perception.

chromoscopy, the procedure for testing color vision.

chromosomal, of or pertaining to chromosomes.

chromosome, one of the rod- or thread-shaped bodies containing chromatin that carry the genes and are present, in a fixed number for each species, in all the cell nuclei of plants, animals, and humans.

chronic, long-lasting or recurring frequently over a long period of time; of a disease or ailment of long duration or repeated occurrence, as differentiated from acute; as, chronic arthritis.

chyle, the milklike fluid found in the intestinal lymph vessels, produced during digestion of fats.

chylopoiesis, the production of chyle.

chylothorax, accumulation of chyle in the pleural cavities.

chylous, pertaining to chyle.

chyme, the semiliquid mass into which food is converted by gastric secretion during digestion.

chymify, to convert or be converted into chyme.

cicatrix, a scar.

cicatrize, 1. to induce the formation of a cicatrix. 2. to become healed, leaving a scar.

cilia, the hairs that grow from the margin of the eyelids; eyelashes.

ciliary, 1. belonging to the eyelids or eyelashes. 2. pertaining to or performed by bibratile cilia; as, ciliary motion.

cillosis, twitching of the eyelid.

cinchona, any of the trees or shrubs constituting the genus **Cinchona** and cultivated for the bark, which yields quinine and other alkaloids.

cinchonine, an alkaloid obtained from the bark of several species of **Cinchona,** along with quinine, and one of the medicinal active principles of this bark, used to reduce fever.

cinchonism, a disturbed condition of the body characterized by dizziness, ringing of the ears, temporary deafness, and headache, the result of overdoses of cinchona or quinine.

cinnamon, the inner bark of a tree of the laurel family, used as a spice or in medicine as a cordial or carminative.

circadian rhythm, rhythmic changes that occur during a period of 24 hours. See **biological clock.**

circulation, the continuous movement of blood through the vessels of the body maintained by the pumping action of the heart.

circulatory, pertaining to circulation.

circumcise, to cut off the foreskin of the penis.

circumcision, the act of circumcising.

cirrhosis, a disease consisting of diminution and deformity of the liver, often seen in alcoholics.

cirrhotic, affected with or having the character of cirrhosis.

cirsotome, instrument for cutting varicose veins.

cirsotomy, multiple surgical incisions of veins as treatment of a varicosity.

citric acid, the acid derived from lemons and similar fruits or obtained by the fermentation of carbohydrates, used to flavor foods, beverages, and pharmaceuticals and to condition water.

clamp, a surgical device to grasp, compress, or support tissue or a vessel.

clap, see **gonorrhea.**

claudication, lameness, limping.

claustrophobia, pathological fear of narrow spaces or closed rooms.

clavicle, a bone of the pectoral arch; either of two slender bones each articulating with the sternum and a scapula and forming the anterior part of a shoulder; the collarbone.

clavicular, pertaining to the clavicle.

clavus, a horny growth on the skin; a corn.

cleft palate, a congenital malformation in which more or less of the palate is lacking, so as to leave a longitudinal gap in the upper jaw, often an accompaniment of harelip.

cleidotomy, a surgical operation in which a fetal clavicle is divided to make delivery possible.

climacteric, the **menopause;** also a corresponding period in the male.

climacterical, pertaining to menopause.

clinic, a medical institution in which a group of physicians jointly examine and treat patients.

clinical, 1. pertaining to clinic. 2. based on examination or diagnosis in a clinic. 3. dealing with the study of patients as opposed to laboratory experiment.

clinician, a physician who studies diseases at the bedside or is skilled in clinical methods.

clitoris, a small erectile organ of the female, located at the anterior part of the vulva, and homologous to the penis of the male.

cloaca, a cavity at the posterior end of the embryo into which urinary, digestive, and reproductive ducts open.

clonic, convulsive, with alternate relaxation.

clonic spasm, a spasm in which the muscles or muscular fibers rapidly contract and relax alternately, as in epilepsy.

Clostridium, a genus of spore-bearing bacteria, some of which produce gas gangrene of wounds and tetanus.

clot, a coagulated mass of soft or fluid matter, as of blood or lymph.

clotting, to coagulate, as soft or fluid matter, into a thick, inspissated mass. Blood clotting insures the stoppage of blood flow.

cloudy swelling, a degeneration of tissues that become swollen during the course of an illness.

clubfoot, a short misshapen foot of congenital origin.

clubfooted, having a clubfoot.

clubhand, a misshapen hand of congenital origin.

clump, an aggregation of particles such as red blood cells or bacteria that have undergone agglutination.

clumping, see **agglutination.**

coagulability, the capacity of being coagulated.

coagulant, an agent that produces coagulation.

coagulase, any of several antibody-producing enzymes causing coagulation of the blood.

coagulate, to change from a fluid into a substance of glutinous consistency; to curdle, congeal, or clot.

coagulation, the process of clotting.

coagulum, a blood clot or clump.

coarctate, pressed together; compressed; contracted.

coarctation, 1. compression or narrowing of a vessel or canal. 2. shriveling. 3. a stricture.

coarctotomy, surgical incision to divide a stricture.

cobalt 60, a heavy radioactive isotope of cobalt, having a mass number of 60 and used as a source of gamma rays, chiefly in radiotherapy.

cocaine, a bitter crystalline alkaloid obtained from coca leaves, used in medicine as a local anesthetic and as a narcotic.

cocainism, 1. addiction to the habitual use of cocaine. 2. the general breakdown due to excessive or habitual use of cocaine.

cocainize, to treat with or affect by cocaine.

coccidioidomycosis, a fever and pulmonary disease or sometimes a skin infection in the form of lesions, occurring in man and some animals, and caused by inhaling the spores of the fungus **Coccidiodes immitis.**

coccidium, any individual organism of an order of protozoans that are usually intestinal parasites.

coccoid, 1. resembling or pertaining to a coccus. 2. berrylike. 3. spherical, as certain microorganisms.

coccus (plural cocci), a globular or spherical bacterium, as in staphylococcus, micrococcus.

coccygeal, pertaining to the coccyx.

coccygectomy, surgical removal of the coccyx.

coccygodynia, pain in the region of the coccyx.

coccyx, a small triangular bone forming the lower extremity of the spinal column, consisting of four ankylosed rudimentary vertebrae.

cochlea, a bony structure in the internal ear, so called from its resemblance to a snail shell.

coconscious, pertaining to a mental process apart from but influencing the stream of consciousness, often characterized by unintended utterances or hallucinations.

codeine, a white, crystalline, slightly bitter alkaloid, obtained from opium, used in medicine as an analgesic, a sedative, and a hypnotic.

coeliac, see **celiac.**

cohabit, to dwell or live together as husband and wife: often applied to persons not legally married, and suggesting sexual intercourse.

cohabitation, the living together of a man and a woman.

cohere, to stick or cleave together.

coherence, a cleaving together.

coherent, sticking together.

cohesion, the act or state of cohering, uniting, or sticking together.

coition, a coming together; copulation.

coitus, sexual intercourse.

colchicine, the compound colchicine tannate, used to alleviate the symptoms of gout.

colchicum, a drug obtained from a genus of liliaceous plants, **Colchicum,** used in the treatment of gout.

cold, a viral infection of the upper respiratory passages, popularly believed to be caused by exposure to cold, characterized by catarrh, hoarseness, and coughing.

cold sore, a vesicular eruption about the mouth often accompanying a cold or a febrile condition.

cold sweat, a chill characterized by perspiration, often induced by a state of nervousness.

colectomy, complete or partial removal of the large intestine or colon.

colic, 1. a painful spasm of the intestines, esp. of the colon, sometimes accompanied by fever or inflammation. 2. pertaining to the colon.

colicroot, either of two North American liliaceous herbs, **Aletris farinosa** and **Aletris aurea,** having a root reputed to relieve colic.

colitis, inflammation of the colon.

collagen, the protein that makes up the major portion of the white fiber in connective tissues, particularly in the skin, bones, and tendons.

collapse, a more or less sudden failure of the vital powers; a sudden and complete failure of any kind; a breakdown.

collarbone, see **clavicle.**

colliculus, any small anatomical eminence.

collodion, a solution that dries to a flexible adhesive film, often used to seal slight wounds.

colloid, a gelatinous or homogenous substance found normally in the thyroid and in some diseased tissues.

collutorium, a gargle or mouthwash.

collyrium, a lotion for the eye; eyewash.

coloboma, a congenital defect of the eye or any portion of it, usually a cleft or fissure of the iris.

colocynth, a purgative derived from the fruit of a Mediterranean plant of the gourd family.

colon, the portion of the large intestine from the cecum to the rectum.

color-blind, 1. incapable of accurately distinguishing colors. 2. having an imperfect perception of colors.

color blindness, total or partial inability to distinguish colors, arising from some defect in the eye.

colostomy, 1. a surgical procedure that forms an artificial anus by making an incision from the colon through the wall of the abdomen. 2. the opening that results from this operation. 3. the act of bringing together two separate parts of the intestine.

colostrum, the first milk secreted in the breasts after childbirth, containing a large amount of protein and immunizing factors for the newborn.

colotomy, surgical incision of the colon.

colpitis, inflammation of the vagina.

colpocele, a hernia protruding into the vagina.

colpocystocele, prolapse of the urinary bladder into the vagina.

colpohysterectomy, surgical removal of the womb through the va-

gina.

colpoplasty, surgical plastic repair of the vagina.

colpoptosis, prolapse of the walls of the vagina.

colporrhaphy, surgical suture to narrow the vagina.

colposcope, instrument for examining the vagina.

coma, a state of prolonged unconsciousness, usually due to disease or injury, from which it is difficult or impossible to rouse a person; stupor.

comatose, 1. pertaining to coma. 2. drowsy. 3. lethargic.

comedo, a hardened plug of sebum in a skin duct; a blackhead.

comminute, to reduce to minute particles; to pulverize.

comminution, the act of comminuting or reducing to a fine pulver or to small particles; pulverization.

commissure, 1. a joint, seam, or suture. 2. a connecting band of nerve tissue.

communicable, capable of being communicated or imparted, as, a communicable disease.

compatible, referring to the formation of a mixture that is not separated or changed by chemical interaction.

complemental, supplying something to remedy a deficiency.

complement fixation, in immunological experimentation, a process involving the addition of complement to a substance produced by the union of an antigen and its antibody.

complex, a group of ideas or mental processes that have been inhibited or restrained and that are regarded as the causative agent in the production of certain abnormal mental states.

complexion, the color or hue of the skin, particularly of the face.

component, an ingredient of a mixture.

compos mentis, of sound mind.

compound, 1. composed of two or more parts, elements, or ingredients. 2. something formed by compounding or combining parts, elements, or ingredients.

compound fracture, a fracture in which a bone is broken and the fracture exposed by laceration of the tissues.

comprehension, the capacity of the mind to understand.

compress, a soft pad, usually of cloth, used as a means of applying pressure, moisture, cold, heat, or medication.

compressed-air sickness, see **caisson disease.**

compulsion, 1. the act of compelling or the state of being compelled. 2. an irresistible impulse to carry out an act.

compulsive, dictated by irresistible psychological urges.

compulsively, by or under compulsion.

compunction, an uneasiness of mind or conscience; regret for wrongdoing or for causing pain.

concave, 1. hollow and curved or rounded, as the inner surface of a spherical body. 2. a concave surface, line, or segment. 3. an arch or vault. 4. a cavity.

concavity, 1. a concave surface, or the space contained in it. 2. a depression.

concavo-concave, concave or hollow on both surfaces, as a lens.

concavo-convex, 1. concave on one side and convex on the other. 2. pertaining to a lens in which the concave face has a greater degree of curvature than the convex face, the lens being thinnest in the middle.

conceive, 1. to become pregnant with. 2. to form a notion or idea in the mind.

concentration, 1. an increase of the proportion of a substance dissolved in a liquid. 2. medicine strengthened by evaporation. 3. the ability to fix the attention.

concentric, having a common center, as circles or spheres.

conception, 1. the act of conceiving, or the state of being conceived. 2. the inception of pregnancy. 3. a notion or idea.

concha, 1. any structure resembling a shell. 2. the outer ear. 3. one of the three bones in the nasal cavity.

concretion, a tophus or other hard inorganic mass found in the body; a calculus.

concupiscence, ardent sexual longing; physical desire; lust.

concussion, 1. shock occasioned by the impact of a collision. 2. injury to the brain or spine from a blow or fall.

conditioned reflex, an automatic response to a particular stimulus, induced by training.

condom, a thin rubber sheath worn over the penis during sexual intercourse as a contraceptive and to prevent venereal disease.

condylar, pertaining to a condyle.

condyle, a protuberance on the end of a bone serving to form an articulation with another bone.

condylectomy, surgical removal of a condyle.

condyloma, a wartlike growth of the skin, usually in the area near the genitalia or anus.

confabulate, to engage in fantasy to replace memory loss.

confabulation, a mental disorder in which the patient invents events, usually to replace lost memory.

confined, in childbirth.

confinement, the state of being confined; lying-in for childbirth.

confusion, perturbation of mind.

congenital, existing from birth; relating to characteristics dating from birth that are not hereditary.

congest, to cause an unnatural accumulation of blood in the vessels of an organ or part.

congestion, an inflammation or excess of fluid in an organ or part.

congestive, pertaining to or characterized by congestion.

conjugal, of, pertaining to, or of the nature of marriage.

conjugant, one of a pair of conjugating sex cells or organisms.

conjugate, joined together or operating as if joined, esp. in a pair; coupled.

conjugated protein, a compound consisting of a protein combined with a nonprotein, as hemoglobin.

conjunctiva, the mucous membrane that lines the inner surface of the eyelids and covers the anterior surface of the eyeball.

conjunctivitis, inflammation of the conjunctiva.

connective tissue, tissue that connects, supports, or surrounds other tissues or organs and occurs in various forms throughout the body.

consanguine, of the same blood.

consanguineous, of the same blood; related by birth; akin; pertaining to consanguinity; related, as having had the same ancestor.

consanguinity, the condition of being of the same blood; relationship by blood; kinship.

conscience, a part of the superego.

conscious, aware of one's own existence, emotions, and thoughts, or of external objects and conditions.

consciousness, the state of being conscious.

consciousness-expanding, causing the mental state of perception or awareness to be greatly intensified. as: LSD is a consciousness-expanding drug.

consolidation, the act of becoming solid or compact, as in lobar pneumonia, where the lobe of the lung that was inflamed and has collapsed is referred to as being consolidated.

constipation, the state of being constipated; a condition of the bowels marked by irregular or difficult evacuation.

constitution, the physical character of the body as to strength or health, character or condition of mind, disposition, temperament.

constitutional, a walk or other exercise taken for the benefit of health.

consumption, tuberculosis; progressive wasting of the body, esp. from tuberculosis of the lung.

consumptive, 1. pertaining to or of the nature of tuberculosis. 2. disposed to or affected with consumption. 3. one who suffers from tuberculosis.

contact, a carrier of contagious disease.

contact lens, a small prescription lens to correct vision, which is applied directly to the surface of the cornea and held in place by surface tension of the eye fluid.

contagion, 1. a communication of disease by direct or indirect contact. 2. a disease so communicated. 3. the medium by which a contagious disease is transmitted.

contagious, causing or involving contagion.

contagium, the medium by which a contagious disease is communicated, as a virus.

continence, self-restraint, esp. in regard to sexual passion or indulgence.

contortion, a writhing, esp. spasmodic; distortion; a distorted form.

contraception, the deliberate prevention of conception or impregnation.

contraceptive, 1. tending or serving to prevent conception or impregnation. 2. pertaining to contraception. 3. a contraceptive agent or device.

contractile, able to contract or shorten.

contraction, 1. the act of contracting, drawing together, or shrinking. 2. the act of shortening, narrowing, or lessening dimensions by causing the parts to approach nearer to each other. 3. the state of being contracted.

contracture, the permanent shortening of a muscle caused by spasm, scar, or paralysis.

contraindicate, of a symptom or condition, to give indication against the advisability of a particular remedy or treatment.

contraindication, the evidence that a particular remedy or treatment of a condition is inadvisable or dangerous.

contralateral, pertaining to the opposite side of the body.

contuse, 1. to wound or injure by bruising. 2. to injure without breaking the flesh.

contusion, 1. a severe bruise. 2. a hurt or an injury as to the flesh or some part of the body without breaking of the skin, as by a blunt instrument or a fall.

convalesce, to grow better after sickness; to recover health.

convalescence, 1. the gradual recovery of health and strength after illness. 2. the state of a person renewing his vigor after sickness or weakness.

convalescent, 1. recovering health and strength after sickness or debility. 2. one who is recovering his health after sickness.

convex, denoting a surface that is curved or rounded outward, as the exterior of a sphere or circle.

convexity, 1. state of being convex. 2. the exterior surface of a convex body.

convexo-concave, 1. con-vex on one side and concave on the other, as a lens. 2. pertaining to a lens in which the convex face has a greater degree of curvature than the concave face, the lens being thickest in the middle.

convexo-convex, curved outward on two opposite faces.

convolute, to coil up; to form into a twisted shape.

convolution, a sinuosity, esp. one of the sinuous folds or ridges of the surface of the brain.

convulsant, a drug or medicine that causes spasms.

convulse, 1. to affect with successive violent and involuntary contractions of the muscles. 2. to affect with irregular spasms. 3. to cause to laugh violently.

convulsion, 1. a violent and involuntary spasmodic contraction of the muscles. 2. an affliction marked by such contractions. 3. a violent fit of laughter.

convulsive, 1. tending to convulse. 2. of the nature of or characterized by convulsion. 3. affected with convulsion.

coprolalia, a morbid, obsessive compulsion to use obscene words.

coprolite, a roundish, stony mass of petrified fecal matter.

coprophagy, the eating of excrement.

coprophilia, pathological attraction to feces.

coprophobia, morbid disgust of feces.

coprostasis, see **constipation.**

copulate, to unite in sexual intercourse.

copulation, the act of copulating; coition.

coracoid, referring to a bone or bony process of the scapula.

Coramine, a drug used as a respiratory stimulant (trademark).

cord, a cordlike structure, as, the spinal cord or the vocal cords.

cordate, heart-shaped.

corium, the sensitive vascular layer of the skin beneath the epidermis.

corn, a hard excrescence or induration of the skin on the toe or some other part of the foot, often painful, caused by the pressure of shoes.

cornea, the transparent anterior part of the external coat of the eye, covering the iris and pupil.

corneal, pertaining to the cornea.

cornification, the process of becoming hard as in a corn or in structures such as horns, etc.

corona, the upper portion or crown of a part, as of the head or a tooth.

coronal, referring or pertaining to a suture extending across the skull between the frontal bone and the parietal bones.

coronary arteries, the two arteries encircling the upper part of the heart.

coronary occlusion, blockage of one of the

coronary arteries.

coronary thrombosis, clotting of blood in one of the arteries of the heart.

coroner, an officer, as of a county or municipality, whose chief function is to investigate, by inquest before a jury, any death not clearly due to natural causes.

corpulence, obesity or fatness.

corpulent, large or bulky of body; portly; stout; fat.

corpus, the body; the principal part of a bodily organ.

corpuscallosum, the large band of nervous tissue joining the two cerebral hemispheres in the brain.

corpuscle, 1. a minute particle. 2. a minute body forming a more or less distinct part of an organism. 3. a cell, esp. one having a distinct function and form, as red and white blood cells.

corpuscular, relating to a corpuscle.

corpus luteum, the yellowish endocrine tissue formed in the ovary by rupture of a Graafian follicle after ovulation which, during pregnancy, secretes the hormone progesterone.

corrode, 1. to eat away by degrees. 2. to wear away or diminish by chemical action.

corrosion, the process of corroding.

corrosive, having the power to corrode.

cortex, the outermost section of an organ, as of the

brain or the adrenal glands.

cortical, belonging to, consisting of, or resembling the cortex.

corticosterone, a steroid hormone of the adrenal cortex.

cortin, a hormone secreted by the adrenal cortex.

cortisone, a steroid hormone of the adrenal cortex, now synthetically produced. It can be administered orally or intramuscularly to cause remission, but not cure, of various collagen diseases.

coryza, acute inflammation of the mucous membrane of the nasal cavities; head cold.

costa, a rib or riblike part.

costal, pertaining to the ribs.

costive, having the bowels bound; constipated.

costoclavicular, pertaining to the ribs and clavicle.

costovertebral, pertaining to the ribs and vertebrae.

costotome, a surgical instrument, as a knife or shears, for cutting through a rib or cartilage.

costotomy, surgical removal of a rib or part of one.

cough, 1. expulsion of air from the lungs marked by sudden loud noise. 2. an illness characterized by such a condition.

counterirritant, an agent for producing irritation in one part of the body to counteract irritation or relieve pain or inflammation elsewhere.

course, the menses.

cowpox, a disease that causes vesicles or blisters on the teats of a cow; the fluid or virus contained therein is capable of immunizing man against smallpox.

coxa, the joint of the hip.

coxalgia, pain in the hip.

cramp, 1. an involuntary, spasmodic, painful contraction of a muscle or muscles, as from a slight strain or sudden chill. 2. a sudden, violent abdominal pain.

cranial index, the ratio of the full breadth of the skull to its length, multiplied by 100.

cranial nerve, one of the nerves that originate in the brain and come through openings in the skull.

craniolgy, the science that deals with the size, shape, and other characteristics of the skull.

craniometry, the science of the measurement of skulls.

cranioplasty, plastic surgery on the skull.

craniopuncture, puncture of the skull.

cranium, 1. the skull. 2. the part of the skull that encloses the brain.

crapulence, 1. drunkenness. 2. the sickness occasioned by intemperance.

crapulous, 1. drunk. 2. ill as a result of intemperance. 3. associated with drunkenness.

creatine, a colorless, crystalline substance that can

be isolated from various organs and body fluids. Combined with phosphate to phosphocreatine, it is an energy-storing substance found esp. in muscle juice and in blood.

cremaster, one of the fascialike muscles in the scrotum suspending and enveloping the testicles.

cremate, to consume by fire; burn, esp. to reduce a corpse to ashes.

cremation, the burning of a corpse to ashes.

cremationist, one who advocates cremation instead of burial of the dead.

crematorium, a place for the burning of corpses.

crepitant, crackling.

crepitate, 1. to crackle. 2. to make a grating sound, as heard on the movement of the ends of a broken bone or, in certain diseases, as the rale heard in pneumonia.

cresol, any one of three colorless, poisonous isomeric phenols, occurring in coal tar and wood tar, and mainly used as a disinfectant.

crest, a prominence, ridge, or ridgelike formation, esp. one on a bone.

cretin, a person afflicted with cretinism.

cretinism, a chronic disease, caused by absence or deficiency of the normal thyroid secretion, characterized by physical deformity, stunted growth, idiocy, and in many cases, goiter.

cribriform, having the form of a sieve; perforated with many small openings.

cribriform plate, a bone in the skull perforated with many small openings through which nerve filaments pass.

crick, a painful muscle spasm, esp. on the neck or back.

cricoid, ring-shaped.

cricoid cartilage, the lowermost ring-shaped cartilage of the larynx.

cripple, 1. one who has lost or never enjoyed the use of his limbs. 2. a partially disabled or lame person.

crisis, the stage in a disease that indicates recovery or death.

critical, pertaining to the crisis or turning point of a disease.

crotch, the part of the human body where the legs are joined.

croup, an inflammation of the respiratory passages characterized by highly labored breathing and a hoarse, rasping cough.

crown, 1. the part of a tooth that appears beyond the gum. 2. to cover the top of a tooth with a false crown.

crowning, that stage in delivery when the baby's head appears at the opening of the birth canal.

crural, pertaining to the leg.

crus, that part of the leg between the femur or thigh and the tarsus or ankle.

crust, see scab.

crutch, a support with a crosspiece at one end to fit under the armpit to assist a lame or infirm person in walking.

cryanesthesia, the inability to sense cold.

crymotherapy, see **cryotherapy.**

cryosurgery, surgery with special instruments using extreme cold to destroy or remove diseased tissue.

cryotherapy, treatment of disease by means of cold.

crypt, 1. a follicle. 2. a glandular cavity.

cryptogenic, of obscure or unknown origin, as a disease.

cryptorchidism, failure of the testicles to descend into the scrotum.

cryptorchism, see **cryptorchidism.**

crystalline, pure; clear; transparent; pellucid.

crystalline lens, the lens of the eye.

crystalluria, the appearance of crystals in the urine.

crystal violet, a chloride used in diagnostic medicine as a stain and an acid-base indicator.

cubital, or or pertaining to the forearm.

cubitus, 1. elbow. 2. forearm. 3. ulna.

cuboid, referring or pertaining to the outermost bone of the distal row of tarsal bones.

Culex, a genus of malaria-carrying mosquitoes.

culture, the cultivation of microorganisms, as bacteria, for scientific study or medicinal use.

cumulative, increasing in

effect by accumulation or successive additions, as of drugs.

cupule, a cup-shaped structure or part.

curare, a blackish, resinlike substance obtained from tropical plants, used by South American Indians as arrow poison. Used in surgery for arresting the action of the motor nerves.

curettage, scraping with a curette.

curette, a scoop-shaped surgical instrument for removing or scraping away foreign matter and granulations from the walls of a body cavity, as the uterus.

curie, the official international unit of radioactivity.

cusp, a point or pointed end; a point, projection, or protuberance, as on the crown of a tooth.

cuspid, a cuspidate tooth; a canine tooth. (Canine teeth are the four teeth, two in each jaw, that have conical crowns.)

cuspidate, having a cusp or cusps; ending in a cusp or sharp point, as a canine tooth.

cutaneous, of, pertaining to, or affecting the cutis or skin.

cuticle, 1. the epidermis. 2. nonliving skin that frames the nails of fingers and toes.

cutis, the corium, or true skin, beneath the epidermis.

cyanocobalamin, vitamin B_{12}.

cyanopia, vision in which

all objects appear to be blue in color.

cyanosed, affected with cyanosis.

cyanosis, blueness or lividness of the skin, as from imperfectly oxygenated blood.

cyanotic, pertaining to cyanosis.

cyclomate, a nonnutritive artificial sweetener.

cycle, a sequence of events or symptoms, usually recurring at regular intervals.

cyclic, pertaining to cycles.

cyclitis, inflammation of the ciliary body of the eye.

cycloplegia, paralysis of the ciliary muscles of the eye.

cyclothymia, a mild psychosis of the manic-depressive type in which the personality alternates between depressed and elated states.

cyclothyme, a person afflicted with cyclothymia.

cyclotron, an instrument for smashing the atom.

cyesis, see **pregnancy.**

cyst, 1. a bladder, sac, or vesicle. 2. a closed bladderlike sac containing fluid or semifluid morbid matter.

cystadenoma, a growth containing an adenoma and cysts.

cystalgia, pain in the urinary bladder.

cystectomy, surgical excision of a cyst or bladder.

cystic, 1. pertaining to a cyst. 2. of or pertaining to the urinary bladder or gallbladder.

cystic fibrosis, a heredi-tary disease appearing in childhood involving the pancreas and lungs.

cystitis, inflammation of the bladder.

cystocele, a hernia or rupture formed by the protrusion of the urinary bladder into the vagina.

cystocolostomy, the surgical formation of a permanent communication between the colon and the gallbladder.

cystoid, resembling a cyst, but having no membrane; bladderlike.

cystolith, a stone in the urinary bladder.

cystolithectomy, surgical removal of a calculus from either the urinary bladder or gallbladder.

cystoplasty, plastic surgery upon the bladder.

cystoscope, an instrument for examining the interior of the bladder.

cystoscopy, examination of the bladder by means of a cystoscope.

cystospasm, a spasmodic contraction or cramp of the urinary bladder.

cystostomy, surgical incision of the urinary bladder to make a temporary opening.

cytoarchitecture, the cell structure of a bodily tissue or part.

cytoblast, a cell nucleus.

cytochemistry, the science of the structure and chemistry of living cells.

cytochromes, a class of iron-containing proteins found in cells of animals and plants dependent upon oxygen.

cytogenesis, the origin of development of cells.

cytokinesis, cytoplasmic changes during fertilization and cell division.

cytology, the scientific study of the structure, functions, and life cycle of cells.

cytolysis, the dissolution or degeneration of cells.

cytoplasm, the living substance of protoplasm of a cell exclusive of the nucleus.

cytotropic, 1. drawn toward or having an attraction for cells, as various viruses. 2. of or pertaining to the propensity of cells to be drawn toward or to move away from each other, singly or in groups.

cytotropism, the tendency of cells to move.

dacryocele, protrusion of a tear sac.

dacryocyst, the tear sac.

dacryocystalgia, pain in the tear sac.

dacryocystitis, the inflammation of a tear sac.

dacryocystotomy, surgical incision of a tear sac.

dacryolith, stony concretion in the tear duct.

dacryorrhea, excessive flow of tears.

dactyl, a finger or toe.

dactylar, pertaining to a finger or toe.

dactylate, resembling a finger or toe.

dactylitis, inflammation of the bones of a finger or toe.

dactylology, 1. the art of communicating ideas or thoughts by the fingers. 2. the language of the deaf and dumb.

dactylomegaly, abnormally large fingers or toes.

dactylospasm, cramp in a finger or toe.

daltonism, color blindness, esp. the inability to differentiate between red and green.

dandruff, a scurf that forms on the scalp and is shed in small scales or particles.

dandy fever, see **dengue.**

dartos, the muscular tissue beneath the skin of the scrotum, which is able to tighten up the organ, as in cold weather.

Darwinian, 1. of or pertaining to the naturalist Charles Darwin or to his doctrine. 2. a believer in Darwinism.

Darwinism, the doctrine, promulgated by Darwin, of the origin and modifications of species on the basis of the survival of the fittest.

DDT, abbreviation for dichlorodiphenyltrichloroethane, a powerful synthetic insecticide.

deaf, lacking the sense of hearing, either wholly or in part.

deaf-mute, a person who is both deaf and dumb, esp. one whose dumbness dates from birth or early life.

deafness, the loss of ability to hear, which can vary in degree.

deallergize, see **desensitize.**

deaminate, to remove an amino group from a compound.

death rattle, a rattling sound made by a person immediately before dying, caused by air passing through mucus in the throat.

debilitate, to weaken; to enfeeble.

debilitation, the act of weakening; the state of enfeeblement.

debility, a state of general bodily weakness; feebleness.

debridement, the surgical removal of foreign matter or contaminated tissue from a wound to prevent the spread of infection.

decalcification, the loss or removal of lime or calcium salts from bones.

decalcify, to deprive, as a bone, of lime or calcareous matter.

decant, 1. to pour off gently, without disturbing sediment. 2. to pour from one vessel to another.

decapitate, to cut off the head. 2. to kill by beheading.

dechloridation, removal of sodium chloride from the body by a reduction or by restricting the dietary intake of salt.

dechlorination, see **dechloridation.**

decibal, a unit for measuring the volume of sound.

decidua, a membrane arising from the alteration of the upper layer of the mucous membrane of the uterus after reception of the fertilized ovum, which is cast off at parturition.

decidual, of or pertaining to the decidua.

deciduate, characterized by or having a decidua.

deciduoma, a uterine tumor.

deciduous, falling off or shed at a particular stage of growth, as teeth.

declinator, a surgical instrument used to retract or hold apart tissue or parts from the immediate operation field.

decline, a gradual decrease of physical powers.

decoct, to extract the strength or flavor from a medicinal preparation by boiling.

decoction, 1. the act of decocting. 2. an extract obtained by decoction. 3. a liquid in which a substance, usually animal or vegetable, has been boiled, and which thus contains the soluble constituents or principles of the substance.

decolorant, a substance having properties that bleach or remove color.

decoloration, the removal of color; abstraction or loss of color.

decolorization, the process of depriving of color.

decompensation, the inability of a diseased organ to compensate for its deficiency, esp. the loss of compensation in the functioning of the heart.

decompose, 1. to separate into constituent parts or elementary particles. 2. to decay or rot; putrefy. 3.

to become resolved into constitutent elements.

decompress, to release from pressure or compression, as in an air lock or decompression chamber.

decompression, 1. the process of decreasing or removing air pressure from a chamber. 2. an adjustment to normal atmospheric pressure after high-altitude flight or a deep-water dive. 3. the technique or operation used to reduce pressure upon an organ.

decongestant, an agent or drug that relieves congestion, esp. in the mucous membrane of the nose.

decontaminate, to purify; to free from harmful substances as poisonous gas, radioactivity.

decortication, removal or stripping off of the surface layer of an organ, as the removal of the capsule of the kidney.

decrepit, wasted or worn by the infirmities of old age.

decrepitude, 1. the state of being decrepit. 2. weakened, as from the infirmities of old age.

decrudescence, decline in severity of a disease.

decubital, pertaining to decubitus.

decubitus, see **bedsore.**

decussate, to cross, as nerves in the body.

decussation, the crossing of two lines, rays, or nerves, which meet in a point and then diverge.

defecate, to void excrement from the bowels.

defect, a flaw; blemish; imperfection; deformity.

defective, 1. marked by a subnormal condition, either mental or physical. 2. one who is physically or mentally deficient.

defeminization, loss of secondary feminine sexual characteristics, usually as a result of hormonal defects.

deferent, serving to convey away; as, a deferent duct.

deferentitis, an inflammation of the vas deferens.

defervescence, a lowering of fever.

defibrillation, stopping of the normal rhythm of the heart.

deficiency disease, a disease caused by a dietary insufficiency, as of vitamins, minerals, or other essential elements.

deflection, an unconscious diversion of ideas from conscious attention.

deform, to disfigure; to render ugly or unpleasing.

deformity, 1. the state of being deformed. 2. a misformed or misshapen part of the body.

degenerate, 1. to decline in physical, mental, or moral qualities. 2. one who has retrograded from a normal type or standard, as in morals or character. 3. one exhibiting certain morbid physical and mental traits and tendencies, esp. from birth. 4. one given to sexual perversion.

degeneration, 1. the process of degenerating. 2. a process by which normal tissue is converted into or replaced by tissue of an inferior quality, as, fatty degeneration. 3. the morbid condition produced by such a process.

deglutition, the act of swallowing.

degradation, the act of degrading; the state of being degraded.

degust, to taste.

degustation, the act of tasting.

dehiscence, the bursting open, esp. of a wound.

dehumanization, degeneration of the qualities that differentiate a human being from an animal.

dehumanize, 1. to deprive of the character of humanity. 2. to deprive of tenderness or softness of feeling. 3. to bring about a loss of individuality.

dehydrate, to lose water or moisture.

dehydration, the loss or removal of water.

dehypnotize, to bring out of a hypnotic state.

déjà vu, the feeling of having experienced at a prior time something actually being experienced for the first time.

dejecta, see **excrement.**

dejection, 1. the state of being downcast. 2. depression of mind. 3. lowness of spirits. 4. excrement.

deleterious, injurious; pernicious; harmful to health or well-being.

delinquency, antisocial behavior.

delinquent, 1. failing in or neglectful of duty or obligation. 2. guilty of a misdeed or offense. 3. being antisocial.

deliquesce, to melt gradually and become liquid by attracting and absorbing moisture from the air, as certain salts, acids, and alkalis.

deliquescence, 1. the process of deliquescing. 2. the resulting liquid.

delirious, characteristic of or pertaining to delirium.

delirium, a more or less temporary disorder of the mental faculties, as in fevers and intoxication, characterized by restlessness, excitement, delusions, and hallucinations.

delirium tremens, a violent delirium caused by excessive consumption of alcohol.

deliver, to give birth.

delivery, the state of being delivered of, or giving birth to, a child; parturition.

delomorphous, having a definite shape or form.

deltoid, a large triangular muscle covering the joint of the shoulder and serving to raise the arm laterally.

delusion, an abnormal phenomenon in which a belief is held despite the presence of evidence sufficient to destroy it.

delusional, characterized by delusions.

demented, mad; insane; out of one's mind.

dementia, any condition of

deteriorated mentality, esp. a decline in the appropriateness of emotional responses and in intellectual powers.

dementia praecox, see **schizophrenia.**

demineralization, abnormal loss of mineral salts from the body.

demonophobia, irrational fear of demons.

demoniac, 1. one seemingly possessed by a demon or evil spirit. 2. a lunatic.

demulcent, a medicine that lessens the effects of irritation, as mucilaginous substances.

demyelinated, pertaining to nerve fibers from which the myelin sheaths have been removed.

denature, 1. to render unfit for human consumption without impairing usefulness for other purposes, as alcohol. 2. to change the nature of.

dengue, an infectious, eruptive, usually epidemic fever of warm climates, characterized esp. by severe pains in the joints and muscles; breakbone fever.

dental, 1. of or pertaining to the teeth. 2. of or pertaining to dentistry.

dental floss, a soft thread, sometimes coated with wax, used to clean between teeth.

dentalgia, see **toothache.**

dental hygienist, one who assists a dentist in the minor functions of dentistry, such as cleaning teeth and taking X rays.

dental technician, a specialist who makes dental appliances.

dentate, toothed; notched.

dentation, a projection in the shape of a tooth.

denticle, a small tooth or projecting point.

dentifrice, a powder, paste, or liquid used in cleaning teeth.

dentin, the hard calcareous tissue beneath the enamel and the cementum of a tooth, enclosing the pulp, and composing the greater part of the tooth.

dentine, see **dentin.**

dentist, one who cares for and treats the teeth, gums, and oral cavity.

dentistry, the profession that deals with the diagnosis, prevention, and treatment of oral malformations and diseases affecting the teeth and their related structures.

dentition, 1. the process of cutting teeth in infancy. 2. the period during which the teeth develop. 3. the tooth system, including number, kind, and arrangement of teeth, that is peculiar to man and other animals.

dentoid, resembling a tooth.

denture, false teeth; one or more artificial teeth used to replace natural teeth.

denudation, the act of denuding; denuded or bare condition.

denude, to make bare or naked; to strip.

deodorant, 1. an agent for destroying odors. 2. a

preparation for checking or masking body odors.

deodorize, to rid of odor or smell, esp. of fetid odor resulting from impurities.

deossification, loss of mineral matter from bones; absorption of bone.

deoxidize, to deprive of oxygen, or reduce from the state of an oxide.

deoxygenate, to remove oxygen from.

deoxyribonucleic acid, see **DNA.**

depersonalization, a mental disorder in which the patient feels he has lost his personality or personal quality.

depersonalize, to deprive of personality or personal quality.

depigmentation, loss of pigment.

depilate, to strip of hair.

depilation, loss or removal of hair.

depilatory, 1. a cosmetic employed to remove superfluous hair from the human skin. 2. having the power to remove hair from the skin.

deplete, to empty or relieve, as by bloodletting or purging.

deplumation, loss or falling out of eyelashes because of disease.

deposit, see **sediment.**

depraved, corrupted; perverted; immoral.

depravity, 1. the state of being depraved. 2. an act or practice exhibiting corrupted morals.

depressant, 1. having the quality of depressing or

lowering activity; sedative. 2. a depressant substance or agent; a sedative.

depressed, 1. dispirited; discouraged; sad; languid; dull. 2. below the normal level, as in a depressed fracture of the skull in which a fragment of bone is driven below its normal level and into the brain.

depression, 1. a hollow. 2. the state or feeling of being depressed in spirits. 3. a low state of strength.

depressomotor, 1. causing a retardation of motor activity, as, depressomotor nerves. 2. a depressomotor agent, as bromine.

depurate, to free from impurities; to purify; to clarify.

deradenitis, inflammation of a lymph gland in the neck.

derange, to unsettle the reason of; to make insane.

deranged, disarranged; disordered; insane.

derangement, a disorder; a mental disorder.

derma, 1. the corium, or true skin, beneath the epidermis. 2. the skin in general.

dermal, pertaining to the skin.

dermatitis, inflammation of the derma.

dermatogen, a cellular layer at the top of a root or stem from which the epidermis is produced.

dermatoid, resembling skin; skinlike.

dermatology, the science of the skin and its diseases.

dermatologist, a physician specializing in dermatology.

dermatome, a surgical instrument used in skin grafting for cutting skin.

dermatomycosis, any skin disease caused by a fungus, such as athlete's foot.

dermatophobia, pathological fear of having or contracting a skin disease.

dermatophyde, a parasitic plant infesting the skin, hair, and nails of men and animals, giving rise to various forms of skin disease, as ringworm.

dermatoplasty, the replacement of skin by skin grafting; plastic surgery.

dermatosis, any disease of the skin.

dermis, see **derma.**

dermoid, see **dermal** and **dermatoid.**

desensitize, 1. to make less sensitive. 2. to remove the sensitivity or reactivity, as of an organ or tissue, to an outside stimulus by means of desensitizing injections.

desiccant, a medicine or application having drying qualities.

desiccate, to dry; to remove moisture from; to dehydrate, as food.

desiccation, the process of drying.

desiccator, 1. one who or that which desiccates. 2. an apparatus for drying fruit or milk. 3. an apparatus for absorbing the moisture present in a chemical substance.

desmitis, inflammation of a ligament.

desmoid, 1. resembling a ligament; ligamentous. 2. resembling a bundle, as applied to certain fibrous tumors.

desmology, the science of tendons and ligaments.

desmotomy, surgical incision to separate ligaments.

desquamate, to shed in scales, as the epidermis in certain diseases; to scale or peel off.

desquamation, shedding or peeling of the skin.

deteriorate, 1. to grow worse or inferior in quality, value, or character. 2. to be impaired in quality. 3. to degenerate. 4. to decompose.

detoxicate, see **detoxify.**

detoxify, to remove poisonous qualities or effects from.

detritus, any disintegrated material, waste product, or substance.

detrude, to thrust down or away; to push down.

detrusion, the act of detruding; ejection.

detrusor, anything serving to expel something, as the detrusor muscle of the urinary bladder that helps to expel urine.

detumescence, the subsidence of a swelling.

deuteranope, a person who has deuteranopia.

deuteranopia, a type of color blindness in which a person cannot distinguish green and red.

deviate, a person or thing differing from a norm.

deviated septum, the deflection, congenital or acquired by injury, of the cartilaginous partition between the nostrils.

devitalize, to deprive of vitality; to weaken.

devolution, degeneration, as opposed to **evolution.**

dexter, pertaining to or situated on the right side.

dexterity, 1. the quality of being dexterous. 2. manual adroitness or skill. 3. adroitness in the use of the body generally. 4. mental adroitness or skill; cleverness. 5. right-handedness.

dexterous, having skill with the hands; having dexterity.

dextrad, to the right, as opposed to **sinistrad.**

dextrocardia, a condition in which the heart lies more to the right side of the chest than somewhat to the left as is usual.

dextroglucose, see **dextrose.**

dextrose, 1. the sugar found in blood and in many plants. 2. corn sugar.

dextrosuria, the presence of dextrose in the urine.

diabetes, any one of various diseases, most of them characterized by abnormal urinary conditions. Without qualification, the term diabetes refers to diabetes mellitus.

diabetes mellitus, a chronic disease characterized by excessive sugar in the blood and in-termittent or continued presence of sugar in the urine, increased excretion of urine and accompanying thirst, and often by increased appetite plus weight loss; alleviated by regular injection of insulin.

diabetes insipidus, a disease characterized by chronic excretion of large amounts of unconcentrated urine and extreme thirst, alleviated by a pituitary hormone extract.

diabetic, 1. of, pertaining to, or affected with diabetes. 2. a person suffering from diabetes.

diagnose, 1. to ascertain the cause, as of an illness or disease, by studying symptoms. 2. to determine the nature or cause, as of a malfunction, by means of scientific analysis.

diagnosis, identification of diseases by their distinctive marks or symptoms; the conclusion reached.

diagnostic, distinguishing; characteristic; indicating the nature of a disease.

diagnostics, that branch of medicine dealing with the diagnosis of diseases.

dialysis, the act or process of separating the crystalloid elements of a body from colloid by diffusion through a membrane.

dialyze, to separate by a dialyzer.

dialyzer, the parchment, or septum, stretched over a ring used in the process of dialysis.

diameter, any straight line

passing through the center of a circle or other curvilinear figure, terminated by the circumference, and dividing the figure into two equal parts, as the pelvic diameter.

diapedesis, the process by which the blood passes through the capillary walls into the tissues.

diaper rash, red spots or patches on the skin of babies caused by irritation from wet diapers.

diaphanous, 1. almost totally transparent. 2. translucent. 3. extremely delicate in form.

diaphoresis, profuse sweating.

diaphoretic, an agent that increases sweating.

diaphragm, 1. a partition or septum. 2. the partition separating the chest cavity from the abdominal cavity. 3. a device placed over the uterine cervix for contraception.

diarrhea, an ailment characterized by abnormally frequent and fluid evacuation of the intestines.

diarrhoea, see **diarrhea.**

diarthrosis, a joint in which the bones revolve freely in every direction, as in the shoulder joint.

diarthrodial, pertaining to diarthrosis.

diastase, an enzyme found in barley and oats after germination and in the digestive juice, which converts starch into sugar.

diastasis, 1. dislocation or separation of bones with-

out fracture. 2. pertaining to the heart, the rest period between the diastole and the systole.

diastole, 1. the normal rhythmic dilatation of the heart, esp. that of the ventricles. 2. any of various other rhythmical dilatations.

diastolic, pertaining to the diastole of the heart.

diathermic, having the property of radiant heat; relating to diathermy.

diathermic surgery, surgery performed by the use of a high-frequency electric arc to cut living tissue and thus avoid excessive bleeding.

diathermy, the application of electric current to produce heat on tissues below the skin for therapeutic purposes.

diathesis, 1. predisposition to certain diseases rather than to others. 2. the tendency to a particular mental development.

dichotomize, 1. to divide into parts. 2. to divide into pairs.

dichotomous, 1. divided or dividing into two parts. 2. characterized by or involving successive division or branching into two parts. 3. pertaining to dichotomy.

dichotomy, division into two parts or categories.

dichromatism, a form of color blindness in which only two of the three primary colors are perceived.

dicrotic, pertaining to dicrotism.

dicrotism, a condition in which there are two arterial beats for one heartbeat.

Dicumarol, a substance found in clover and hay and also prepared synthetically, used to prevent clotting of the blood (trademark).

didelphic, relating to or having a double womb.

didymitis, inflammation of the testicle.

dienestrol, a synthetic female ovarian hormone, used for estrogen therapy.

diencephalon, the posterior part of the prosencephalon, or forebrain. brain.

diet, 1. a person's regular food and drink. 2. a course of food and drink prescribed, as for health reasons, and limited in kind and quantity. 3. to eat according to rules prescribed, esp. in order to lose weight.

dietetic, pertaining to diet.

dietetics, the science of nutrition.

dietician, one skilled in dietetics; one who arranges diets.

diet kitchen, a kitchen for preparing and dispensing special diets, in a hospital.

differential, 1. of or pertaining to difference or diversity. 2. exhibiting or depending upon a difference or distinction between things, individuals, or groups.

differential blood count, the counting under a mi-

croscope of the number of white and red blood cells in a blood sample.

differential diagnosis, a diagnosis arrived at by comparing two or more similar diseases.

differentiation, 1. the act or process of differentiating, or the resulting state. 2. the modification of cells, tissues, and body parts as they develop into mature structure and function.

diffuse, spreading widely, horizontally, and irregularly.

diffusion, a spreading or scattering.

digest, to convert, as food or drink, in the alimentary canal into a form absorbable by the body tissues.

digestion, the process that food undergoes, primarily through the action of enzymes in the alimentary canal, whereby it is prepared for absorption into and nourishment of the body tissues.

digestive, pertaining to digestion.

digit, 1. a finger or toe. 2. the breadth of a finger, or 3/4 inch.

digital, 1. of or pertaining to digits. 2. resembling a finger or toe.

digitalin, 1. a white, crystalline powder, a glucoside of digitalis used in medicine. 2. any of several mixtures of glucosides extracted from digitalis.

digitalis, 1. any of several Eurasian herbs of the figwort family, esp. the common foxglove. 2. the dried and powdered leaf of foxglove containing several important glucosides and serving as a powerful heart stimulant and a diuretic.

digitalize, to administer digitalis in the treatment of heart disease.

digitalization, 1. the process of administering digitalis in the course of treatment. 2. the physiological effect induced by this.

digitate, possessing digits or digitlike appendages.

digitoxin, a bitter, odorless, white, highly poisonous powder, the most active glucoside of digitalis, used as a heart stimulant.

dilatation, 1. a pathological enlargement, as of an organ or passageway. 2. an induced, temporary enlargement of an opening or passageway, as to aid examination. 3. the establishment of or restoration to normal size of an abnormally small canal or orifice.

dilate, to expand or swell, esp. by filling.

dilated, expanded from a side, or in all directions; broadened.

dilative, tending or causing to dilate.

dilator, an implement used to dilate an opening or canal of the body.

dilute, 1. to render liquid or more liquid, esp. by mixing with water. 2. to weaken by an admixture.

dilution, 1. the act of diluting. 2. weakening the strength of a solution.

diminution, the act, fact, or process of diminishing; lessening; reduction.

dimple, a small natural depression in the cheek or other part of the body.

diopter, in lenses, the unit of refractive power, being that of the reciprocal of the focal lens. One diopter is the unit of measurement of the focus of a lens.

dioptometer, an instrument that measures the eye's accommodation and refraction.

dioptric, 1. of or pertaining to dioptrics. 2. assisting vision by refracting light, as a lens.

dioptrics, the branch of optics that deals with refraction of light.

dioxide, an oxide consisting of two atoms of oxygen per molecule, as carbon dioxide.

diphase, having two phases.

diphtheria, an epidemic inflammatory disease of the air passages, and esp. of the throat, characterized by the formation of a false membrane; now controlled by vaccine injections.

diphtheritic, connected with, relating to, or formed by diphtheria.

diphyodont, having two successive sets of teeth.

diplegia, paralysis of two similar parts on either side of the body, as two legs or two arms.

diplococcus, a form of parasitic bacteria occurring in pairs.

diploe, the cancellate bony tissue between the hard inner and outer walls of the bones of the cranium.

diploic, pertaining to the diploe.

diploid, having the two sets of chromosomes characteristic of a somatic cell.

diplophonia, the simultaneous production of two different voice tones from the larynx, caused by paralysis of one of the vocal cords.

diplopia, double vision.

dipsomania, an irresistible, generally periodic, craving for intoxicating liquor.

dipsophobia, pathological fear of alcohol.

disaccharide, any of a class of sugars yielding two monosaccharide molecules upon hydrolysis.

disarticulate, 1. to take apart at the joints. 2. to come apart at the joints.

disarticulation, surgical removal of a limb by cutting through the joint.

disc, see **disk.**

discharge, the flowing away or emission from the body of a secretion or excretion, which may be composed of pus, blood, mucus, feces, urine, etc.

disease, an impairment of the functioning of a system of the body, or an organ or part thereof.

disinfect, to cleanse of infection by destroying or inhibiting the activity of disease-producing microorganisms.

disinfectant, a chemical substance or other agent, such as ultraviolet light, used to disinfect inanimate objects.

disinfestation, rendering free from infesting insects or parasites; delousing.

disjoint, 1. to separate at the joints. 2. to put out of joint; to dislocate. 3. to separate bones from their joint.

disk, any thin, flat, circular plate or organ, as one of the fibro-cartilaginous plates between the vertebrae of the spinal column.

dislocate, 1. to move out of place. 2. to wrench out of proper position or joint, esp. a bone.

dislocation, the act or result of dislocating.

disorganize, 1. to disturb or destroy the organic structure or orderly arrangement of. 2. to throw into confusion or disorder.

disorganization, 1. the act of disorganizing. 2. the state of being disorganized.

disorient, to cause to lose one's bearings; to confuse.

disorientation, 1. the state of being disoriented. 2. temporary or permanent loss of the perception of space, time, or identity.

dispensary, 1. a place in which medicines are dispensed. 2. a charitable establishment where medicines and medical advice are given gratis or for a nominal fee.

disposition, 1. a natural tendency or aptitude. 2. susceptibility to disease.

dissect, to anatomize; to divide, separate, or cut apart, esp. a body for scientific investigation and study.

dissection, the act of dissecting; the state of being dissected.

dissector, one who dissects; an anatomist.

disseminate, to spread or scatter widely.

dissemination, the act of disseminating.

dissolution, the act of dissolving; liquefaction; a breaking up.

distal, 1. applied to the end of a bone, limb, or organ farthest removed from the point of attachment. 2. situated at the extremity. 3. most distant from the center.

distemper, 1. one of several highly contagious diseases of animals, esp. one affecting young dogs. 2. to derange the bodily function or mental state of.

distend, to stretch or swell by force from within; to dilate; to expand; to swell; of the bladder or the lungs, to puff out.

distill, to concentrate or purify by distillation.

distillation, 1. the process of purification or refinement of a substance. 2. the separation of different substances.

districhiasis, the growing of two hairs from one follicle.

distrix, the splitting of the ends of hair.

dither, a state of great agitation, excitement, or confusion.

diuresis, an excessive flow of urine.

diuretic, a medicine that increases the secretion of urine.

diurnal, belonging to the period of daylight, as distinguished from night; happening every day.

diver's paresis, an occupational disease taking the form of paralysis, occurring in caisson disease or bends.

diverticular, pertaining to a diverticulum.

diverticulitis, inflammation of the diverticulum.

diverticulosis, the presence of many diverticula in the colon without symptoms.

diverticulum, a blind, tubular sac or process branching off from a canal or cavity.

divulsion, 1. the act of pulling or tearing apart. 2. violent separation. 3. laceration.

divulsor, a device for dilation of a part, esp. the urethra.

dizygotic, describing fraternal twins.

dizzy, 1. having a sensation of whirling with instability or proneness to fall; giddy. 2. mentally confused or dazed.

dizziness, the state of being dizzy.

DNA, deoxyribonucleic acid, a compound found in chromosomes consisting of a long chain molecule comprising many repeated and varied combinations of four nucleotides, one of which is the sugar deoxyribose; subdivisions of the molecule are believed to be the genes.

doctor, a person licensed to practice medicine; a physician, dentist, or veterinarian.

dolichocephalic, long-headed; having a breadth of skull small in proportion to the length from front to back.

dolichocranic, having a skull with a cranial index of less than 75; proportionately smaller in breadth than in length.

dolor, grief; sorrow; lamentation.

dolorous, expressing pain or grief; sorrowful; doleful.

dolorific, causing pain.

domatophobia, pathological fear of being in a house; a form of claustrophobia.

dominant, 1. prevailing. 2. designating a generic character or trait that overshadows the effect of recessive characters in an organism.

donor, a person who gives or donates, as a person furnishing blood for transfusion or biological tissue or organ for transplant.

dope, a slang expression for stupefying or stimulating drugs.

doraphobia, pathological aversion to touching skins or fur.

dormancy, state of being dormant.

dormant, 1. sleeping; lying asleep or as if asleep. 2. inactive.

dorsalgia, back pain.

dorsalis, relating to the back.

dorsolateral, of or pertaining to the back and sides.

dorsoventral, extending from the dorsal to the ventral side of the body.

dorsum, 1. the back, as of the body. 2. the back or outer surface of an organ or part of the body.

dosage, 1. the administration of medicine in dosages. 2. the amount of medicine administered.

dose, a quantity of medicine prescribed to be taken at one time.

dosimeter, an apparatus for measuring minute doses of radiation or X rays.

dosimetry, the determination of doses of medicine or radiation.

dotage, feebleness or imbecility, particularly in old age; childishness of old age; senility.

dotard, one whose intellect is impaired by age.

double vision, 1. the seeing of two images of one object at the same time.

douche, 1. a jet or current of water or the like applied to a particular part or cavity of the body for hygienic or medicinal purposes. 2. an instrument for administering it.

dragée, a sugar-coated medicine.

drainage, a slow draining of fluids, as from wounds, with a tube or other appliance.

dream, to have vivid images and thoughts during sleep.

dressing, that with which something is dressed, as bandages for a wound.

drip, 1. to fall in drops. 2. to cause liquid medicaments, blood, plasma, and the like to fall in drops. 3. a device for administering fluid slowly and continuously, esp. in a vein. 4. the material so injected.

drivel, to let saliva flow from the mouth; to slaver.

dropsy, an abnormal collection of serous fluid in any cavity of the body or in cellular tissue. See **edema.**

drug, any medicinal substance for internal or external use given for the purpose of treatment or prevention of disease or for diagnosis; also for relieving pain.

druggist, a pharmacist; the operator or owner of a drugstore.

drum, see **eardrum.**

duct, a tube, canal, or vessel conveying a bodily fluid, esp. a glandular secretion.

ductless glands, see **endocrine glands.**

ductule, a small duct.

dumb, mute; without the power of speech.

duodenal, pertaining to the duodenum.

duodenectomy, surgical excision of the duodenum or part of it.

duodenitis, inflammation of the duodenum.

duodenostomy, surgical formation of an artificial opening into the duodenum through the abdominal wall.

duodenum, the first portion of the small intestine, extending from the stomach to the jejunum.

dural, pertaining to the dura mater.

dura mater, the tough, fibrous membrane forming the outermost of the three coverings of the brain and spinal cord.

dwarf, a human being much smaller than the ordinary stature or size.

dwarfism, the state of being a dwarf.

dynamometer, an instrument for measuring force or power; also for measuring muscular strength.

dysacousia, discomfort caused by loud noises; hypersensitivity of the sense of hearing.

dyscrasia, a generally faulty or disordered condition of the body.

dysenteric, pertaining to dysentery.

dysentery, an infectious disease characterized by inflammation and ulceration of the lower portion of the bowels, with diarrhea that becomes mucous and hemorrhagic.

dysfunction, abnormal or impaired functioning, as of an organ.

dysgenics, the scientific study of factors that cause degeneration in the type of offspring produced.

dysgerminoma, a malignant, slow-growing tumor of the ovary or testicle.

dysgraphia, inability to write, usually caused by a disorder of the brain.

dyskinesia, a number of diseases causing impairment of voluntary movements.

dyslexia, a term for a variety of writing, reading, and learning disorders.

dysmenorrhea, excessively painful or difficult menstruation.

dyspepsia, impaired digestion.

dyspeptic, pertaining to, subject to, or suffering from dyspepsia.

dysphagia, difficulty in swallowing.

dysphasia, impairment of speech caused by a disease of the nervous system.

dysphoria, a general feeling of anxiety, depression, and restlessness.

dysplasia, 1. abnormal development or growth, as of cells, organs, or tissues. 2. abnormality in anatomic structure due to such growth.

dyspnea, labored or difficult breathing; shortness of breath, sometimes accompanied by pain.

dystrophic, pertaining to dystrophy.

dystrophy, 1. faulty nutrition or abnormal development. 2. any of several neuromuscular ailments marked by degeneration or weakness of muscle.

dysuria, see alginuresis.

ear, the organ of hearing and equilibrium, composed of the external ear, a cartilaginous funnel for collecting sound waves and directing them inward; the middle ear, called tympanum or drum; and the internal ear, or labyrinth.

earache, pain in the ear.

eardrum, the tympanic membrane that separates the middle ear from the external ear.

earlobe, the soft, pendent part of the ear.

earwax, a yellowish waxlike secretion from certain glands in the external auditory canal, acting as a lubricant and arresting the entrance of dust.

eburnation, degeneration of bone and cartilage, caused by osteoarthritis, which makes them become harder and denser.

ecbolic, a substance that produces or hastens labor or abortion by causing the womb to contract.

eccentric, 1. deviating from the usual practice; odd; peculiar in behavior. 2. not concentric; being away from the center. 3. peripheral.

eccentricity, behavior that deviates from the usual; oddity; whimsicality.

ecchondroma, a cartilaginous tumor.

eccrine, pertaining to secretion.

eccrinology, the study of secretion and secretory glands.

eccyesis, extrauterine pregnancy.

echidnin, poisonous snake

venom.

Echinococcus, a genus of tapeworms that in the larval stage invade tissues and form cysts, esp. in the liver.

echinosis, a change in the blood corpuscles by which they lose their smooth outline.

echolalia, 1. an infant's normal imitation of sounds made by others. 2. uncontrollable repetition of another person's words.

eclampsia, a form of toxemia, marked by convulsions of recurrent nature, and occurring during pregnancy or childbirth.

ecmnesia, loss of memory of recent events, occurring in senility.

ecological, pertaining to ecology.

ecologist, a specialist in ecology.

ecology, the branch of sociology concerned with human populations, their environment, spatial distribution, and resulting cultural patterns.

ecphoria, recall of memory; reestablishment of memory.

ecphyma, an excrescence, as a wart.

ectiris, the outermost portion of the iris.

ectoblast, see **ectoderm**.

ectoderm, the outer primary layer of cells in the embryo, as opposed to endoderm.

ectogenous, capable of developing outside of the host, as certain pathogenic bacteria.

ectomere, any of the cells formed from the fertilized egg that eventually make up the ectoderm.

ectomorph, 1. a type of body structure characterized by linearity and leanness, developed by the relative dominance of tissues derived from the ectoderm, the outermost of the three cell layers of the embryo. 2. a person having this type of body structure.

ectomorphic, of, pertaining to, or characteristic of ectomorphs.

ectoparasite, an external parasite, opposed to endoparasite.

ectopia, malposition of an organ or structure.

ectopic, in an abnormal position.

ectopic pregnancy, a pregnancy occurring in the abdomen or a fallopian tube instead of in the womb.

ectoplasm, the outer portion of the cytoplasm in a cell.

ectopotomy, surgical removal of a fetus developing outside the uterus in an ectopic pregnancy.

ectoretina, the outermost layer of the retina.

ectotoxemia, blood poisoning caused by introduction of a poison into the blood.

ectromelia, congenital absence of a limb or part of a limb.

ectropic, see **eversion**.

ectropion, eversion of an edge or part, esp. of an eyelid.

eczema, an inflammatory disease of the skin attended by itching and the exudation of serous matter.

eczematoid, resembling eczema.

eczematous, pertaining to eczema.

edeitis, see **vulvitis.**

edema, a swelling caused by excessive accumulation of fluid in a serous cavity or connective tissue.

edematous, pertaining to edema.

edentulous, without teeth.

educational psychology, the branch of psychology that investigates educational problems through psychological methods and concepts.

edulcorate, to free from acids, salts, or impurities by washing.

effect, a result; a consequence; the end result.

effector, a motor nerve that transforms nerve impulses into physical action.

effeminate, 1. having qualities unsuitable to a man. 2. womanish.

efferent, conveying outward from a central organ or a point, esp. conveying impulses from a nerve center to an effector.

effervesce, 1. to bubble, hiss, and froth, as when the gaseous part escapes from a liquid. 2. to show signs of excitement.

effervescence, 1. the bubbling, frothing, or sparkling of a fluid when some part of the mass flies off in a gaseous form. 2. strong manifestation of feelings.

effete, lacking vitality; exhausted.

effleurage, deep and gentle stroking movements given in massage.

efflorescence, a redness, rash, or eruption of the skin.

effluvium, something flowing out in a subtle or invisible form; emanation, esp. a noxious or disagreeable exhalation.

effusion, 1. the escape of any fluid from the vessel containing it into a cavity of the body. 2. the escaping fluid itself.

egersis, extreme alertness; abnormal wakefulness.

egest, to discharge from the body; void; excrete.

egesta, matter egested from the body; excrement.

egestion, the process of egesting; the voiding of the refuse of digestion.

egg, the roundish reproductive body in a membrane, produced by the female, consisting of the ovum or female reproductive cell together with its appendages.

ego, 1. that part of the psyche that is conscious, experiencing and reacting to the outside world and thus acting as mediator between the id's unconscious primitive impulses and society's expectations. 2. egotism; vanity; self-esteem; self-concept.

egocentric, 1. self-centered. 2. regarding oneself as the center of all things, esp. in relation to the world.

ego ideal, a desired and actively sought standard of personal excellence, derived from the total of positive identifications with parents or other esteemed persons.

egoism, the habit of valuing everything only in reference to one's personal interest; pure selfishness; self-conceit.

egoist, a self-centered or selfish person; a conceited individual.

egoistic, characterized by or proceeding from egoism or selfishness.

egomania, egotism developed to an abnormal degree.

egotism, 1. the practice of too frequently using the word I; hence, a practice of speaking or writing too much about oneself. 2. an objectionable degree of pride. 3. a passionate and exaggerated love of self, bringing one to refer all things to oneself and to judge everything by its relation to one's interest or importance.

egotist, a conceited, self-centered, boastful person.

egotistical, pertaining to egotism.

eidetic, of, referring to, or composed of visual images that can be reproduced from memory with almost photographic accuracy.

eighth nerve, the acoustic nerve; the eighth cranial nerve.

ejaculate, to eject semen.

ejaculation, the sudden discharge of semen by the male reproductive organs.

ejaculatio precox, premature ejaculation.

elastin, the protein or albuminoid that constitutes the basic substance of elastic tissue as found in tendons and cartilage.

elbow, the outer part of the bend or joint of the arm.

Electra complex, the unresolved, usually unconscious, libidinal feelings of a daughter toward her father, accompanied by jealousy of the mother.

electroanalysis, chemical analysis by electrolysis.

electroanalytical, pertaining to electroanalysis.

electroanesthesia, local or general anesthesia induced by an anesthetizing agent injected by electricity.

electrocardiogram, the record produced by an electrocardiograph.

electrocardiograph, an electric instrument used in medical diagnosis to detect and record the heartbeat.

electrocardiography, the study and recording of electrocardiograms.

electrocatalysis, chemical decomposition of compounds by means of electricity.

electrocautery, cauterization by means of an instrument with a platinum wire tip that can be heated by electricity and used to burn small growths or to coagulate small blood vessels.

electrocoagulation, coagulation of tissues by high-frequency electric current.

electrocute, to execute or kill by means of an electric current or shock.

electroencephalograph, a device for recording the spontaneous electrical activity of the brain by means of leads attached to the skull.

electroencephalography, the study and recording of electroencephalograms.

electrohemostasis, the stopping of bleeding by means of high-frequency electric current.

electrolysis, 1. the decomposition of a chemical compound by an electric current. 2. the destruction of tumors or hair roots by an electric current.

electrolyte, a substance whose solutions are capable of conducting electric current, esp. a compound that decomposes by electrolysis.

electrolytic, pertaining to electrolysis or to an electrolyte.

electromyogram, the record produced by electromyography.

electromyography, the study and interpretation of an electromyogram, which is a graphic record of the contraction of a muscle after electrical stimulation.

electronarcosis, see **electroanesthesia.**

electrophoresis, the movement of particles suspended in a fluid under the influence of an electric field.

electroshock, the treatment of a mental disorder by electric shock administered to the brain.

electrosurgery, the use of electricity in surgery.

electrotherapy, the treatment of disease by the use of brief, nonconvulsive electric shocks.

electuary, a medicinal paste usually composed of a powder mixed with honey or syrup.

elephantiasis, a chronic disease, caused by lymphatic obstruction by filarial worms, characterized by enormous enlargement of the parts affected and hardening and fissuring of the skin, which becomes like an elephant's hide.

elinguation, surgical removal of the tongue from the oral cavity.

elixir, an aromatic, sweetened alcoholic liquid containing medicinal agents.

emaciate, 1. to cause to lose flesh gradually. 2. to become lean from loss of appetite or other cause.

emaciation, the process of making or becoming lean or thin in flesh; the state of being reduced to leanness; wasting.

emaculation, the removal of spots from the skin.

emasculate, 1. to castrate.

2. to deprive of masculine vigor. 3. to render effeminate.

embalm, to protect a dead body from decay by treatment with drugs and chemicals; to preserve from decay.

embalmer, one who embalms.

embalmment, the act of embalming.

embedding, a process by which a piece of tissue is placed in paraffin or celloidin to support it during the cutting into sections for microscopic examination.

embolectomy, surgical removal of an embolus.

embolic, 1. of or pertaining to an emboly. 2. pertaining to an embolus or to embolism.

embolism, the blockage of a blood vessel by an embolus; broadly, an embolus.

embololalia, the inclusion of meaningless words or phrases in the speech.

embolus, an abnormal particle circulating in the bloodstream, as an air bubble or blood clot.

emboly, the intrusion or growth of one part into another, as in the invagination of the blastula wall by gastrula formation.

embrocate, to moisten and rub with a liniment or lotion.

embrocation, 1. the act of embrocating a bruised or diseased part of the body. 2. the liquid used for this. 3. a liniment or lotion.

embryo, a multicellular organism in the process of development from the fertilized ovum, up to the end of the second month after conception.

embryogeny, 1. the formation and development of embryos. 2. the study of such formation and development.

embryology, the science of the development process of embryos.

embryonic disk, 1. the blastodisc or blastoderm. 2. the homologous disk of cells of the blastocyst from which the embryo develops.

embryonic layer, the germ layer.

embryonic membrane, an extraembryonic structure in vertebrates, mainly nutritive and protective, which lies outside the embryo proper but is derived from the zygote.

emesis, see **vomiting.**

emetic, 1. inducing vomiting, as a medicinal substance. 2. an emetic medicine or agent.

emetine, an alkaloid with emetic and other medicinal properties, used chiefly in the treatment of amoebic dysentery.

emissary veins, small veins that pierce the bones of the skull and carry blood from the dural sinuses within the skull to the veins on the surface of the skull.

emission, release of fluid, such as semen, from the body.

emmenagogue, a medicine taken to promote the

menstrual discharge.

emmenia, the monthly menstrual flow.

emmetropia, the normal refractive condition of the eye, in which rays of light are accurately focused on the retina and there is perfect vision.

emmetropic, relating to emmetropia.

emollient, 1. softening; making supple; relaxing; soothing to the skin. 2. a medicine that softens and relaxes inflamed tissues.

emotion, 1. an affective state of consciousness in which joy, sorrow, fear, hate, or the like is experienced. 2. any agitated or intense state of mind, usually with concurrent physiological changes.

emotional, 1. pertaining to or characterized by emotion. 2. attended by or producing emotion. 3. appealing to emotions.

empathy, 1. mental entrance into the feeling or spirit of another person or thing. 2. appreciative perception or understanding.

emphysema, distention or puffiness caused by the presence of air in body tissues or organs; esp. a disease of the lungs characterized by a thinning and loss of elasticity of the lung tissues.

emphysematous, pertaining to emphysema.

empiric, relying on experience and observation.

empirical, 1. pertaining to experiments or experience. 2. depending upon experience or observation alone, without regard to science and theory.

emplastrum, a preparation for external application, a plaster, that adheres to the skin.

empyema, a collection of pus in certain cavities of the body, esp. in the chest cavity.

emulsify, to make or form into emulsion.

emulsion, a mixture of two immiscible liquids kept in suspension one within the other, as butterfat in milk.

enamel, the smooth, hard substance that covers the crown of a tooth, overlying the dentine.

enanthesis, a skin eruption or rash caused by specific internal diseases, such as typhoid fever or syphilis.

enarthrosis, a ball-and-socket joint.

encanthis, a new, tiny growth at the inner angle of the eye.

encapsulate, 1. to enclose in or as in a capsule. 2. to become enclosed in or as in a capsule.

encarditis, see **endocarditis.**

enceinte, pregnant; with child.

encephalagia, headache.

encephalatrophy, cerebral atrophy; wasting away of brain tissue.

encephalic, belonging or relating to the brain or to other structures within the cranial cavity.

encephalitis, inflammation of the brain.

encephalitis lethargica, see **sleeping sickness.**

encephalogram, an X-ray photograph of the brain.

encephalography, the technique or act of taking X-ray photographs of the brain, usually after replacing some of the cerebrospinal fluid with oxygen or another gas.

encephalograph, an encephalogram; an electroencephalograph.

encephaloid, resembling brain tissue.

encephaloma, a growth in the brain.

encephalomalacia, cerebral softening, usually resulting from cutting off of the blood supply.

encephalomeningitis, inflammation of the covering of the brain.

encephalomyelitis, inflammation of the brain and spinal cord.

encephalon, the brain.

encephalopathy, any malfunction of the brain.

encondrosis, a benign cartilaginous tumor of a bone.

encyst, to enclose or become enclosed in a cyst, sac, or vesicle.

endamoeba, parasitic amoebas that cause amoebic dysentery.

endangeitis, inflammation of the endangium.

endangium, the innermost layer of a blood vessel.

endarteritis, inflammation of the inner layer of the wall of an artery.

endbrain, see **telencephalon.**

endemic, 1. of a disease peculiar to a people, locality, or region. 2. a disease to which inhabitants of a particular region are subject.

endemiology, the science of endemic diseases.

endermic, acting on or through the skin, as a medicine.

endoblast, see **endoderm.**

endocardial, relating to the endocardium.

endocarditis, inflammation of the endocardium.

endocardium, a colorless transparent membrane that lines the interior of the heart.

endocervical, pertaining to the endocervix.

endocervisitis, inflammation of the mucous lining of the neck of the uterus.

endocervix, the lining of the neck of the uterus.

endochondral, from within a cartilage.

endocolitis, inflammation of the mucous lining of the colon.

endocolpitis, inflammation of the mucous lining of the vagina.

endocranial, 1. within the cranium. 2. pertaining to the endocranium.

endocranium, the tough fibrous membrane covering the brain, known as the dura mater; the inner surface of the cranium.

endocrine, pertaining to the endocrine glands and their secretions.

endocrine glands, ductless glands, as the thyroid, suprarenal, or pituitary glands, which produce and release hormones directly into the blood or lymph.

endocrinology, the science that deals with the endocrine glands and their relation to bodily changes and disease.

endocrinopathy, any disease caused by a disorder of an endocrine gland or glands.

endocystitis, inflammation of the mucous lining of the urinary bladder.

endoderm, the innermost of three germ layers of an embryo from which is derived the epithelium of the digestive and respiratory tracts.

endoenteritis, inflammation of the mucous lining of the intestine.

endogastritis, inflammation of the lining of the stomach.

endodontia, the branch of dentistry specializing in diseases of the tooth's pulp.

endoenzyme, an enzyme that functions inside a cell.

endogenous, 1. of or pertaining to the anabolism of the nitrogenous parts of the cells and tissues. 2. produced from within the body.

endointoxication, poisoning by a toxic substance produced within the body.

endolymph, a limpid fluid in the labyrinth of the ear.

endometrial, pertaining to the endometrium.

endometrioma, a tumor in the lining of the womb.

endometritis, inflamma-tion of the endometrium.

endometrium, the mucous membrane lining the uterus in which the fertilized egg is embedded.

endomorph, 1. a type of body structure characterized by soft roundness, massive digestive viscera, and comparatively weak muscle and bone structure, developed by the dominance of tissues derived from the endoderm, the innermost of the three cell layers of the embryo. 2. a person having this type of body structure.

endomorphic, of, pertaining to, or characteristic of endomorphs.

endoneuritis, inflammation of the endoneurium.

endoneurium, a connective tissue that surrounds nerve fibers.

end organ, any specialized structure that forms the peripheral terminus of a path of nervous conduction.

endoscope, an instrument designed to give a view of some internal part or hollow organ of the body, such as the womb.

endoscopic, pertaining to endoscopy.

endoscopy, examination with an endoscope.

endosteum, the membrane lining the narrow cavity of a bone.

endothelial, pertaining to the endothelium.

endothelioma, a growth formed from endothelial cells.

endothelium, a delicate

membrane lining the heart, blood vessels, and body cavities.

endothermy, surgical diathermy.

endotoxin, the poison liberated at the death and disintegration of a microorganism, such as the typhoid fever agent.

end plate, the ending of a motor nerve, usually embedded in muscle fiber.

enema, 1. the injection of fluid into the rectum for cleansing, diagnosis, etc. 2. the liquid injected.

energy, the actual or potential ability to perform work.

enervate, 1. to deprive of nerve, force, or strength; to weaken. 2. without strength or force; weakened; debilitated.

enflame, see **inflame.**

engorge, to congest with blood.

engorgement, 1. the act of engorging, or the state of being engorged. 2. congestion with blood.

engram, a lasting subconscious memory of a physical experience.

engramme, see **engram.**

enophthalmos, recession of the eyeball into the orbital cavity; sunken eye.

ensiform, sword-shaped, said of a cartilage at the lower part of the sternum or breastbone.

enteral, having reference to the enteron or alimentary canal.

enteralgia, pain in the intestines, cramps, or colic.

enterectomy, surgical removal of a portion of the intestine.

enteric, belonging or relating to the intestines.

enteric fever, see **typhoid.**

enteritis, inflammation of the intestines, esp. the small intestine.

enterococcus, a streptococcus usually found in the intestine.

enterocolitis, inflammation of the small and large intestines.

enterocolostomy, a surgical operation by which the small and large intestines are joined together.

entero-enterostomy, a surgical operation to form a communication between two loops of the intestine after a diseased intermediate portion has been removed.

enterogastritis, inflammation of the intestines and of the stomach.

enterogenous, pertaining to the intestine.

enterohepatitis, an infectious disease affecting the intestines and liver.

enterolith, an intestinal stonelike body.

enterologist, a specialist in intestinal disorders.

enterology, the science of the intestinal tract and its diseases.

enteromegaly, abnormal enlargement of the intestines.

enteron, the alimentary canal, specifically the digestive tract, of the fetus or embryo.

enteropathy, any disorder of the intestines.

enteroplasty, plastic surgery to repair the intestine.

enteroplegia, paralysis of the intestines.

enterospasm, intestinal spasms; colic.

enterostenosis, stricture of the intestinal tube or prolapse of abdominal organs.

enterostomy, an incision of the intestine through the abdominal wall, to permit drainage or feeding.

entoderm, see **endoderm.**

entopic, 1. pertaining to the interior of the eye. 2. opposed to ectopic.

entropion, inversion of the edges of the lower eyelid.

enucleate, 1. to remove, as a kernel, tumor, or eyeball from its enveloping cover. 2. to deprive of the nucleus.

enuresis, incontinence or involuntary discharge of urine.

environment, all the physical, social, and cultural factors and conditions influencing the existence or development of an organism or group of organisms.

enzyme, a large class of protein substances produced by living cells, essential to life by acting as catalysts in the metabolism of the organism.

enzymology, the branch of science that deals with the nature and activity of enzymes.

eosin, a red crystalline powder, used primarily to dye fabrics and to stain specimens for microscopic examination.

eosinophil, a microorganism, cell, or substance readily stained by eosin.

Epanutin, a drug used in the treatment of epilepsy (trademark).

epencephalon, the rhombencephalon, or hindbrain. See **metencephalon.**

ependyma, the membrane lining the cerebral cavities and the central canal of the spinal cord.

ephedrine, a crystalline alkaloid found in species of **Ephedra** or synthesized, used medicinally in the treatment of colds, asthma, and hay fever.

epiblast, see **ectoderm.**

epiboly, the surrounding of a group of cells by another more rapidly dividing group.

epicardia, the abdominal portion of the esophagus, extending from the diaphragm to the stomach.

epicardiac, pertaining to the epicardium.

epicardium, the inner serous layer of the pericardium, lying directly upon the heart.

epicranium, the soft part covering the cranium.

epicritic, relating to cutaneous sensitivity to very small variations in heat, cold, or pain stimuli.

epidemic, 1. common to or affecting a whole people, or a great number in a community at the same time, as a contagious disease; widely prevalent. 2. an occurrence of an epidemic disease. 3. any outbreak that spreads or increases rapidly.

epidemiology, the science concerned with the study and control of epidemic diseases.

epidermal, pertaining to the epidermis.

epidermatoplasty, the grafting of skin.

epidermis, the outer, non-vascular, nonsensitive layer of the skin, covering the true skin or cutis.

epidermitis, inflammation of the epidermis.

epididymis, an elongated oblong body, chiefly convoluted tubes, resting upon and alongside the testicle.

epididymitis, inflammation of the epididymis.

epidural, located upon or over the dura mater.

epigastric, pertaining to or lying upon the upper and anterior part of the abdomen.

epigastrium, the region over the pit of the abdomen, just below the chest plate.

epiglottic, pertaining to the epiglottis.

epiglottis, a thin cartilaginous plate behind the tongue, which covers the glottis like a lid during the act of swallowing and thus prevents food or drink from entering the larynx.

epilate, to remove hair with the roots.

epilation, removal of hair with the roots.

epilatory, a chemical agent that destroys hair.

epilepsy, a chronic nervous disease characterized by brief convulsive seizures and loss of consciousness.

epileptic, 1. pertaining to, or affected with, epilepsy. 2. one affected with epilepsy.

epileptoid, similar to epilepsy.

epileptiform, resembling an epileptic attack.

epimysium, the sheath of a muscle formed by connective tissue.

epinephrine, an adrenal gland hormone that raises blood pressure, having among its many medicinal uses those of heart stimulant and muscle relaxant in asthma.

epinephritis, inflammation of an adrenal gland.

epineurium, the dense sheath of connective tissue that surrounds the trunk of a nerve.

epiphenomenon, a secondary or additional symptom or complication arising during the course of an illness.

epiphora, excessive flow of tears caused by a disorder of the lacrimal glands.

epiphyseal, referring to epiphysis.

epiphysis, 1. a part or process of a bone separated from the main body of the bone by a layer of cartilage, which finally becomes united with the bone through further ossification. 2. the pineal body of the brain.

epiphysitis, inflammation of the epiphysis.

epiploic, pertaining to the

omentum.

episiotomy, surgical incision of the vaginal opening in order to avoid extensive tearing in childbirth.

epistasis, the suppressive action one gene exercises over the effect of another not allelomorphic to it.

epistaxis, bleeding from the nose.

episternum, the uppermost of the three parts of the sternum.

epithelial, pertaining to the epithelium.

epithelioma, a malignant growth consisting chiefly of epithelial cells; a kind of skin cancer.

epithelium, any tissue that covers an external or internal surface, or lines a cavity or the like, which performs protective, secreting, or other functions, as the epidermis or the lining of the blood vessels.

Epsom salt, hydrated magnesium sulfate, used in medicine as a cathartic.

equilibrium, 1. equal balance between opposing forces. 2. a state of rest due to the action of counteracting forces. 3. mental balance.

erectile, capable of being distended with blood and becoming rigid, as tissue.

erection, a distended and rigid state of an organ or part that contains erectile tissue, esp. of the penis or the clitoris.

erector, a muscle that raises or erects another body part.

eremophobia, pathological fear of being alone.

erepsin, a proteolytic mixture containing peptidases, found in intestinal secretions.

erethism, an abnormal excitement or irritability in any organ.

ereuthrophobia, pathological fear of blushing.

ergograph, a device for measuring and recording muscular work performed.

ergometer, a device for measuring the work performed by a set of muscles.

ergonovine, a crystalline alkaloid made from ergot, used esp. to prevent hemorrhage after childbirth or abortion.

ergosterol, a sterol obtained from ergot or yeast, which is converted to vitamin D by ultraviolet radiation, and is used to prevent or cure rickets.

ergophobia, pathological dread of working.

ergot, a drug derived from a fungus and used in medical practice and midwifery.

ergotamine, an alkaloid extracted from ergot, used chiefly in treating migraine and in stimulating labor contractions.

ergotism, a disease resulting from the consumption of food prepared from rye and other cereals affected with the ergot fungus.

ergot poisoning, poisoning resulting from eating bread made with diseased grain or from taking an overdose of the drug ergot.

erogenous, inducing sexual desire; sexually excitable, as, the body's erogenous zones.

erotic, 1. pertaining to or prompted by sexual desire. 2. increasing sexual desire. 3. moved by sexual desire. 4. an erotic person.

eroticism, 1. a sexual quality. 2. use of sexually stimulating themes in art, literature, and drama. 3. a condition of sexual excitement. 4. an unusually insistent sexual desire.

erotomania, abnormally strong sexual desire.

erotopath, a sex pervert.

erotophobia, a morbid fear of sex.

erubescence, 1. the act of turning red. 2. redness of the skin or the surface of anything. 3. blushing.

eruct, to eject, as wind from the stomach; to belch.

eructation, the act of belching wind from the stomach; a belch.

eruption, 1. the breaking out of a rash. 2. a rash or exanthema.

eruptive fever, any fever that produces a rash on the skin.

erysipelas, an infectious disease characterized by fever and inflammation, affecting subcutaneous tissue and caused by a specific streptococcus.

erysipeloid, an inflammatory skin disease resem-

bling erysipelas.

erythema, abnormal redness of the skin caused by local congestion, as in inflammation.

erythrism, abnormal or excessive redness, as of hair.

erythroblast, one of the nucleated cells found in bone marrow from which the red blood cells are formed.

erythrocyte, a mature red blood corpuscle.

erythrocytometer, an instrument for counting red blood cells.

erythrocytosis, an abnormal increase in the number of red blood cells.

erythroderma, any skin disease causing abnormal redness of the skin.

erythromycin, an antibiotic used in treating amoebic and other diseases, produced by the actinomycete **Streptonyces erythraeus.**

erythropoiesis, the production of red blood corpuscles.

eschar, a crust or scab on the skin caused by burns or caustic applications.

esophagismus, spasms of the esophagus.

esophagitis, inflammation of the esophagus.

esophagoscope, an instrument used to examine the esophagus.

esophagospasm, see **esophagismus.**

esophagotomy, surgical incision of the esophagus.

esophagus, the muscular tube extending from the

pharynx to the stomach, through which food passes; the gullet.

esophoria, inward turning of the eye; squinting inward.

esophoric, pertaining to esophoria.

esotropia, a convergent squint; crossed eyes.

estivo-autumnal fever, see **malaria.**

estradiol, a hormone used to treat estrogen deficiency and some menopausal and postmenopausal symptoms.

estriol, an estrogenic substance found in the urine of pregnant women.

estrogen, a female hormone that induces estrus, causes sexual receptivity, and promotes the development of secondary sex characteristics in the female.

estrone, a female sex hormone used in treating estrogen deficiency and some menopausal and postmenopausal symptoms.

estrous, of or pertaining to the estrus.

estrous cycle, the complete cycle of reproductive changes in the female, running from the start of one period of estrus to the start of the next.

estrus, the point of highest sexual excitability in the female, during which conception is possible.

ethmoid, 1. noting or pertaining to a bone of the skull situated at the root of the nose and containing numerous perforations for the filaments of the olfactory nerve. 2. the ethmoid bone.

ethmoidal, pertaining to the ethmoid bone.

ethmoidectomy, surgical excision of ethmoid cells.

ethmoiditis, inflammation of the ethmoid bone or of ethmoidal cells.

ethmoid sinuses, cavities in the ethmoid bone.

etiology, the study of causation in the fields of pathology, biology, philosophy, and physics.

eugenic, pertaining to or bringing about improvement in the type of offspring produced.

eugenicist, 1. one versed in eugenics. 2. an advocate of eugenic measures.

eugenics, 1. the science of improving the qualities of the human species. 2. the science of bringing about an improved type of offspring of the human species.

eugenist, see **eugenicist.**

eunuch, a castrated male; a male deprived of testes.

euphoria, a feeling of well-being not always justified by physical health; a mood of elation.

euphoric, relating to euphoria.

eustachian tube, the tube between the middle ear, or tympanum, and the pharynx.

eustachitis, inflammation of the eustachian tube.

euthanasia, a painless putting to death of persons having an incurable disease; an easy death. Also called mercy killing.

evacuant, 1. promoting evacuation, esp. from the bowels. 2. diuretic. 3. an evacuant medicine or agent.

evacuate, to make empty, or expel the contents of, as, to evacuate the stomach by an emetic.

evacuation, the act or process of evacuating.

evert, to turn outward or inside out, as, eversion of the eyelid.

eversion, the turning outward or inside out.

eviscerate, to remove the viscera from; disembowel.

evolution, development from a rudimentary to a more complex state; in modern use, the fact or doctrine of the descent of all living things from a few simple forms of life, or from a simple form.

evulsion, the act of plucking or pulling out; forcible extraction.

exacerbate, 1. to increase the violence, intensity, or bitterness of, as a disease or unfriendly feeling. 2. to irritate, exasperate, or embitter.

exacerbation, an increase of the severity of a disease; aggravation of symptoms of a disease.

exaltation, elation of mind or feeling, sometimes abnormal in character.

exanthema, 1. an eruption or rash on the skin. 2. an eruptive disease, esp. one attended by fever, as smallpox or measles.

exanthrope, any external

cause or source of a disease.

exarteritis, inflammation of the outer coat of an artery.

excipient, a more or less inert substance, as sugar or jelly, used as a medium or vehicle for the administration of an active medicine.

excise, 1. to cut out or off; to remove by cutting, as in surgery. 2. to delete or expunge.

excision, the act of cutting out or off; resection.

excitable, 1. able to react to stimulus or to be aroused to activity by a stimulus. 2. capable of being excited.

excitant, something that excites; a stimulant.

excite, to produce a reaction in or increase the activity of, as of a nerve or muscle.

excitement, the act of exciting; the state of being excited.

excitor, a nerve whose stimulation produces greater action.

excoriate, 1. to break or wear off the cuticle of. 2. to abrade a part of the skin so as to reach the flesh.

excoriation, the act of excoriating.

excrement, refuse matter discharged from the body after digestion.

excreta, excreted matter; the excretions of the body, as sweat or urine.

excrete, to separate and expel from the blood or tissues, as waste or harmful matter.

excretion, 1. the act of excreting. 2. the substance excreted, as sweat, urine, etc.

excretory, pertaining to or concerned with excretion.

excruciate, to cause extreme pain to; to torture; to cause extreme mental agony to.

excruciating, extremely painful; intensely distressing; torturing; agonizing.

exenterate, 1. to surgically excise the contents of a body cavity, as of the pelvis. 2. to eviscerate.

exenteration, 1. surgical removal of the contents of a body cavity; evisceration. 2. removal of a fetus in embryotomy.

exfoliation, the scaling off of dead tissue.

exfoliative, causing exfoliation.

exhale, 1. to breathe out; to eject breath or vapor. 2. to expel or let out of the lungs.

exhalant, 1. having the quality of exhaling or emitting. 2. a duct having the function of exhaling.

exhausted, completely consumed, spent, or drained; greatly fatigued.

exhaustion, the act or process of exhausting, or the state of being exhausted.

exhibit, to administer, as a remedy.

exhibitionism, a form of sexual perversion marked by a usually compulsive display of the sex organs.

exhibitionist, a person addicted to exhibitionism.

exhume, to dig up after burial; to disinter.

exocrine, pertaining to the external secretion of a gland.

exodontia, the branch of dentistry that deals with tooth extraction.

exoenzyme, an enzyme that functions outside the cell that produces it.

exoergic, of or pertaining to a reaction accompanied by a release of energy.

exophthalmos, protrusion of the eyeball from the eye socket, usually caused by excessive activity of the thyroid gland.

exophoria, outward turning of the eye; squinting outward.

exostosis, any abnormal protuberance or enlargement of a bone or tooth.

exoteric, developed outside the body.

exotoxin, a soluble toxin formed within and secreted by a microorganism which itself is not toxic.

expectant, see **pregnant.**

expectorant, 1. having the quality of promoting discharges from the mucous membrane of the lungs or trachea. 2. a drug that promotes such discharges.

expectorate, to eject from the trachea or lungs; to discharge, as phlegm or other matter, by coughing, hawking, and spitting.

expiration, 1. the act of

breathing out; emission of breath. 2. close, end, conclusion, or termination. 3. expiry.

expire, 1. to emit breath. 2. to die. 3. to come to an end.

exploration, examination of a wound or an organ.

explore, to examine closely, as in probing an organ.

expulsion, the act of driving out or expelling.

exsanguinate, to render bloodless; to drain the blood from.

exsanguine, see **anemic**.

exscind, to cut out or off.

exsiccate, to dry; to dehydrate.

extirpate, to eradicate; to destroy totally; to exterminate.

extirpation, total removal, as of a part.

extrasystole, an abnormal contraction of the heart causing a brief interruption of the heartbeat.

extrauterine, situated or taking place outside the uterus, as an extrauterine pregnancy.

extravasate, to force or let out of the proper vessels, as blood into surrounding tissue.

extravasation, 1. the act of extravasating. 2. the state of fluid being forced or let out of the ducts of the body that contain it; effusion.

extravascular, being outside of the blood vessel or vascular system.

extreme unction, a sacrament of the Roman Catholic Church involving the anointing with oil of a person on the point of death.

extremity, the end part of a limb, or the limb itself, esp. the human hand or foot.

extrinsic, originating from outside the part where it occurs or which it affects, esp. of a muscle.

extroversion, the act or characteristic of directing one's interest primarily toward what is outside the self; the state of being extroverted.

extrovert, one whose interest and attention is directed primarily toward what is outside the self; one who relates to the external or objective; loosely, one who is outgoing, active, expressive, and gregarious.

extrude, to thrust out; to expel.

extrusion, the act of extruding, or the fact of being extruded.

extrusive, tending to extrude; pertaining to extrusion.

exuberant, full of joyful enthusiasm; high-spirited; unrestrained.

exude, to ooze; to seep out gradually, as sweat through the pores.

exudation, 1. the act or process of exuding. 2. an exuded substance.

eye, the organ of sight, one of a pair of globular bodies each consisting of a cornea, an iris, a pupil, a lens, a retina, and various muscles, nerves, and blood vessels and set in an orbit or socket in the skull. The eye is divided by the iris into two chambers, an anterior and a posterior chamber, both of which are filled with a watery substance called aqueous humor. There is a much larger cavity behind the lens that is filled with a jellylike substance called vitreous humor.

eyeball, the ball or globe of the eye.

eye bank, a place where corneas removed from newly dead persons are stored until needed for transplantation to restore the sight of those with corneal defects.

eyebrow, the arch or ridge forming the upper part of the orbit of the eye, or the fringe of hair growing upon it.

eyecup, a device for applying lotions to the eye, consisting of a cup or glass with a rim shaped to fit snugly about the orbit of the eye.

eyedropper, a dropper for administering eye drops.

eyedrops, drugs used for the treatment of eye diseases.

eyeglasses, see **spectacles.**

eyelash, 1. one of the many hairs that edge the eyelid. 2. (pl.) the entire fringe of these hairs.

eyelid, the portion of movable skin that serves as a cover for the eyeball.

eyeshot, range of vision.

eyesight, 1. the ability to see. 2. vision. 3. the extent of vision.

eyestrain, discomfort or fatigue of the eyes due to excessive or incorrect use or to uncorrected visual defects.

eyetooth, one of the two upper canine teeth.

eyewash, a lotion to cleanse or treat the eye.

face, the front part of the head, including the forehead, chin, cheeks, eyes, nose, and mouth.

facet, a flat smooth surface of a bone.

facial, 1. of or pertaining to the face. 2. a facial massage or beauty treatment.

facies, 1. a specific surface of the body. 2. facial appearance indicative of a disease.

facioplasty, plastic surgery of the face.

facioplegia, facial paralysis.

factitious, contrived rather than spontaneous; artificial.

factitious fever, a fever produced artifically, usually by the use of a drug.

faeces, see **feces.**

faint, 1. to become temporarily unconscious. 2. a loss of consciousness. 3. on the verge of losing consciousness. 4. indistinct or lacking brightness; feeble; weak.

falcate, curved like a sickle; hooked.

fallectomy, the surgical excision of part of the fallopian tube.

fallopian tube, either of a pair of slender tubes that convey the ova from the ovaries to the cavity of the uterus.

fallostomy, surgical opening of a fallopian tube.

fallotomy, a division of the fallopian tubes by surgery.

false rib, a rib that is not directly attached to the sternum.

falter, 1. to stagger, stumble, or totter. 2. to speak hesitatingly; to stammer.

familial, pertaining to or common to a family, as a disease to which a family is prone.

family, 1. the unit consisting of parents and their children. 2. persons related by blood or marriage. 3. descendants of a common progenitor.

fantasy, 1. the usually pleasant process of subjectively solving complex problems by imagining them in concrete symbols and images. 2. the images themselves.

faradism, 1. induced electricity. 2. its application for therapeutic purposes.

faradize, to stimulate or treat, as a muscle, with induced electric currents.

farcy, see **glanders.**

farinaceous, containing or yielding farina or flour; starchy; mealy.

farsighted, seeing more clearly at a distance than close at hand.

fascia, 1. a band or sheath of connective tissue investing, supporting, or binding together internal organs or parts of the body. 2. a bandage.

fascicle, a small cluster of

nerve fibers within the central nervous system.

fascicular, pertaining to or forming a fascicle; fasciculate.

fasciculi, a fascicle, as of nerve fibers or muscle fibers.

fasciectomy, surgical excision of strips of fascia.

fasciola, a bundle or small group of nerve or muscle fibers.

fascioplasty, plastic surgery on a fascia.

fasciotomy, surgical incision and separation or division of a fascia.

fascitis, inflammation of a fascia.

fastigium, the period of highest fever or greatest infection during the course of an illness.

fat, 1. a soft solid organic compound composed of carbon, hydrogen, and oxygen. 2. a solid glycerol ester of higher fatty acids. 3. the tissues of animals and men that contain principally an oily or greasy substance. 4. fleshy; corpulent; obese.

fatigue, 1. weariness from bodily labor or mental exertion; lassitude or exhaustion of strength. 2. a temporary loss or diminution in a bodily organ because of continued stress.

fauces, the passage that links the mouth and the pharynx, lying between the soft palate and the base of the tongue.

faucial, pertaining to the fauces.

faucitis, inflammation of

the fauces.

faveolus, a small depression or pit, esp. on the skin.

favus, a fungus-borne disease, attacking the scalp of humans and characterized by yellowish dry incrustations resembling a honeycomb.

febrifacient, causing or producing fever.

febrifuge, 1. serving to dispel or reduce fever. 2. a febrifuge medicine or agent. 3. a cooling drink.

febrile, feverish.

fecal, relating to feces.

feces, excrement; the waste products of the body discharged from the anus.

feculent, containing feces.

fecund, abundantly productive in children, prolific.

fecundate, 1. to make fruitful or prolific. 2. to impregnate. 3. to fertilize.

fecundation, see **fertilization.**

feebleminded, deficient in mentality.

fellatio, stimulation of the penis by oral means.

felon, an acute and painful inflammation of the deeper tissues of a finger or toe, usually near the nail.

feminism, in a male, the presence of feminine characteristics.

feminize, to acquire a feminine or effeminate character.

femoral, pertaining to the femur.

femur, a bone in the leg, extending from the hip to the knee.

fenestra, a natural perforation, esp. one in the bone between the typanum and the inner ear.

fenestration, surgical formation of an opening in the bone between the middle and inner ear.

fennel, a herb of the parsley family bearing aromatic seeds used in cooking and medicine.

ferment, any of various agents or substances, as yeast, enzymes, or certain bacteria, capable of producing chemical changes, as effervescence or decomposition, in other substances.

fermentation, the act or process of fermenting.

ferric, of or containing iron.

ferriferous, producing or yielding iron.

ferrous, pertaining to, obtained from, or containing iron.

ferruginous, 1. containing iron. 2. colored like iron rust.

fertile, able to produce offspring; prolific.

fertility, the state of being fertile; the ability to produce offspring.

fertilization, fecundation; the union of a sperm cell and an ovum.

fester, 1. to suppurate; to form pus; to putrefy. 2. the act of festering.

fetal, pertaining to or having the character of a fetus.

fetation, the development of a fetus; pregnancy.

feticide, the destruction of a fetus.

fetid, having an offensive

smell.

fetish, any object or any part of the body, not of the generative system, that arouses sexual interest.

fetishism, belief in the potency of an object, esp. one associated with a beloved person, to stimulate sexual desire.

fetor, any strong offensive smell; stench.

fetus, an unborn human from after the third month of pregnancy until birth.

fever, 1. an abnormal increase in body temperature. **2.** any disease having high temperature as a principal symptom. **3.** agitation or excitement by anything that strongly affects the passions. **4.** contagious zeal.

fever blister, an eruption around the mouth that may accompany a cold or fever.

feverish, 1. having fever, esp. a slight degree of fever. **2.** of, indicating, or pertaining to fever. **3.** tending to cause fever.

feverous, see **feverish**.

fiber, one of the threadlike elements composing the tissue of muscles and nerves.

fibril, a small or very fine fiber or filament.

fibrillar, of, pertaining to, or composed of fibers or fibrils.

fibrillation, 1. the twitching of certain muscle fibers without coordination or control. **2.** erratic and irregular contractions of heart muscle fibers resulting in abnormally rapid heartbeats.

fibrin, a fibrous, elastic, insoluble protein, formed by the interaction of fibrinogen with the enzyme thrombin, which promotes clotting to prevent blood loss.

fibrinogen, a globulin in the blood that is a soluble protein and assists in producing fibrin for the clotting of blood.

fibrinogenous, producing fibrin.

fibroadenoma, a benign tumor, often found in the breasts of young women, composed of glandular and fibrous tissue.

fibroblast, any cell from which connective tissue develops.

fibrocystic, a fibrous degeneration that produces cysts.

fibroid, 1. resembling or formed of fibrous tissue. **2.** a fibroid tumor.

fibroma, a benign tumor or growth of fibrous matter.

fibromatosis, a condition characterized by simultaneous development of many fibromas.

fibrosarcoma, a malignant tumor containing much connective tissue.

fibrosis, abnormal increase of fibrous tissue in an organ.

fibrositis, inflammation of fibrous tissue anywhere in the body. Also called muscular rheumatism.

fibrous, containing, consisting of, or resembling fibers.

fibrovascular, composed of a fibrous tissue that

conveys fluid from one part to another.

fibula, the outer and lesser bone of the lower leg.

filaria, a type of threadworm.

filarial, pertaining to filaria.

filariasis, any disease due to one of the filariae, esp. elephantiasis, which is caused by filariae gaining entrance to the lymphatic ducts and causing inflammation, fibrosis, and blockage of the lymph flow that results in swelling of the area.

filiform, threadlike; filamentous.

finger, any of the terminal members of the hand other than the thumb.

fingernail, the hard protective growth at the end of each of the fingers of the hand.

first aid, emergency aid or treatment given to the victim of an accident or sudden illness before regular medical services can be obtained.

first cranial nerve, see **olfactory nerve.**

fissure, 1. any cleft or groove in an organ, as in the brain. 2. to cleave or make a fissure in. 3. to crack or fracture.

fist, 1. the hand closed tightly, with the fingers doubled into the palm. 2. a grasp or hold.

fistula, an abnormal duct or passage caused by injury or disease, as one leading from an abscess to the body surface or from one cavity or hollow organ to another.

fistulous, pertaining to a fistula.

fit, 1. an attack or manifestation of a disease characterized by loss of consciousness or by convulsions. 2. an uncontrollable attack of any physical disturbance, as a fit of coughing. 3. an intensive but brief surge or occurrence of something, as a fit of enthusiasm or activity. 4. an uncontrolled expression of emotion.

fixate, 1. to develop a fixation. 2. to suffer abatement at a particular stage of sexual or emotional development.

fixation, an attaching or arresting of emotional and psychosexual development at an early or infantile stage, often caused by a childhood trauma.

flabby, hanging loosely or limply, as flesh or muscles.

flaccid, not firm; lacking vigor.

flagellum, a long, lashlike appendage in certain reproductive bodies, bacteria, and protozoa.

flail joint, a joint with abnormal mobility.

flatfoot, a condition in which the arch of the foot is flattened so that the entire sole rests upon the ground.

flatulence, see **eructation.**

flatulent, affected with or caused by gases generated in the alimentary canal.

flatus, an accumulation of gas in the stomach, intestines, or other body cavity.

flavedo, yellowness, as of the skin; jaundice.

fleam, a sharp surgical instrument for opening veins; a lancet.

flection, 1. the act of bending a limb of the body. 2. the bending of a limb by exercising the flexor muscle. 3. a curved or bowed part.

Fletcherism, the practice of chewing food until it is reduced to a liquefied mass, advocated as a health measure.

flexible, capable of being bent; easily bent or pliant.

flexion, see flection.

flexor, a muscle that serves to flex or bend a joint of the body.

flexure, a curved structure in the body.

floating kidney, a kidney that has become loose and displaced in the abdomen.

floating rib, one of the lowest pairs of ribs, not attached to the breastbone or other ribs.

flooding, profuse bleeding from the womb.

flora, the normal bacterial content of a part, such as intestinal, vaginal, or skin flora.

fluid dram, see fluidram.

fluid ounce, a unit of liquid capacity equal to one-sixteenth pint.

fluidram, a unit of liquid capacity equal to one-eighth part of a fluid ounce.

fluke, any of several trematode flatworms, parasitic in man.

fluoridation, the addition of a fluoride to drinking water to prevent tooth decay.

fluoride, a compound of fluorine with another element or radical.

fluorine, an extremely reactive nonmetallic element, a light-yellow corrosive gas, found naturally in combination in minerals, such as cryolite.

fluoroscope, an instrument that permits direct observation on a fluorescent screen of the shadows produced by X-rays or other radiation passing through an opaque object.

fluoroscopic, pertaining to the fluoroscope or to fluoroscopy.

fluoroscopy, examination by means of a fluoroscope.

fluorosis, chronic fluorine poisoning.

flush, suffusion with a reddish color; blushing.

flutter, to be agitated or upset; to beat irregularly, as the heart.

flux, an evacuation of fluid matter from the body, esp. an abnormal discharge from the bowels.

focus, 1. that part of the body in which a disease develops or is localized. 2. a point at which rays of light, heat, or the like converge.

folic acid, a member of the vitamin B complex, found in green plants, fresh fruits, liver, and yeast, used for treatment of nutritional anemia.

follicle, a small cavity, sac, or gland.

follicle-stimulating hormone, a pituitary hormone that stimulates production of Graafian follicles in the female and spermatozoa in the male.

follicular, 1. pertaining to, consisting of, or like a follicle; provided with follicles. 2. affecting or originating in a follicle.

folliculate, provided with or consisting of a follicle.

folliculin, a female hormone produced by the ovarian follicles.

folliculitis, inflammation of a follicle.

fomentation, 1. the application of warm liquids to relieve pain. 2. that which is applied as a lotion or poultice.

fomes, any substance capable of transmitting infectious diseases.

fontanel, one of the spaces, covered with a membranous structure, between certain bones of the fetal or young skull.

food poisoning, an acute gastrointestinal ailment caused by food chemically contaminated by insecticides or bacterial toxins.

foot, the terminal part of the vertebrate leg, on which the body stands and moves.

foot-and-mouth disease, a highly contagious, febrile disease of cattle and other hooved animals, marked by blisters in the mouth and around the hooves, teats, and udder. The disease can be transmitted to man.

footdrop, failure of the foot to be maintained in a normally flexed position, usually caused by paralysis of certain leg muscles.

foramen, a small natural opening or perforation, such as an opening by which nerves or blood vessels obtain a passage through bones.

foramen magnum, the occipital bone opening and passageway of the spinal cord that unites with the medulla oblongata.

faraminate, perforated; full of holes.

forceps, an instrument, as pincers or tongs, for seizing and holding objects, as in surgical operations.

forearm, the part of the arm between the elbow and the wrist.

forebrain, 1. the anterior of the three major divisions of the embryonic brain. 2. the diencephalon and telencephalon, the segments of the adult brain that develop from this tissue.

forehead, the part of the face above the eyes.

forensic medicine, medical knowledge as applied to issues involved in civil and criminal law, esp. in the proceedings in a court of law.

foreskin, the fold of skin that covers the glans of the penis; the prepuce.

formaldehyde, a colorless, water-soluble, poisonous

gas with a pungent odor, used, usually in solution, in the manufacture of synthetic resins and other organic compounds and as a preservative and disinfectant.

formalin, an aqueous solution of formaldehyde.

forme fruste, a disease that appears in an atypical and indefinite form.

formication, a sensation as if ants were crawling across the skin, one of the more common side-effects of cocaine withdrawal in addicts.

formula, 1. a prescription. 2. the constituents of a medicine.

formulary, 1. a book listing pharmaceuticals and medical formulas. 2. pertaining to a formula or formulas. 3. prescribed.

fornicate, to commit fornication.

fornication, sexual intercourse, with mutual consent, between two persons not married to each other.

fornix, any of various arched or vaulted structures, as an arching fibrous formation in the brain.

fossa, 1. a depression. 2. one of various hollows in the body. 3. a furrow.

fossette, a deep corneal ulcer of small circumference.

foundling, a child found after being abandoned by its parents.

fourchette, a small fold of membrane forming the posterior margin of the vulva.

fovea, a pit or cuplike depression.

foxglove, any flowering plant of the genus **Digitalis** from which a drug is derived to treat heart disease.

fracture, the breaking of a bone or cartilage and the resulting condition.

fraenum, see frenum.

fragile, brittle; easily broken; delicate; frail.

frail, lacking physical strength and robust health.

frailty, the condition or quality of being frail.

fraternal twin, one of a pair of twins each originating from separately fertilized ova, consequently having different hereditary features and not necessarily being identical or of the same sex.

freckle, a brownish spot on the skin, particularly on the face, neck, or hands, often caused by exposure to the sun, but sometimes of congenital origin and an inherited factor.

fremitus, palpable vibration, as of the walls of the chest.

frenum, a ligament or fold of membrane that checks or restrains the motion of a part, as the one that binds down the under side of the tongue.

frenzy, 1. violent mental agitation resembling temporary madness. 2. wild excitement or enthusiasm. 3. delirium.

frenzying, affecting with or driving to frenzy; rendering frantic.

Freudian, of or pertaining to the physician, psycho-analyst, and psycho-pathologist Sigmund Freud, or his close associates or doctrines.

friable, easily crumbled or pulverized.

frigid, 1. abnormally unresponsive or indifferent to sexual intercourse. 2. without sympathy, passion, or sensitivity.

frigidity, inability to respond to sexual stimuli.

frontal, noting or pertaining to the forehead or the bone or pair of bones forming the forehead.

frontal bone, a membrane bone in the skull, one of a pair forming the forehead.

frontal lobe, the anterior or upper division of the cerebral hemisphere.

frostbite, damage to tissues in any part of the body occasioned by exposure to severe cold, resulting in inflammation and sometimes gangrene.

frottage, arriving at an orgasm by pressing up behind someone in a crowd and rubbing against that person.

frotteur, one who practices frottage.

fructose, see **levulose.**

fugue, a mental state in which the person shows rational behavior but has a complete loss of memory for the behavior when he recovers from the fugue state.

fulguration, destruction, esp. of tissue of an abnormal growth, by electricity.

fulminant, of a disease, showing rapid development or progression.

fulminating, rapid and severe.

fumigant, any chemical compound or vapor used to fumigate.

fumigate, to expose to fumes or vapors, esp. for disinfection or for destruction of vermin.

functional, 1. affecting only the functions and not the structure of an organ. 2. pertaining to the special function of an organ.

functional disease, a disease in which there is a pathological change in the function of an organ but no structural alteration in the tissues involved, as opposed to organic disease.

functionalism, the point of view that considers mental phenomena as useful activities or processes in terms of need, effect, or achievement.

fundus, the bottom of a hollow organ, or the part opposite to or remote from an aperture.

fungal, pertaining to or of the nature of a fungus.

fungicide, 1. a chemical agent that eradicates fungi. 2. a chemical that prevents future fungoid growths.

fungoid, 1. resembling a fungus. 2. characterized by spongy growths resembling fungi.

fungus, 1. any of the Fungi,

a group of parasitic and saprophytic plants. 2. a spongy growth.

funiculus, a part of the body resembling a cord, as the umbilical cord, spermatic cord, and small bundles of nerve fibers.

funny bone, the part of the elbow where the ulna nerve passes by the internal codyle of the humerus, which when struck causes a peculiar tingling sensation in the arm and hand.

furfur, see **dandruff.**

furfuraceous, scurfy; scaly or flaky, as with dandruff.

furuncle, a boil or inflammatory sore.

furunculosis, the condition marked by the tendency toward or presence of furuncles.

fusiform, spindle-shaped; rounded and tapering from the middle toward each end.

gag, 1. to hold open, as the jaws with an instrument, in a surgical operation. 2. to cause to vomit. 3. to choke or prevent passage through.

gait, a characteristic manner of walk.

galactacrasia, an abnormal composition of the breast milk.

galactemia, a milky condition of the blood.

galactic, 1. pertaining to milk. 2. increasing the flow of milk.

galactophagous, feeding upon milk.

galactophore, a milk duct.

galactophoritis, inflammation of a milk duct.

galactorrhea, 1. excessive production of milk. 2. continuation of flow of milk after nursing has ended.

galactostasis, cessation or stagnation of milk in the breast.

gall, see **bile.**

gallbladder, a small membranous sac, shaped like a pear, which receives and stores bile from the liver.

gallstone, a stony particle or small stonelike mass formed in the gallbladder or biliary passages.

galvanism, the application of voltaic or battery current to the body for therapeutic purposes.

galvanocautery, cauterization of tissue by means of an instrument with a platinum loop that is heated by galvanic current.

galvanolysis, see **electrolysis.**

galvanometer, an instrument for detecting the existence and determining the strength and direction of an electric current.

galvanoscope, see **galvanometer.**

gambier, an astringent extract obtained from the leaves and young shoots of a tropical Asiatic vine and used in medicine.

gamete, either of the two reproductive germ cells that unite to form a new organism; the name given to the male or female reproductive cell.

gametocyte, a gamete-producing cell.

gametogenesis, the creation of gametes.

gametophore, a part or structure producing gametes.

gamic, sexual.

gamma globulin, a protein separated from blood and containing antibodies, used in inoculation against measles, poliomyelitis, and infectious hepatitis.

gamma rays, penetrating rays emitted by radioactive material and reducing the energy of the cell nucleus, used in radiotherapy.

gamogenesis, sexual reproduction.

ganglial, pertaining to ganglion.

gangliectomy, surgical excision of a ganglion.

ganglion, 1. an encysted tumor or enlargement in connection with the sheath of a tendon. 2. any aggregation of nerve cells or mass of gray matter forming a nerve center external to the central or cerebrospinal nervous system.

ganglionectomy, see **gangliectomy.**

ganglionic, pertaining to a ganglion.

ganglionitis, inflammation of a ganglion.

gangrene, the dying of tissue, as from interruption of circulation; mortification.

gargarism, see gargle.

gargle, 1. a liquid preparation for washing the mouth and throat. 2. to wash or rinse the mouth or throat with a liquid preparation kept in motion by air expelled from the lungs.

gargoylism, a usually congenital condition characterized by mental deficiency and dwarfism.

garrot, see **tourniquet.**

gastral, pertaining to the stomach or digestive tract.

gastralgia, pain in the stomach, esp. neuralgic pain.

gastrectomy, excision of the stomach or a portion of it.

gastric, of or pertaining to the stomach.

gastric juice, an acidic digestive fluid containing enzymes and hydrochloric acid, secreted by glands in the mucous membrane of the stomach.

gastric ulcer, an open sore on the mucous membrane of the stomach, usually caused by excessively acidic gastric juice.

gastrin, a hormone inducing secretion of gastric juices.

gastritis, chronic inflammation of the stomach, esp. of the mucous membrane.

gastrocele, hernia of the stomach.

gastrocnemius, the large muscle in the calf of the leg.

gastrocolic, pertaining to both stomach and colon.

gastrocolic reflex, nerve stimulus causing the

peristaltic wave in the colon when food enters the stomach.

gastrocolitis, inflammation of the stomach and colon.

gastrocolostomy, surgical formation of a permanent connection between the stomach and the colon.

gastroduodenal, relating to the stomach and the duodenum.

gastroduodenitis, inflammation of the stomach and the duodenum.

gastroenteric, pertaining to the stomach and the intestine.

gastroenteritis, inflammation of the lining of the stomach and the intestine.

gastroenterology, the branch of medicine relating to the psychology and pathology of the stomach and the intestines.

gastroenteroptosis, displacement of the stomach and the intestines downward.

gastroenterostomy, a surgical joining of the small intestine with the wall of the stomach in order to bypass a diseased duodenum.

gastroesophagal, pertaining to the stomach and the esophagus.

gastrointestinal, relating to or affecting the stomach and the intestines.

gastrojejunal, pertaining to the stomach and the jejunum.

gastrojejunostomy, the joining of the jejunum with the stomach by surgery.

gastrologist, a physician specializing in gastrology.

gastrology, the science of the structure, functions, and diseases of the stomach.

gastromalacia, abnormal softening of the stomach walls.

gastronephritis, simultaneous inflammation of stomach and kidneys.

gastro-oesophageal, see **gastroesophagal.**

gastroparalysis, paralysis of the stomach.

gastropathy, any disorder or disease of the stomach.

gastrophrenic, relating to the stomach and the diaphragm.

gastroplegia, see **gastroparalysis.**

gastroptosis, abnormal dropping of the stomach.

gastroptyxis, surgical reduction of a dilated stomach.

gastropyloric, pertaining to the stomach and the pylorus.

gastrorrhagia, bleeding from the stomach.

gastroscope, an instrument for inspecting the interior of the stomach.

gastroscopy, examination of the stomach with a gastroscope.

gastrotomy, incision of the abdomen or the stomach.

gathering, see **abscess.**

gatophilia, pathological love for cats.

gatophobia, pathological aversion to cats.

gauze, a loosely woven cotton bandage applied to wounds.

gavage, forced feeding by

means of a flexible stomach tube and force pump.

gelsemium, the root of the yellow jasmine, or the tincture from it, used as a drug.

gene, the element or unit of a chromosome that carries and transfers an inherited characteristic from parent to offspring and determines the development of some particular character or trait in the offspring.

gene mutation, a significant alteration in an organism resulting from a chemical rearrangement within the molecules of a gene.

genetic, 1. pertaining to the science of genetics. 2. pertaining to genes.

geneticist, a specialist in the science of genetics.

genetics, 1. the science of the hereditary and evolutionary similarities and differences of related organisms, as produced by the interaction of the genes. 2. the inherited features and characteristics of an organism or group or type of organisms.

genial, of or pertaining to the chin.

genic, pertaining to or resulting from a gene or genes.

geniculate, 1. having kneelike joints. 2. bent at an angle like the knee.

genital, pertaining to procreation, or to the sexual organs.

genitalia, see **genitals.**

genitals, the organs of the system of reproduction, esp. the external organs.

genitourinary, noting or pertaining to the genital and urinary organs.

gentian, the root of **Gentiana lutea** or a preparation of it used as a tonic or an aid to digestion.

gentian violet, a dye used as a biological stain, as an acid-base indicator, and medicinally as a fungicide and bactericide.

genu valgum, see **knock-knee.**

genu varum, see **bowleg.**

geophagy, the practice of eating earthy substances such as chalk or clay.

geriatric, pertaining to old age.

geriatrics, the area of medicine that deals with the diseases of old age and the problems and care of aging persons.

germ, 1. a disease-producing microorganism. 2. an embryo in its early stages.

German measles, an infectious virus disease, less severe than measles, with such symptoms as fever, rash, and sore throat, and potentially damaging to an unborn child if the mother contracts the disease early in pregnancy.

germ cell, 1. a cell capable of sexual reproduction. 2. sperm or egg cell.

germicidal, destructive to germs.

germicide, a substance that destroys germs.

germinal, pertaining to or of the nature of a germ or

germ cell.

germinal disc, 1. a blastodisc. **2.** the part of a fertilized egg containing the first visible traces of the embryo proper.

germinal vesicle, the nucleus of an ovum before the polar bodies are formed.

germ layer, any one of the three embryonic cell layers: ectoderm, endoderm, mesoderm.

germ plasm, that part of the protoplasm of a cell containing the chromosomes and genes by which hereditary characteristics are transmitted.

gerontology, see **gerlatrics.**

gestate, to carry in the womb during pregnancy.

giantism, see **gigantism.**

giddiness, the state of being giddy.

giddy, 1. having a sensation of whirling or reeling. **2.** affected with vertigo; dizzy.

gigantism, excessive growth of the body or parts of the body, most often caused by malfunction of the pituitary gland.

gingiva, see **gum.**

gingival, pertaining to the gums.

gingivitis, inflammation of the gum tissues.

girdle, the pelvic or pectoral arch.

glabella, the flat area of the face between the eyebrows.

glabrous, 1. smooth. **2.** having a surface devoid of hair or pubescence.

gland, 1. an organ by which certain constituents are separated from the blood for use in the body or for ejection from it, or by which certain changes are produced in the blood or lymph. **2.** any of various organs or structures likened to true glands, as, a lymph gland.

glanders, a dangerous and contagious disease, chiefly of horses but capable of being transmitted to man, characterized by glandular swelling, nasal discharge, and lesions of the lungs.

glandular, 1. consisting of a gland or glands. **2.** pertaining to glands.

glandular fever, see **mononucleosis.**

glans, the head of the penis, glans penis; or of the clitoris, glans clitoridis.

Glauber's salt, a colorless, crystalline sodium sulfate, used mainly in medicine as a cathartic.

glaucoma, a disease of the eye characterized by increased intraocular pressure and progressive loss of vision.

gleet, 1. a transparent mucous discharge from the urethra, an effect of gonorrhea. **2.** a thin fluid running from a sore.

glenoid, 1. shallow or slightly cupped, as the articular cavities of the scapula and the temporal bone. **2.** pertaining to such a cavity.

glia, see **neuroglia.**

gliadin, any simple vegetable protein or globulin

found in gluten, the protein of wheat and rye, used in the synthesis of spinal anesthetics and other drug preparations.

glioma, a tumor arising from and consisting largely of neuroglia.

globin, a protein formed in the decomposition of hemoglobin.

globulin, any of several simple proteins that are insoluble in water, soluble in dilute solutions of salt, and coagulated by heat, as, gamma globulin.

globus hystericus, the sensation of a permanent lump in the throat occurring in certain cases of hysteria or other neuroses.

glomerule, a compact cluster, as of capillary blood vessels.

glomerulitis, an inflammation of glomeruli.

glomus, the primitive glomerule present in the embryonic kidney.

glossa, see **tongue.**

glossal, concerning the tongue.

glossectomy, surgical removal of the tongue.

glossitis, inflammation of the tongue.

glottic, relating to the glottis.

glottis, the opening at the upper part of the windpipe and between the vocal cords, which, by its dilatation and contraction, contributes to the modulation of the voice.

glucoprotein, see **glycoprotein.**

glucose, a sugar found in

three forms, most commonly as dextrose, which occurs in many fruits, animal tissues, and fluids and is formed by the hydrolysis of carbohydrates.

glucoside, see **glycoside.**

glucosuria, the presence of glucose in the urine.

glutamic acid, an amino acid that occurs in all complete proteins, used in the form of monosodium glutamate as a salt substitute and flavor intensifier.

gluteal, pertaining to the buttocks.

glutei, the muscles that form the buttocks.

gluten, the protein in flour and bread.

gluteus, any of several muscles of the buttocks.

glycemia, a condition in which sugar or glucose is found in the blood.

glycerin, see **glycerol.**

glycerol, an odorless, colorless, syrupy, sweettasting liquid compound of the alcohol class, obtained by saponification of fats and oils, used esp. as a solvent.

glycine, a colorless, sweet, crystalline amino acid, used chiefly in biochemical research, medicine, and organic synthesis.

glycogen, a white, amorphous, tasteless storage form of carbohydrate found mainly in the liver and muscles.

glycogenesis, the transformation of glucose or other sugars in the body into glycogen.

glycolysis, the breakdown of carbohydrates by enzymes in a living organism.

glycolytic, pertaining to glycolysis.

glycoprotein, any of a group of conjugated proteins containing a protein plus a carbohydrate, as mucin.

glycoside, any of a group of organic compounds, found abundantly in plants, which hydrolyze into sugars and other organic substances.

glycosuria, see **glucosuria.**

goiter, a morbid enlargement of the thyroid gland, forming a protuberance on the side or front part of the neck.

goitre, see **goiter.**

goitrous, pertaining to goiter; affected with goiter.

gomphosis, an immovable peg-and-socket articulation, as the root of a tooth in the jaw socket.

gonad, 1. a male or female reproductive gland that produces gametes, sperm, or ovum. 2. a testis or an ovary.

gonadal, relating to a gonad.

gonadotrophic, relating to gonadotrophin.

gonadotrophin, a substance that stimulates the sex glands.

gonococcal, relating to the gonococcus.

gonococcus, the bacterium that causes gonorrhea.

gonogenesis, the process of maturation of the germ cells.

gonorrhea, a contagious, inflammatory ailment of the male urethra or the female vagina, caused by the gonococcus and accompanied by secretions of mucus and pus.

gonorrheal, relating to gonorrhea.

gooseflesh, a rough condition of the skin, resembling that of a plucked goose, induced by cold or fear.

gout, a disease caused by defective metabolism and characterized by inflamed joints, esp. the big toe, and excessive uric acid in the bloodstream, affecting mainly males.

gouty, 1. of or like gout. 2. causing gout. 3. resulting from gout. 4. marked by gout.

graft, a portion of living skin, muscle, bone, nerve, or other tissue transplanted by surgery from one body or part of a body to another.

gramicidin, a powerful germicide.

gram-negative, denoting an inability, usually of bacteria, to hold the violet dye used for classification purposes in Gram's method.

gram-positive, denoting the ability of an organism to hold the violet dye used in Gram's method of typing bacteria.

Gram's method, a method in which an organism is stained, treated with solution, and classified according to its ability to retain the stain. The staining is done with a mixture of iodine and potassium iodine.

grand mal, a severe variety of epilepsy marked by convulsions, stupor, and unconsciousness.

granulation, 1. a process by which minute granular projections form on healing sores. 2. the granular projections themselves.

granulation tissue, tissue formed in the process of healing, which is made up of minute projections of flesh and causes a granular appearance.

granulocyte, a white blood cell whose cytoplasm contains granules.

granuloma, a mass or growth of granulation tissue occurring during the process of infection.

granulomatous, characterized by granulation tissue.

gravel, 1. small crystals or calculi in the kidneys or bladder. 2. the disease occasioned by such concretions.

gravid, pregnant.

gravida, a pregnant woman.

gray matter, nerve tissue, as of the spinal cord and brain, made up of both nerve cells and nerve fibers, brownish gray in color.

greensickness, an anemic condition occurring in young women and girls, characterized by a yellow-greenish skin pallor.

gripe, to produce pain in the bowels of, as if by con-

striction.

grippe, see **influenza.**

gristle, see **cartilage.**

gristly, consisting of or like gristle.

groin, the fold or hollow on either side of the body where the thigh joins the abdomen.

growing pains, dull, indefinite pains in the limbs during childhood and adolescence, commonly associated with the process of growing.

growth, 1. the act, process, or manner of growing. 2. an abnormal tissue development, as a tumor.

gullet, the passage by which food and liquid are taken into the stomach; the esophagus.

gum, the fleshy tissue that covers the necks of the teeth and the parts of the jaws in which the teeth are set.

gumboil, a boil or small abscess on the gum.

gumma, a soft tumor that can appear anywhere on the body, characteristic of the tertiary stage of syphillis.

gummatous, affected with gumma; of the nature of gumma.

gustation, the sense of taste.

gustatory, of or pertaining to tasting.

gut, 1. the intestinal canal from the stomach to the anus. 2. an intestine.

gutta, a drop or something droplike.

gutta-percha, the coagulated, milky juice of various Malaysian trees used for electrical insulation and in dentistry.

guttate, spotted, as if discolored by drops or having droplike spots.

gymnophobia, pathological aversion to seeing a naked body.

gynecologist, one who specializes in gynecology.

gynecology, the aspect of medical science that deals with the functions and diseases peculiar to women, esp. of the organs of reproduction.

gynecomastia, abnormally large mammary glands in the male.

gynephobia, pathological fear of the company of women.

gyrus, a ridge or raised convolution, as on the surface of the brain.

habit, 1. a disposition or involuntary tendency to act constantly in a certain manner, usually acquired by frequent repetition. 2. an addiction or usage, as the habit of smoking.

habit spasm, a spasmodic movement of groups of muscles that has become involuntary, as eye-blinking, coughing, etc.

habitual, 1. formed or acquired by habit, frequent use, or custom. 2. constantly practiced.

habituate, to accustom; to make familiar by frequent use or practice; to familiarize.

habitus, the physical appearance of a person that

indicates a tendency to certain diseases.

hack, 1. to emit short, frequent coughs. 2. a short, broken cough.

hair, one of the fine filaments that grow from the skin.

halation, blurring of vision because of strong light shining directly in one's eyes.

half-life, the length of time in which one-half of the radioactive atoms present in a substance decay; knowledge of this is necessary to calculate dosages in radiotherapeutics.

half-wit, a feebleminded person; one who lacks mental acuity.

halide, a compound, usually of two elements only, of which one is a halogen.

halisteresis, lack of calcium in bones.

halite, natural sodium chloride; rock salt.

halitosis, condition of having foul or offensive breath.

halitus, see breath.

hallucinate, to affect with hallucination.

hallucination, an apparent perception, as by sight or hearing, for which there is no real external cause, as distinguished from illusion.

hallucinogen, a chemical substance or drug such as LSD or mescaline that causes hallucinations.

hallucinogenic, pertaining to a hallucinogen.

hallucinosis, a disordered mental condition marked

by hallucinations.

hallux, the big toe.

hallux valgus, a displacement of the big toe toward the other toes.

hallux varus, displacement of the big toe away from the other toes.

halogen, any of the elements astatine, chlorine, iodine, bromine, and fluorine, and sometimes the radical cyanogen, which form a salt by direct union with a metal.

halogenate, 1. to treat or combine with a halogen. 2. to add a halogen to, esp. to an organic compound.

haloid, 1. resembling common salt in composition. 2. formed by the combination of a halogen and a metal.

halothane, a fluorinated hydrocarbon used as a general anesthetic.

ham, 1. the part of the leg behind the knee. 2. the back of the thigh together with the buttocks; the area of the thigh from the buttock to the back of the knee, in which region the hamstring muscles are located.

hamamelis, see **witch hazel.**

hamartoma, a mass of cells resembling a tumor resulting from faulty development of the embryo, as a nevus.

hamartophobia, pathological fear of making a mistake.

hammer, see **malleus.**

hammer finger, a deformity of a finger due to loss of power of extension, causing permanent flexion; dropfinger.

hammer toe, a deformity of a toe due to abnormal flexion or loss of power of extension.

hamstring, any of the tendons of the hamstring muscle that serve to bend the knee and turn the foot.

hamulus, a small hook or hooklike process.

hand, the extremity of the arm, consisting of the palm, four fingers, and thumb.

hangnail, a small piece of skin, partly detached, at the base or side of a fingernail.

haphephobia, pathological aversion to being touched by another person.

hard-of-hearing, of, concerning, or possessing an impaired sense of hearing.

harelip, 1. a congenital division or vertical fissure of the upper lip, often extending to the palate. 2. the deformed lip itself.

hartshorn, 1. antler of the stag, once used as an ammonia source. 2. ammonium carbonate or sal volatile.

hashish, the flowering tops and leaves of the hemp, **Cannabis sativa,** which is drunk, chewed, or smoked for its narcotic and intoxicating effect. See also **cannabis.**

haunch bone, see **ilium.**

hawk, 1. to cough up, as phlegm. 2. to use a cough

for clearing the throat.

hay fever, an allergy to the pollen of various plants, marked by sneezing, inflamed eyes, and other symptoms similar to those of a cold.

head, the upper part of the human body, joined to the trunk by the neck.

headache, a pain in the head.

head cold, a variation of the common cold characterized by congestion of mucous membranes of the nasal passages and related tissues.

head shrinker, slang, psychiatrist.

heady, 1. apt to affect the mental faculties. 2. strongly intoxicating.

heal, to make hale, sound, or whole; to cure of a disease or wound and restore to health.

health, the sound condition of a living organism; absence of ailments or defects.

healthy, 1. enjoying or being in good health; hale or sound. 2. indicative of or pertaining to good health or a sound mentality.

hear, to perceive by the auditory sense.

hearing, 1. the act of perceiving sound. 2. the faculty or sense by which sound is perceived. 3. reach of sound, earshot.

hearing aid, a small, inconspicuous amplifying device, worn to correct or improve faulty hearing.

heart, the hollow muscular organ that circulates blood throughout the body by means of rhythmic contractions and dilations.

heart attack, a sudden impairment in the heart's ability to function, often caused by an embolism or by high blood pressure.

heartbeat, the dual sound of the diastole and the systole made by the rhythmical contraction and dilation of the ventricles of the heart as blood is forced through its chambers.

heart block, an impairment of the ventricular beat of the heart.

heartburn, a burning sensation in the thorax and stomach, sometimes accompanied by a slight eructation of acid-tasting fluid. Also called cardialgia.

heart disease, an abnormality of the heart impairing its normal functioning.

heart failure, cessation of the beat of the heart.

heart-lung machine, an apparatus used to maintain circulation and oxygenation of the blood while the heart is stopped during open-heart surgery.

heart murmur, an abnormal heart sound, usually audible with the aid of a stethoscope, and usually indicating a structural or functional defect.

heat exhaustion, a physical condition caused by extended exposure to high temperature combined with exertion, and marked by faintness, nausea, and profuse sweating.

heat prostration, see **heat exhaustion**.

heat rash, see **prickly heat**.

heatstroke, a state of collapse, usually accompanied by high fever, brought on by exposure to heat, as of the sun or a furnace; also called sunstroke.

hebephrenia, a type of schizophrenia, occurring more often in the teen and preteen period of youth, with disorders characterized by delusions, hallucinations, and childish, regressive behavior.

hebephrenic, pertaining to hebephrenia.

hebetude, dullness; lethargy; stupidity.

hebosteotomy, surgical enlargement of the pelvic diameter to aid childbirth.

hectic fever, a fluctuating fever characteristic of pulmonary tuberculosis.

hedonophobia, pathological fear of pleasure.

helical, of, pertaining to, or shaped like a helix.

helicoid, helixlike; coiled or curving, as a spiral.

heliotherapy, treatment of disease by exposure to sunlight.

helix, the whole circuit of the external ear.

helminth, 1. a worm. 2. an intestinal worm, as the tapeworm or roundworm.

helminthiasis, an unhealthy condition of the body caused by worms.

helminthic, 1. pertaining to worms. 2. pertaining to that which expels worms.

helminthicide, a medicine that kills worms.

helminthology, the study and treatment of helminths, esp. of parasitic worms.

helminthophobia, pathological fear of worms or delusion of having worms.

heloma, a corn or callosity.

helosis, the condition of having corns.

helotomy, surgical removal of corns.

hemacytometer, see **hemocytometer**.

hemadostenosis, the contraction of blood vessels.

hemal, 1. of or pertaining to the blood or blood vessels. 2. noting, pertaining to, or situated on that side of the spinal column containing the heart and great blood vessels.

hemangioma, see **nevus**.

hemarthrosis, bleeding into a joint, usually as the result of an injury.

hematein, a reddish-brown crystalline substance, useful as a stain in microscopic investigation.

hematemesis, vomiting of blood.

hematherapy, the treatment of a disease by the infusion of blood or blood plasma.

hematic, 1. of or pertaining to blood. 2. contained in blood. 3. acting on the blood, as a medicine.

hematic abscess, an abscess caused by an infected blood clot.

hematimeter, an instrument used in counting blood corpuscles.

hematin, a reddish pigment containing iron, produced in the decomposition of hemoglobin.

hematinic, 1. a medicine, as a compound of iron, that tends to increase the amount of hematin or hemoglobin in the blood. 2. pertaining to hematin.

hematocrit, 1. a centrifugal device for determining the percentage of red cells in a given amount of whole blood. 2. the volume percentage of red blood cells in blood.

hematogenous, 1. originating in the blood. 2. blood-producing. 3. spread by means of the bloodstream.

hematologic, pertaining to hematology.

hematology, that branch of medicine dealing with the blood and its diseases.

hematoma, a swelling or mass of blood, usually clotted, in an organ or tissue, caused by a ruptured blood vessel due to injury.

hematometra, hemorrhage within the cavity of the womb.

hematomyelia, hemorrhage into the spinal cord.

hematopericardium, hemorrhage into the pericardial sac.

hematoperitoneum, hemorrhage into the peritoneal cavity.

hematophobia, see **hemophobia.**

hematopoiesis, the process of the formation of blood cells.

hematosalpinx, retained menstrual blood in, or hemorrhage into, the fallopian tube.

hematosis, the change that takes place in venous blood as it converts into arterial blood by oxygenation in the lungs.

hematospermia, sperm that contain blood.

hematothorax, blood in the chest cavity.

hematozoon, an animal parasite living in the blood.

hematuria, blood in the urine.

heme, see **hematin.**

hemeralopia, day blindness; a condition of the eyes in which distinct vision is possible only at night or in dim light.

hemianacusia, loss of hearing in one ear.

hemianalgesia, absence of the sense of pain on one side of the body.

hemianesthesia, anesthesia of half of the body.

hemianopia, blindness for half of the visual field in one or both eyes.

hemiatrophy, wasting of a part of one side of the body caused by impaired nutrition.

hemic, of or pertaining to blood.

hemicrania, a headache, usually a migraine, affecting only one side of the head.

hemin, a reddish-brown crystalline compound derived by heating hemoglobin with sodium chloride and acetic acid, used in tests to indicate the presence of blood.

hemiplegia, paralysis of only one side of the body.

hemisphere, either of the two convoluted parts, one on each side, which constitute a great part of the cerebrum.

hemispheric, pertaining to a hemisphere.

hemlock, a plant the extract of which, when drunk, causes drowsiness, nausea, paralysis, and, if not treated, death.

hemocytometer, an instrument used to count blood corpuscles.

hemoglobin, a red respiratory pigment occurring in the red corpuscles of the blood and composed of iron-containing protein matter that carries oxygen from the lungs to the tissues.

hemoglobinic, pertaining to hemoglobin.

hemoglobinometer, a device for measuring the amount of hemoglobin in the blood.

hemolysin, an antibody which, in cooperation with a material in fresh blood, causes the breakdown of red blood corpuscles.

hemolysis, the destruction of red blood cells with liberation of hemoglobin.

hemolytic, pertaining to hemolysis.

hemophilia, an inherited defect of males, transmitted through the mother, which leads to excessive bleeding due to deficiency of a coagulant factor in the blood.

hemophiliac, a person having hemophilia.

hemophilic, evidencing hemophilia.

hemophobia, pathological aversion to the sight of blood.

hemoptysis, spitting up of blood caused by hemorrhage of the larynx, trachea, bronchi, or lungs.

hemorrhage, 1. a rapid and heavy flow of blood from a ruptured blood vessel. 2. to bleed heavily.

hemorrhagenic, producing hemorrhage.

hemorrhagic, pertaining to hemorrhage; bloody.

hemorrhoid, a swelling formed by the dilatation of a blood vessel at the anus.

hemorrhoidal, pertaining to hemorrhoids.

hemorrhoidectomy, the surgical excision of hemorrhoids.

hemosalpinx, see **hematosalpinx.**

hemostasis, 1. the termination of bleeding. 2. retardation of the blood circulation. 3. blood congestion, as in a localized part.

hemostat, an instrument or chemical used to check or arrest hemorrhaging.

hemostatic, causing bleeding to stop.

hemotherapy, see **hematherapy.**

hemothorax, see **hematothorax.**

hemp, see **cannabis.**

henbane, a poisonous viscid Eurasian herb of the

nightshade family, which contains narcotic alkaloids and is in limited cultivation for sedative drugs.

heparin, a complex blood anticoagulant found in various domestic animal tissues, esp. the liver.

heparinize, to treat therapeutically with heparin in order to retard blood coagulation.

hepatic, 1. pertaining to the liver. 2. a medication acting on the liver.

hepatitis, inflammation of the liver.

hepatize, to convert, as spongy lung tissue, into liverlike tissue by congestion.

hepatography, X-ray photography of the liver.

hepatologist, a physician specializing in diagnosis and treatment of diseases of the liver.

hepatology, the branch of medicine concerned with the diagnosis and treatment of diseases of the liver.

hepatoma, a tumor of the liver.

hepatomegalia, see **hepatomegaly.**

hepatomegaly, enlargement of the liver.

herbalist, a healer who specializes in the curative properties of herbs.

herb doctor, see **herbalist.**

hereditary, 1. transmitted from predecessors. 2. descending from genetic inheritance, as opposed to acquired.

heredity, the transmission of characteristics of parents to offspring through chromosomes that bear the genes.

hermaphrodite, an animal or human being having the sexual characteristics of both male and female.

hermaphroditism, the condition of a hermaphrodite.

hernia, the projection of an internal organ or tissue through an abnormal aperture in the wall that encloses it, usually in the abdominal area. See also **rupture.**

hernial, relating to a hernia.

herniated disk, rupture or herniation of a disk between vertebrae, usually occurring between lumbar vertebrae.

herniation, development of a hernia.

heroin, a morphine derivative, being white, odorless, and crystalline, and constituting a dangerously addictive narcotic.

herpes, any of certain inflammations of the skin or mucous membrane characterized by clusters of blisters, which often spread.

herpes simplex, a viral disease marked by clusters of blisters chiefly around the mouth and on the lips.

herpes zoster, see **shingles.**

herpetic, relating to herpes.

herpetiform, resembling herpes.

heterochromatic, referring to heterochromatin.

heterochromatin, a component of chromatin, dense and easily stained, which evidences little genetic activity.

heterogeneous, 1. differing in kind. 2. having dissimilar or incongruous elements, as opposed to **homogeneous.**

heterologous, abnormal; consisting of tissue unlike the normal tissue of a part, as a tumor.

heterology, an abnormality, deviating from the common type, as a tumor.

heterophthalmia, a condition in which the iris of each eye has a different color.

heteroplasty, an operation in which lesions are repaired with grafted tissue taken from another person or organism.

heterosexual, 1. of or pertaining to sexual orientation toward the opposite sex. 2. one who is heterosexual.

heterosexuality, sexual attraction toward the opposite sex.

heterotopy, displacement of an organ or a portion of the body.

heterotropia, inability to have bifocal vision.

heterozygosis, the union of genetically unlike gametes that form a heterozygote.

heterozygote, a person who has one or more unlike pairs of genes.

hexachlorophene, a bactericidal agent used in soaps, cosmetics, and deodorants.

hexamine, a drug used as a disinfectant of the urinary tract.

hiatus, any natural aperture, fissure, or cleft.

hiatus hernia, a hernia in the diaphragm that causes a protrusion of part of the stomach.

hiccup, 1. a quick involuntary intake of breath suddenly checked by closure of the glottis, producing a characteristic sound. 2. (pl.) an attack of such spasms.

hiccupping, 1. making the sound of a hiccup. 2. affected with hiccups.

hidrosis, 1. perspiration, esp. excessive perspiration caused by drugs, disease, or the like. 2. any of certain diseases characterized by sweating.

high, (slang) excited with drink, or drugs.

high blood pressure, abnormally high arterial blood pressure; hypertension.

hilar, concerning or near a hilum.

hilum, the point at which vessels, ducts, or nerves enter a bodily part or emerge from it.

hindbrain, the posterior of the vertebrate brain including, primarily, the pons, cerebellum, and medulla oblongata; rhombencephalon.

hindgut, the posterior of the embryonic alimentary structure, from which the colon and rectum evolve.

hip, 1. the side of the pelvis and upper region of the thigh with their fleshy covering parts. 2. the haunch. 3. the hip joint.

hipbone, see **innominate bone.**

hip joint, the ball-and-socket joint between the hipbone and the femur.

hipped, (slang) having a mental obsession; fanatically interested.

hippocras, a medicinal cordial made of wine infused with spices.

Hippocrates, Greek physician born 460 B.C.

Hippocratic oath, a pledge embodying a code of ethics taken by those about to receive a degree in medicine.

hirsute, 1. hairy. 2. shaggy. 3. of or relating to hair. 4. covered with long, bristly hair.

hirsuties, see **hirsutism.**

hirsutism, abnormal, excessive growth of hair or the presence of hair in unusual places, esp. that which occurs on the face of some women.

histaminase, an enzyme that deactivates a histamine and therefore is used to treat certain allergies.

histamine, a chemical, amine, that occurs naturally in the tissue of the body and is released during allergic reactions. It dilates the capillaries, stimulates gastric secretion, and causes uterine contractions. Histamine can also be produced synthetically.

histogenesis, the origin, development, and differentiation of tissues.

histologist, a person who practices histology.

histology, 1. the science and study of tissues, esp. of their microscopic structure. 2. the structure, esp. the microscopic structure, of a given tissue of an organism.

histolysis, the dissolution and breaking down of organic tissues.

histone, any of a class of protein substances, as globin, having marked basic properties, and, on hydrolysis, yielding amino acids.

histoplasmosis, a usually fatal respiratory disease caused by a fungus.

hives, see **urticaria.**

hoarse, having a husky, harsh, rough, or grating voice, as when affected with a cold.

hoarsen, to make or to grow hoarse.

hoarseness, the state of being hoarse.

Hodgkin's disease, a progressive disease marked by chronic inflammation and enlargement of the lymph nodes and other organs.

homeopath, one who practices homeopathy.

homeopathic, relating to homeopathy.

homeopathy, the system of treating disease by administering minute quantities of drugs which, if given in larger doses to a healthy person, would produce symptoms similar to those of the disease.

homeostasis, the tendency of the physiological system to maintain an environment of organic stability even when its natural function or condition has been disrupted.

homeostatic, pertaining to homeostasis.

homicide, 1. the killing of one human being by another, including acts of manslaughter, murder, accidental killing, and justifiable homicide. 2. a person who kills another.

homoerotic, pertaining to erotic attraction to members of the same sex.

homogeneity, the state or quality of having like characteristics or uniformity of nature, composition, or structure.

homogeneous, of the same kind or nature; essentially alike; uniform in structure; belonging to the same type.

homogenesis, the ordinary course of generation, in which the offspring is like the parents and runs through the same cycle of development.

homogenetic, 1. pertaining to homogenesis. 2. having a common origin. 3. derived from the same structure, however modified.

homogenous, see **homogeneous.**

homograft, an organ or tissue removed from an individual and grafted to another of the same species.

homologous, pertaining to a bacterium and its relationship to the serum derived from it.

homology, 1. the state of being homologous. 2. sameness of relation. 3. correspondence, or an instance of correspondence. 4. homologous relation or correspondence.

homosexual, one who is characterized by a sexual interest in persons of the same sex.

homosexuality, condition in which sexual desire is directed to a member of the same sex.

hookworm disease, a disease characterized by severe anemia and caused by any of certain bloodsucking nematode worms equipped with mouth hooks, which feed on the lining of the intestines of men and animals.

hormone, 1. a secretion of an endocrine gland, distributed in the bloodstream or in bodily fluids to stimulate its specific functional effect in another part of the body. 2. such a substance produced synthetically.

horn, a substance, mainly composed of keratin, of which hair and nails are composed.

horripilation, see **goose flesh.**

horseshoe kidney, a congenital abnormality in which the kidneys are united at their lower ends in the shape of a horseshoe.

host, an organism upon which a parasite is dependent for its existence.

housemaid's knee, an acute or chronic inflammation of the bursa over the kneecap, so called because of its supposed prevalence among housemaids who knelt to do much of their work.

humerus, the long, cylindrical bone of the arm, extending from shoulder to elbow.

humor, any functioning body fluid.

humoral, pertaining to or proceeding from the humors or fluids of the body.

hunchback, 1. a back deformed by a convex curvature of the spine. 2. one who has such a back.

hunchbacked, see **kyphosis.**

Huntington's chorea, an adult form of St. Vitus's dance, an inherited disease of the central nervous system.

hyaline, 1. any of various nitrogenous substances, esp. that which is the main component of hydatid cysts. 2. something glassy or transparent.

hyaline cartilage, the typical translucent form of cartilage, containing little fibrous tissue.

hyaluronic acid, a polymer that apparently holds cells together and lubricates joints, found in tissues, esp. skin, vitreous humor, and synovial fluid.

hyaluronidase, an enzyme that breaks down the molecular structure of hyaluronic acid, thus increasing the permeability of tissues.

hybrid, the offspring of parents of different races or parents who differ in one or more distinct characteristics.

hybridize, to cause to produce hybrids.

hydatid, 1. a fluid-filled cyst formed in the bodies of men and certain animals by the tapeworm larva. 2. an encysted tapeworm larva.

hydatidiform, having the form of or resembling a hydatid.

hydradenitis, inflammation of a sweat gland.

hydragogue, a drug promoting the secretion of water from the kidneys. See also **diuretic.**

hydrarthrosis, serous accumulation in a joint.

hydrate, any of a class of compounds produced when certain substances, as metallic salts, unite with water.

hydrating, combining chemically with water; forming into a hydrate.

hydration, the act of hydrating.

hydremia, excess of watery fluid in the bloodstream.

hydroa, a term for any skin disease characterized by bullous skin eruptions.

hydrobromic acid, a hydrogen bromide in aqueous solution, sometimes used for sedative purposes.

hydrocele, a collection of serous fluid in a saccular body cavity, esp. the scrotum.

hydrocephalic, pertaining

to hydrocephalus.

hydrocephalus, an accumulation of serous fluid within the cavity of the cranium, esp. in infancy, causing enlargement of the head.

hydrochloric acid, an aqueous solution of hydrogen chloride, a strong, fuming, highly corrosive acid, used in medicine, industry, and research.

hydrocortisone, an adrenal cortical steroid hormone, used in medicine as an anti-inflammatory acid in treating arthritis and other conditions.

hydrolysis, chemical decomposition in which a compound is divided into other compounds by taking up the elements of water.

hydrolyte, a compound subject to hydrolysis.

hydrolyze, to go through or cause to go through the process of hydrolysis.

hydrometer, a device for measuring the specific gravity of fluids.

hydronephrosis, swelling of the kidney by urine because of an obstruction to its outflow.

hydroperitoneum, accumulation of fluid within the abdominal cavity.

hydrophobia, 1. rabies, an infectious disease of certain animals caused by a virus and transmitted to man by the bite of the infected animal. 2. pathological fear of water.

hydrophobic, 1. pertaining to hydrophobia. 2. having

no affinity for water.

hydrops, see dropsy.

hydrotherapy, the scientific treatment of disease by means of water.

hydrothorax, the presence of excess serous fluid on one or both pleural cavities.

hydroureter, swelling of the ureter with fluid due to an obstruction.

hydruria, excessive discharge of urine.

hygiene, the system or practice of principles or rules designed for promotion and maintenance of health and cleanliness.

hygienic, pertaining to hygiene.

hygienics, the science of health and cleanliness.

hygienist, one trained in hygiene.

hygrometer, an instrument for measuring the degree of moisture of the atmosphere.

hygroscope, an instrument for indicating the presence and approximate amount of moisture in the atmosphere.

hygroscopic, 1. pertaining to the hygroscope. 2. capable of absorbing moisture from the atmosphere.

hymen, the mucous membrane situated at the entrance of the vagina.

hyoid, referring to a U-shaped movable bone between the root of the tongue and the larynx.

hyoscine, see Scopolamine.

hyoscyamine, a poisonous alkaloid obtained from

henbane and other solanaceous plants, used as a sedative, mydriatic, antispasmodic, and analgesic.

hyperacidity, excessive acidity, as of the gastric juice.

hyperacousis, abnormal perception of the sense of hearing.

hyperactive, overly or abnormally active.

hyperactivity, abnormal and excessive activity.

hyperacuity, abnormal perception of senses, such as hearing or sight.

hyperalgesia, excessive sensibility to pain.

hyperbaric chamber, the airtight chamber through which oxygen is forced under pressure to reach the heart and lungs of a patient, as in open-heart surgery.

hyperchromic, an anemia characterized by an increase of hemoglobin in each red blood cell and a general decrease in the number of red blood cells.

hyperemesis, excessive vomiting.

hyperemesis gravidarum, excessive morning sickness during pregnancy.

hyperemia, congestion with blood in a localized area.

hyperesthesia, extreme sensitivity to pain, touch, cold, or heat.

hyperglycemia, an excessive increase of sugar in the blood, as in diabetes.

hyperhidrosis, excessive sweating.

hyperinsulinism, an excessive amount of insulin in the blood.

hyperinvolution, the reduction of an organ to a smaller than normal size, esp. after hypertrophy, as hyperinvolution of the uterus after pregnancy.

hyperirritability, abnormally excessive reaction to stimulation.

hyperkeratosis, excessive development of the horny tissue of the skin.

hypermetropia, see **hyperopia.**

hypermyotonia, increased muscle tone.

hypernephroma, a malignant tumor of the kidney.

hyperopia, a defect of the eyesight in which the focus falls behind the retina, with the result that distant objects are seen more sharply than those nearby.

hyperosmia, an abnormally acute sense of smell.

hyperparathyroidism, overactivity of the parathyroid glands.

hyperpiesia, abnormally high blood pressure.

hyperpituitarism, 1. extreme activity of the pituitary gland, with an excessive quantity of growth hormone produced. **2.** the resultant irregularity, as gigantism.

hyperplasia, excessive increase in the number of normal cells in the tissue of an organ, resulting in an increase of its size.

hyperpnea, increased respiratory rate; overbreathing or panting.

hyperpyretic, relating to hyperpyrexia.

hyperpyrexia, an excessive degree of fever.

hypersecretion, an abnormal increase in secretion.

hypersensitive, 1. excessively sensitive. 2. reacting abnormally to a drug or other substance. 3. allergic.

hypersensitiveness, the state of being hypersensitive.

hypertension, a condition characterized by high blood pressure, esp. in the arteries.

hyperthermia, an abnormal rise of body temperature without presence of infection.

hyperthyroidism, 1. excessive activity of the thyroid gland. 2. the resulting abnormal conditions, as rapid heartbeat and increased metabolism.

hypertonia, an excessive degree of tone or tension, esp. of the muscles.

hypertonic, pertaining to hypertonia.

hypertoxic, excessively poisonous.

hypertrichiasis, excessive growth of hair.

hypertrichosis, see **hypertrichiasis.**

hypertrophic, relating to hypertrophy.

hypertrophy, an abnormal growth of tissue caused by enlargement of each of the cellular parts without an increase in the number of cells.

hypervitaminosis, a condition caused by excessive amounts of vitamins.

hypesthesia, diminished capacity for sensation.

hyphidrosis, diminution in the amount of perspiration.

hypnagogic, relating to the condition of drowsiness that precedes sleep.

hypnoanalysis, treatment conducted while the subject is under hypnosis.

hypnogenesis, induction of the hypnotic state.

hypnoidal, referring to a mental condition similar to light hypnosis, but usually caused by some means other than hypnosis.

hypnolepsy, see **narcolepsy.**

hypnopaedia, a teaching procedure designed so that a person can learn while asleep by listening to specially adapted recording devices.

hypnophobia, pathological fear of falling asleep.

hypnopompic, referring to the state of drowsiness associated with awakening from sleep.

hypnosis, a condition or state, allied to normal sleep, that can be artificially induced and is characterized by marked susceptibility to suggestion and considerable loss of willpower and sensation.

hypnotherapy, treatment of mental or physical disease by hypnotism.

hypnotic, 1. pertaining to hypnosis or hypnotism. 2. susceptible to hypnotism, as a person. 3. inducing sleep. 4. an agent or drug that produces sleep. 5. a sedative. 6. a person under the influence of hypnotism. 7. one subject to hypnotic influence.

hypnotism, 1. the induction of hypnosis. 2. the science dealing with the induction of hypnosis.

hypnotist, one who hypnotizes.

hypnotize, to put into a hypnotic state.

hypoblast, see **endoderm.**

hypochondria, a morbid condition, characterized by depressed spirits and fancies of ill health.

hypochondriac, 1. a person suffering from or subject to hypochondria. 2. pertaining to or afflicted with hypochondria.

hypochondriacal, pertaining to the hypochondria, the parts of the abdomen left and right of the epigastrium and above the lumbar regions. See **hypochondrium.**

hypochondriasis, an abnormal concern for one's health, accompanied by imaginary ailments.

hypochondrium, the part of the abdomen beneath the lower ribs on each side of the epigastrium.

hypoderm, see **hypoblast; hypodermis.**

hypodermic, 1. characterized by the introduction of medical preparations under the skin. 2. pertaining to parts under the skin. 3. lying under the skin, as tissue.

hypodermic injection, the

forceful implanting of fluid by inserting a syringe under the skin.

hypodermic needle, the hollow needle that is part of a hypodermic syringe.

hypodermic syringe, a device composed usually of a hollow glass barrel and a hollow needle used to inject fluid into or under the skin.

hypodermis, a layer of tissue or cells lying beneath the skin.

hypogastric, pertaining to the hypogastrium.

hypogastrium, the frontal lower and middle part of the abdomen.

hypoglossal, situated under the tongue, wholly or in part.

hypoglossal nerve, either of the pair of cranial nerves that give rise to the movements of the tongue.

hypoglycemia, a deficiency of sugar in the blood.

hypohydrosis, abnormally diminished perspiration.

hypomania, a mild degree of mania.

hypomenorrhea, regular menstrual periods, but deficient flow.

hypomorph, a mutant gene, less effective than its equivalent ancestral gene.

hypophyseal, relating to the pituitary gland.

hypophysectomy, surgical excision of the pituitary gland.

hypophysis, see **pituitary gland.**

hypophysitis, inflammation of the pituitary gland.

hypopituitarism, a condition caused by a diminished secretion of the pituitary gland.

hypoplasia, arrested growth of an organ or part, causing it to be undersized or immature.

hypopyon, presence of pus in the interior chamber of the eye in front of the iris but behind the cornea.

hyposecretion, abnormally lowered amount of secretion.

hyposensitize, 1. to lessen sensitivity. 2. to reduce the allergic reaction.

hypostasis, 1. a sediment or deposit, as from urine. 2. the settling of a fluid, as blood, in a bodily part.

hypostatize, to treat or regard as a distinct substance or reality.

hypotension, a condition marked by unusually low blood pressure.

hypotensive, denoting hypotension.

hypothalamus, the part of the posterior section of the forebrain, or diencephalon, that composes the floor of the third ventricle.

hypothermal, having subnormal temperature.

hypothermia, a condition marked by subnormal body temperature.

hypothyroidism, a condition caused by deficient activity of the thyroid gland.

hypotonia, diminished muscle tone or activity.

hypotonic, having an inadequate degree of tension, as the muscles.

hypovitaminosis, a condition caused by lack of vitamins.

hysterectomy, surgical removal of the uterus.

hysteria, a psychoneurotic disorder characterized variously by violent emotional outbreaks, irrationality, simulated bodily symptoms due to autosuggestion, and impairment of motor and sensory functions.

hysteric, one subject to hysteria.

hysterics, a fit of hysteria; an uncontrollable outburst.

hysterogenic, producing hysteria.

hysteroid, producing hysteria.

hystero-oophorectomy, surgical removal of the womb and one or both ovaries.

hysterotomy, excision of the uterus; a caesarean operation.

Iatric, pertaining to a physician or to medicine.

Iatrogenic, caused by the mannerisms or treatment of a physician, as imaginary illness of the patient brought about unintentionally by the physician.

Iatrology, medical science.

ichor, a watery, acrid discharge from an ulcerated wound.

ichthammol, see **Ichthysol.**

Ichthyol, a dark-brown syrupy compound, used

as an astringent, antiseptic, and alterative, esp. for skin diseases, as to relieve pruritus (trademark).

ichthyophobia, abnormal aversion to fish.

ichthyosis, a hereditary skin disorder marked by a thick, scaly skin surface.

icteric, affected with or relating to jaundice.

icteroid, resembling jaundice.

icterus, see **jaundice.**

ictus, a seizure, stroke, or fit.

id, a part of the psyche, constituting the unconscious, which is the source of instinctual or libidinal energy.

ideate, 1. to form an idea or thought. 2. to imagine. 3. to conceive. 4. to form ideas. 5. to think.

ideation, 1. the faculty of the mind for forming ideas. 2. the establishment of a distinct mental representation or image of an object.

identical twin, either of a pair of twins originating from a single fertilized ovum, each being of the same sex and having the same hereditary features, distinguished from **fraternal twin.**

idiocy, 1. the condition of being an idiot. 2. mental deficiency.

idiopathic, pertaining to idiopathy.

idiopathy, 1. a disease of unknown or obscure cause. 2. a primary or spontaneous disease.

idiosyncrasy, 1. a personal peculiarity of constitution, temperament, or manner. 2. a quirk. 3. a mental or moral characteristic belonging to and distinguishing an individual. 4. an unusual way of thinking or feeling.

idiosyncratic, relating to idiosyncrasy.

idiot, 1. one who suffers from mental retardation in one of its most severe forms, having a mental age of three years or less. 2. an extremely incompetent or foolish person.

idiot savant, a mentally retarded person who possesses a high degree of some special ability.

ileac, relating to the ileum.

ileectomy, surgical excision of the ileum.

ileitis, inflammation of the ileum.

ileocecal, pertaining to the ileum and the cecum.

ileocecostomy, the joining of the cecum with the ileum by surgery, after a part of the ileum has been removed.

ileocolic, relating to the ileum and the colon.

ileocolostomy, the surgical forming of a passage between the ileum and the colon in order to bypass a diseased cecum.

ileostomy, the surgical creation of a passage through the abdominal wall into the ileum.

ileum, the lower third of the small intestine located between the jejunum and the cecum.

ileus, severe colic caused by intestinal obstruction.

iliac, pertaining to the ilium.

ilium, 1. a bone that forms the upper portion of the innominate bone. 2. the hipbone.

illusion, 1. a perception of a thing that misrepresents it or gives it qualities not present in reality. 2. something that deceives by producing a false impression.

illusory, 1. causing illusion. 2. deceptive. 3. of the nature of an illusion. 4. unreal.

image, the representation in the mind of something once perceived and not now present.

imagination, 1. the act of imagining, or of forming mental images or concepts of what is not actually present to the senses. 2. the faculty of forming such images or concepts.

imago, an idealized conception of a parent or other person loved in childhood, the unaltered concept being retained in adulthood.

imbalance, faulty coordination of glands or muscles, as in the ocular muscles.

imbecile, 1. one who is mentally deficient. 2. a person having an intelligence quotient between 25 and 50 or a mental age of about seven.

imbecility, 1. the condition or quality of being an imbecile. 2. fatuity.

immiscibility, the state of being immiscible.

immiscible, incapable of being mixed; used esp. in referring to liquids, as oil with water.

immix, to mix; to mingle; to blend.

immobile, immovable; not able to move; fixed.

immobility, the state of being immobile.

immobilize, to restrain movement of, as the body or a bodily part, as part of a surgical or corrective procedure.

immune, protected against a disease, poison, or the like, usually by inoculation.

immunity, the state of being immune from or insusceptible to a disease.

immunization, 1. the condition of being immunized. 2. the act of immunizing.

immunize, to render immune.

immunochemistry, a part of the study of immunology dealing with its chemical aspects.

immunogenetic, relating to immunogenetics.

immunogenetics, 1. the study of the genetic aspects of immunity. 2. the study of biological relationships by comparison of serological reactions.

immunogenic, producing immunity to a particular disease.

immunology, the branch of medical science that deals with immunity from disease and the production of such immunity.

immunosuppressive, relating to that which is capable of inhibiting immune responses, such as the rejection by a body of a transplanted organ.

immunotherapy, the prevention or cure of disease through the use of antigens.

immunotoxin, see **antitoxin.**

impacted, of a tooth, so firmly held by the jawbone that it cannot emerge from the gum.

impaction, the state of being impacted.

impalpable, 1. not felt. 2. not easily apprehended or grasped by the mind. 3. incapable of being distinguished or perceived by the touch. 4. intangible.

imparidigitate, having uneven numbers of fingers or toes.

imperceptible, not discernible by the senses or the mind.

imperception, faulty perception.

imperceptive, lacking perception or vision.

imperforate, having no openings or pores.

impermeable, 1. impassable. 2. not permitting the passage of substances, such as fluids, through the pores or interstices.

impetigo, a contagious skin disease, esp. of children, which manifests itself in pustules and eruptions.

impetus, 1. anything that is an incentive to action. 2. stimulus.

implant, 1. tissue grafted into the body. 2. a filled tube, as one containing radium, placed in an organ or tissue for treatment.

implantation, the act of implanting.

impotence, lack of sexual power.

impotent, 1. entirely wanting power, strength, or vigor of body or mind. 2. deficient in capacity. 3. weak. 4. feeble. 5. completely powerless to perform sexual intercourse, specifically in the male.

impregnate, 1. to make pregnant. 2. to fertilize. 3. to fill or saturate with, or cause to absorb, some substance.

impregnation, the act of impregnating.

impression, 1. an effect produced on the senses or mind. 2. a strong effect produced on the intellect, feelings, or conscience. 3. in dentistry, an imprint of the teeth and adjacent tissues taken in a plastic or semisoft material.

impulse, 1. a stimulating or inhibiting wave transferred through nerve fibers. 2. a sudden involuntary inclination prompting to action.

impulsion, 1. impetus. 2. a constraining or inciting action on the mind or conduct. 3. the inciting influence of some feeling or motive. 4. mental impulse.

impulsive, having the power or effect of impelling.

inactivate, 1. to arrest the activity of, as of a serum by means of heat. 2. to render inactive.

inactivation, the process of rendering inactive.

inactive, not active; inert; idle; out of use; indolent; sluggish.

inanition, 1. exhaustion from lack of nourishment. 2. deficiency of vigor. 3. sluggishness or lethargy.

inappetence, lack of appetite, desire, or concern.

inarticulate, unintelligible; unable to use clear or understandable speech; unable to use speech to convey ideas.

in articulo mortis, at the moment of death.

inassimilable, unabsorbable; unable to be used by the body as nutrition.

inborn, innate; inherent; implanted by nature; congenital.

inbreathe, see **inhale.**

inbred, bred within; innate; natural.

inbreed, to cross or mate closely related individuals.

incest, sexual intercourse or marriage between close blood relations.

incidence, the range of occurrence or influence of a thing or the extent of its effects, as, the incidence of a disease.

incipient, 1. in the beginning stage. 2. commencing. 3. beginning to appear.

incise, to cut into, surgically.

incision, 1. a cut, particularly one made in surgery. 2. a gash.

incisive, 1. cutting. 2. pertaining to the incisors.

incisor, one of eight cutting teeth, located in the upper and lower jaws, be-

tween the canines.

inclusion body, a stainable foreign particle contained in a virus-infected cell.

incoherence, the state of being incoherent.

incoherent, disorganized or uncoordinated, without logical connection, disjointed or rambling, as thought or language.

incompatible, undesirable or dangerous when combined, as substances in medications. 2. unable to coexist in harmony.

incomprehensible, 1. not to be grasped by the mind. 2. not to be understood. 3. unintelligible.

incompressible, not able to be pressed together, reduced, or lessened.

incontinence, 1. inability to restrain the passions or appetites, particularly the sexual appetite. 2. inability to restrain natural bodily discharges.

incoordination, inability to coordinate voluntary muscular movements.

incrustation, the forming of a crust over a healing wound.

incubate, to maintain, as bacterial cultures or embryos, in a controlled environment most suitable for development.

incubation, 1. the act or process of incubating. 2. the period of development of a disease between infection and the appearance of symptoms.

incubator, 1. an apparatus for maintaining suitable temperature, humidity, and oxygen for babies born prematurely or otherwise physically subnormal. 2. an apparatus for incubating bacteriological cultures. 3. one who or that which incubates.

incubus, see **nightmare.**

incurable, 1. beyond medical help or skill. 2. a person diseased beyond the possibility of cure.

incus, see **anvil.**

index finger, the finger next to the thumb; the forefinger.

Indian hemp, see **cannabis.**

indigestible, 1. not digestible. 2. digested with difficulty.

indigestion, 1. incapability or difficulty in digesting food. 2. see **dyspepsia.**

indispose, to cause to become sick.

indisposed, mildly ill.

indole, a white or yellow crystalline compound, produced in the intestines as a decomposition of protein, which gives odor and color to the feces.

indolent, 1. causing little or no pain, as an indolent tumor. 2. sluggish.

induce, to bring on, produce, or cause, as, to induce labor in a pregnant woman.

inductive, in embryology, pertaining to the interaction between an embryonic cell and adjacent inductive cells.

indurate, 1. to grow or become hard. 2. to make unfeeling. 3. callous.

induration, the state of

being hardened, unfeeling, or callous.

inebriant, anything that intoxicates.

inebriate, 1. to make drunk; intoxicate. 2. to excite or confuse. 3. a habitual drunkard.

inebriety, drunkenness; intoxication.

in extremis, near death.

infancy, 1. the state or period of being an infant. 2. babyhood. 3. early childhood.

infant, a child during the earliest period of its life.

infanticide, the murder of an infant.

infantile, of or pertaining to infants; infantlike; childish.

infantile paralysis, see **poliomyelitis.**

infantilism, 1. abnormal persistence or recurrence of childish characteristics, physical, emotional, or mental, in an adult, often accompanied by a failure to mature sexually. 2. a lack of mature emotional development.

infarct, a dying portion of tissue whose blood supply has been cut off by the presence of an obstruction, usually an embolus.

infarction, the formation and development of an infarct.

infect, to contaminate with disease-producing germs.

infection, 1. the penetration of body tissue by disease-producing organisms. 2. the area affected by the injurious organisms.

infectious, 1. causing or carrying infection. 2. communicable by infection, as diseases. 3. contagious.

infectious hepatitis, an acute liver inflammation caused by a virus and marked by jaundice, nausea, and abdominal pain.

infectious mononucleosis, an acute, contagious viral disease in which fever and sore throat occur, the lymph nodes enlarge, and mononuclear white blood cells increase abnormally in number.

infecund, unfruitful; barren.

inferior, beneath; lower.

inferiority complex, a condition in which extreme feelings of inferiority, often derived from childhood frustrations, manifest themselves either in the form of aggression or withdrawal and reticence.

infertile, not fruitful or productive; sterile; barren.

infirm, feeble or weak in body or health, esp. from age.

infirmary, a small hospital or dispensary for the care of the sick, injured, or infirm, usually in a school or institution.

infirmity, 1. the state of being infirm; feebleness. 2. debility. 3. a physical or moral malady. 4. a defect or flaw.

inflame, 1. to excite violent passion, feeling, or emo-

tion. 2. to produce inflammation in. 3. to cause swelling, fever, or soreness in.

inflammation, 1. the act of inflaming. 2. a redness and swelling of any part of the body, attended by heat and pain.

inflammatory, tending to cause inflammation, usually accompanied by heat.

influenza, an acute, infectious, and highly contagious disease affecting the respiratory tract, producing symptoms not unlike a severe cold, and caused by viruses; it is frequently epidemic.

influenzal, pertaining to influenza.

infra-axillary, below the armpit.

infraclavicular, below the collarbone.

infracostal, below a rib.

infraction, the incomplete fracture of a bone.

inframammary, below the mammary gland.

infraorbital, below the eye socket.

infrapubic, below the pubis.

infrared, below the red, as the invisible rays of the spectrum lying outside the red end of the visible spectrum.

infrascapular, below the shoulder blade.

infrasternal, below the breastbone.

infundibular, having the form of a funnel.

infundibulum, 1. the funnel-shaped portion of the third ventricle in the brain leading to the pituitary gland. 2. an area in the right ventricle where the pulmonary artery arises. 3. cone-shaped areas in the lungs where the bronchial tubes end. 4. the funnel-shaped opening of a fallopian tube.

infusion, the introduction of a saline or other solution into a vein.

ingest, to put or take into the body, as food.

ingesta, substances ingested.

ingrowing, 1. growing within or inward. 2. growing into the flesh, as a nail.

inguinal, pertaining to or located in the groin.

inhalant, an apparatus or a medicine used for inhaling, as, a nasal inhalant.

inhalation, the act of breathing medicated vapors or gas into nose and lungs.

inhalator, a device used to aid breathing, or to administer a medicine in vapor form.

inhale, to breathe in; to draw in by or as by breathing, as, to inhale air.

inhaler, see **respirator.**

inherit, to derive or acquire, as traits or characteristics, through heredity.

inheritance, traits of one's ancestors genetically transmitted.

inhibit, to restrain; to hinder; to check; to stop or repress.

inhibition, a process that checks or restrains an impulse involving actions

or thoughts.

inhibitor, 1. anything that inhibits. 2. a substance that slows, interferes with, or stops a chemical reaction.

inject, to force fluid into a passage, cavity, or tissue, as, to inject a drug into the body with a syringe.

injection, 1. the act of injecting. 2. a liquid injected into the body, as for medicinal purposes. 3. a shot.

injector, one who or that which injects.

inner-directed, of or referring to a person whose reactions are guided by his own value system rather than by external norms.

innervate, 1. to supply with nerves. 2. to communicate nervous energy to. 3. to stimulate through nerves.

innervation, 1. the communicating of nervous energy by means of nerves. 2. the stimulation of some part or organ through its nerves. 3. the disposition of nerves in a body or some part of it.

innerve, 1. to supply with nervous energy. 2. to invigorate. 3. to animate.

innominate artery, the right artery arising from the arch of the aorta.

innominate bone, either of the two bony masses consisting of the fused iliac, ischial, and pubic bones that make up the sides of the pelvis.

innominate veins, the right and left vein that join to

form the superior vena cava.

inoculant, see **inoculum.**

inoculate, 1. to implant, as virus or bacteria, within a human body to cause a mild disease and thus confer immunity from that disease. 2. to introduce, as microorganisms, into surroundings suitable to their growth, esp. in living organisms. 3. to perform inoculation.

inoculation, 1. the act of inoculating. 2. the injection, esp. of serum.

inoculator, one who or that which inoculates.

inoculum, the prepared material for injections, usually composed of bacteria or viruses.

inoperable, unsuitable for surgical operation, as, an inoperable tumor.

inquest, 1. a postmortem investigation made by a coroner. 2. persons holding such an investigation, esp. a coroner's jury. 3. their final verdict.

insane, 1. not sane or of sound mind. 2. mentally deranged. 3. mad.

insane asylum, a place where mentally deranged persons are confined and treated.

insanitariness, 1. want of sanitation or sanitary regulation. 2. unhygienic condition.

insanitary, 1. not hygienic. 2. unclean. 3. injurious to health.

insanity, 1. the condition of being insane. 2. more or less permanent derangement of one or

more psychical functions.

inseminate, see **impregnate.**

insemination, see **impregnation.**

insensibility, the state of being insensible.

insensible, 1. unconscious; numb to pain. 2. unable to perceive or understand. 3. not susceptible to emotion or passion.

insensitive, without physical sensation or feeling.

insensitivity, the state of being insensitive.

insentient, 1. lacking sensation or feeling. 2. inanimate.

insertion, the manner or place of attachment, as of an organ or muscle.

insidious, operating or proceeding inconspicuously but with grave effect, as, insidious poison or insidious disease.

in situ, in a given or original position.

insobriety, intemperance; drunkenness.

insomnia, inability to sleep, esp. when chronic.

insomniac, one who suffers from insomnia.

inspiration, 1. breathing in. 2. a prompting, esp. to creative action, that arises within the mind.

inspiratory, 1. referring to or assisting in inhalation. 2. pertaining to inspiration.

inspire, 1. to draw into the lungs. 2. to breathe or inhale. 3. to communicate inspiration.

inspissate, to make thick by evaporation.

inspissation, the process

of making dry by evaporation.

instep, the arched part of the upper side of the foot.

instinct, an innate, automatic impulse in humans and animals to satisfy basic biological needs, leading to behavior that is purposeful and directive.

instinctive, spontaneous; unlearned.

instinctual, 1. pertaining to or of the nature of instinct. 2. prompted by or resulting from instinct.

insufflate, 1. to blow, as air or medicinal substances into an opening or cavity or upon a part of the body. 2. to treat by insufflation.

insufflation, the act of insufflating.

insufflator, an apparatus used for insufflation.

insulin, 1. a hormone secreted by the islets of Langerhans in the pancreas, essential to the regulation of carbohydrate metabolism. 2. a preparation of this hormone used in the treatment of diabetes.

insulinemia, presence of an abnormally large percentage of insulin in the blood.

insulin shock, an abnormal condition, likely to cause collapse, which occurs when an overdose of insulin causes a sudden reduction of sugar in the blood.

insuloma, a tumor of the islets of Langerhans in the pancreas.

insusceptibility, see **immunity.**

integument, a covering, as the skin of the body.

integumentary, pertaining to the skin.

intellect, mental capacity to comprehend ideas and relationships and to exercise judgment.

intellection, the act of understanding.

intellective, pertaining to the intellect.

intellectual, relating to the intellect in the exercise of mental faculties; engaged in creative thinking.

intellectualize, to make rational; to regard intellectually.

intelligence, the faculty or ability for comprehending and reasoning with facts, truths, or propositions.

intelligence quotient (I.Q.), a technique for stating a person's general intelligence, reached by dividing his mental age, as determined through intelligence tests, by his chronological age, then multiplying by 100.

intelligence test, one or more standardized graded tests, aimed at measuring an individual's general intelligence or mental ability.

intelligent, having the faculty of understanding and reasoning.

interarticular, between two joints.

interatrial, between the atria of the heart.

interauricular, between the auricles.

interbrain, see **diencepha-**

lon.

intercellular, lying between cells.

interchondral, between cartilages.

interclavicular, between the clavicles.

intercostal, between the ribs.

intercourse, sexual union; copulation.

intercranial, pertaining to the inner part of the skull.

intercurrent, referring to a disease that occurs during the course of another disease.

interdental, between the teeth.

interdigital, between the fingers or toes.

interdigitate, to interlock, as the fingers of both hands.

intermammary, between the breasts.

intermenstrual, between menstrual periods.

intermittent fever, see malaria; undulant fever.

intermittent pulse, a pulse in which a beat is dropped at intervals.

intern, a recent medical graduate acting as assistant in a hospital for the purpose of clinical training.

internal medicine, the branch of medicine concerned with the diagnosis and treatment of nonsurgical diseases.

internist, 1. a physician who treats internal diseases. 2. a specialist in internal medicine.

internuncial, serving as a link between nerve fibers of the brain or spinal cord.

interosseous, between two bones.

interosseus, a muscle lying between bones.

interpalpebral, between the eyelids.

intersexual, 1. occurring between the sexes. 2. having sexual traits intermediate between the two sexes.

interstice, a small opening, hole, or space in a tissue, a series of tissues, or an organ.

interstitial, 1. pertaining to, situated in, or forming interstices. 2. situated between the cellular elements of a structure or part.

interventricular, between two ventricles.

intervertebral, between two (adjacent) vertebrae.

intestinal, of or relating to the intestine.

intestinal juice, the liquid substances secreted into the intestine.

intestine, the lower part of the alimentary canal, extending from the pylorus to the anus. See large intestine, small intestine.

intima, the innermost membrane, coat, or lining of an organ or part, esp. of an artery, a vein, or a lymphatic vessel.

intimal, of or pertaining to the intima.

intolerance, incapacity for bearing, or inability to endure, pain or the effects of a drug or other substance.

intoxicant, that which intoxicates.

intoxicate, to inebriate; to

make drunk.

intoxication, the state of being intoxicated.

intra-abdominal, within the abdomen.

intra-arterial, within the arteries.

intra-articular, within a joint.

intra-atrial, within an atrium.

intra-aural, within the ear.

intracellular, occurring within a cell.

intracranial, within the skull.

intractable, difficult to treat or cure, as illness.

intracutaneous, see **intradermal.**

intracutaneous test, a test for allergic sensitivity made by injecting a diluted antigen into the skin.

intradermal, within the skin or between the layers of the skin, as an injection.

intradural, within the dura mater.

intraglandular, within a gland.

intra-intestinal, within the intestine.

intramammary, within the breast.

intramembranous, within a membrane.

intramolecular, occurring or existing within the molecule.

intramural, within the substance of a wall, as of an organ or cavity of the body.

intramuscular, occurring within, or affecting the interior of a muscle.

intranasal, within the nasal cavity.

intraneural, within a nerve.

intra-ocular, within the eyeball.

intra-oral, within the mouth.

intra-orbital, within the eye socket.

intraosteal, within a bone.

intrapleural, within the pleural cavity.

intrapsychic, arising or occurring within the psyche, mind, or self, as conflicting motives within the same person.

intrathoracic, within the thorax.

intrauterine, occurring or situated within the uterus.

intrauterine device (IUD), a means of continuous contraception placed within the uterus, as a plastic coil.

intravaginal, within the vagina.

intravenous, occurring or introduced within a vein or veins, esp. by means of injection, as, intravenous feeding.

intraventricular, within a ventricle.

intravitam, 1. happening during life. 2. used upon a living subject, as a stain that will not kill living cells.

intrinsic, 1. inherent; essential; belonging to the thing in itself. 2. belonging entirely to or being within a given bodily part, as certain muscles.

intrinsic factor, an element of normal gastric and intestinal mucous membranes or mucosae, essential to the absorption of vitamin B_{12} by the body.

introitus, any opening or

entrance into a canal or cavity.

introject, to incorporate (external influences and esp. the characteristics of other individuals) into one's own pattern of behavior.

introspect, to look into or examine, as one's own feelings or thoughts.

introspection, the observation or examination of one's own mental states or processes.

introversion, 1. the act of introverting. 2. an introverted state. 3. concern and interest directed inward toward oneself, rather than toward the external world.

introvert, one characterized by introversion; broadly, one who is shy or reserved.

intubate, to insert a tube into (a hollow organ or orifice), as into the larynx to aid breathing.

intubation, the process of intubating.

intumesce, to swell; to enlarge or expand, as with heat.

intumescence, a swelling or the process of swelling.

intussuscept, to take within, as one part of the intestine into an adjacent part; invaginate.

intussusception, 1. the taking in of foreign matter, as nutriment, by a living organism and its conversion into living tissue. 2. the reception of one part into another, as when a part of the intestine is in-troduced into an adjacent part, usually causing obstruction.

intussuscipiens, the part of intestine that enters the intussusceptum to form an intussusception.

inunction, the rubbing in of an oil or ointment.

invaginate, 1. to insert or receive as into a sheath. 2. to fold or draw, as a tubular organ, back within itself.

invagination, intussusception, as of a portion of the intestine. 2. the drawing inward of a portion of the wall of a blastula in the formation of a gastrula.

invalid, impaired in health; sick or infirm.

invert, 1. to turn upside down. 2. to invaginate or turn inside out. 3. to put in reverse order or position. 4. one that is inverted or affected by inversion. 5. a homosexual.

invertase, an enzyme, found in some plants and in an animal's digestive tract, which causes the inversion of cane sugar into two simple sugars, glucose and fructose.

invertebrate, of or pertaining to animals without a vertebral column.

in vitro, occurring outside a living organism and in an artificial environment, as tissues cultivated in a test tube.

in vivo, occurring within a living organism.

involuntary, operating or acting independently of will or conscious control.

involuntary   muscle,

smooth muscle, which acts not under the control of the conscious will, as the muscles of the heart, intestines, bladder, etc.

involution, 1. a retrograde change, as the return of an organ to its normal size after enlargement. 2. degeneration. 3. the bodily changes and loss of vigor associated with aging. 4. in embryology, the inward turning of cells to form a gastrula.

iodate, to combine, impregnate, or treat with iodine.

iodide, a compound of iodine with an element or radical; a salt of hydriodic acid, as, hydrogen iodide.

iodine, a nonmetallic element occurring, at ordinary temperatures, as a grayish-black crystalline solid, which changes to a dense violet vapor when heated; used in medicine and photography.

iodism, poisoning from the use of iodine or its compounds.

iodize, to treat or impregnate with iodine.

iodoform, a yellowish crystalline compound, resembling chloroform and used as an antiseptic.

iodol, a crystalline compound containing iodine and used as an antiseptic.

iodopsin, visual violet pigment occurring in retinal cones and important to daylight vision.

ipecac, the dried root of the ipecac shrub of tropical South America. The al-

kaloid obtained from the root is used as an emetic and expectorant.

I.Q. see **intelligence quotient.**

iridemia, bleeding from the iris.

iridotomy, surgical incision of the iris without excising any part of it.

iris, the contractile circular diaphragm forming the colored portion of the eye and containing the pupil in its center.

iritis, inflammation of the iris.

iron, a metallic element widely distributed in nature and important in the diet for prevention of certain forms of anemia.

iron lung, a sealed chamber placed over or around the chest of a patient, which forces respiration by rhythmic changes in air pressure, thus acting as a substitute for normal lung action.

irradiate, 1. to penetrate by radiation. 2. to treat or heal by radiation.

irradiation, the act of irradiating; the condition of being irradiated.

irrational, 1. void of reason. 2. absurd. 3. mentally unstable.

irrespirable, unfit for breathing.

irritability, 1. the state of being irritable. 2. the attribute of organisms and protoplasm to become aroused to distinctive action following a certain stimulus.

irritable, 1. susceptible to,

responding to, or being acted upon by stimuli. 2. subject to excessive reaction or inflammation following certain stimuli or irritants. 3. readily provoked or exasperated; of a fiery temper.

irritant, 1. causing irritation. 2. anything that irritates. 3. something producing irritation, as a poison or chemical agent.

irritate, 1. to excite, as a bodily part, to a particular function. 2. to excite anger in; to provoke; to vex; to inflame.

irritation, a condition of inflammation or unusual sensitivity in a bodily part.

irritative, serving to excite or irritate; produced by an irritant or irritation.

ischemia, localized anemia of tissue, often caused by a blood vessel that contracts, thus restricting arterial inflow.

ischial, relating to the ischium.

ischium, the posterior and inferior part of the pelvic arch at the hip joint.

islets of Langerhans, clusters of endocrine cells, scattered through the tissues of the pancreas, which secretes insulin; also called islands of Langerhans.

isoagglutination, the clumping or grouping of red blood cells that occurs when one animal receives a transfusion from another animal of a like species.

isoagglutinin, an antibody or clotting agent from one

organism that is effective in the cells of other individuals of the same species.

isogamete, a sex cell, or gamete, that cannot be distinguished from a similar gamete with which it pairs and is capable of uniting to form a zygote.

isogamous, having two similar gametes in which no differentiation of sex, size, or structure can be distinguished, and reproducing by the union of such gametes.

isoleucine, an amino acid, considered essential in the diet of humans and animals.

isomer, a compound or nuclide isomeric with one or more other compounds.

isomeric, of compounds or nuclides composed of the same elements in the same proportions by weight and having the same molecular weight, but differing in one or more properties as a result of different spatial arrangements of the atom within the molecule.

isomerism, the fact or condition of being isomeric.

isometric, pertaining to or having equality of measure.

isometric exercise, physical exertion that does not involve motion, muscle tone being achieved by setting one muscle against another muscle.

isometropia, a condition in which the refraction is the same in the two eyes.

isotherm, a line on a chart or map passing through places having a corresponding temperature at any particular time.

isothermal, having equal temperature.

isotonia, of equal tone.

isotonic, 1. noting or pertaining to a solution containing just enough salt to prevent the destruction of the red corpuscles when added to the blood. 2. noting or pertaining to a contraction of a muscle when under a constant tension.

isotope, any of two or more forms of the same element having the same atomic number and nearly the same chemical properties but of different atomic weight.

isotropic, 1. having the same properties in all directions, as elasticity or conduction. 2. lacking well-defined axes.

isthmus, a connecting part, organ, or passage joining structures or cavities larger than itself, as, the isthmus of the fauces.

itch, 1. to have or feel a peculiar irritation of the skin that causes the desire to scratch the part affected. 2. to cause such an irritation. 3. see **scabies.**

jactitation, severe restless tossing of the body in disease.

jaundice, an abnormal physical condition caused by bile pigments in the blood, characterized by yellowness of the skin and sclera of the eye, and by lassitude and loss of appetite.

jaw, one of the two bones or structures, upper and lower, that form the framework of the mouth.

jawbone, a bone of the jaw, esp. the lower jaw or mandible.

jejunal, of or pertaining to the jejunum.

jejune, lacking in nutritive or substantial qualities.

jejunectomy, surgical excision of part or all of the jejunum.

jejunitis, inflammation of the jejunum.

jejunocolostomy, surgical creation of an artificial passage between the jejunum and the colon.

jejunoileitis, a condition in which both the jejunum and the ileum are inflamed.

jejunoileostomy, the joining of the jejunum and the ileum by surgery and removal of the diseased part of the intestine between them.

jejunojejunostomy, a surgical operation in which a diseased part of the jejunum is excised and the cut ends are rejoined.

jejunotomy, surgical incision of the jejunum to remove a foreign body swallowed by the patient.

jejunum, the portion of the small intestine between the duodenum and the ileum.

jerk, 1. a reaction or a reflex to a stimulus. 2. a tic.

joint, 1. the joining of two or

more bones, as in the elbow. 2. a junction connecting two body segments.

jugal, of or pertaining to the bony arch of the cheek.

jugular, of or pertaining to the throat or neck.

jugular veins, the two large veins of the neck that return blood from the neck, face, and brain to the heart.

jugulate, to check or suppress, as disease and the like, by extreme measures, as a tracheotomy.

juice, a natural body fluid, as digestive juices, etc.

julep, a sweetened drink serving as a vehicle for medicine.

Kahn's test, a blood test to detect syphilis.

kainophobia, a pathological fear of new situations and things.

kaolin, a mineral clay that remains white after firing, used as a coating for pills and a component of ointments, lotions, and poultices.

karyogenesis, formation and development of a cell nucleus.

karyokinesis, see **mitosis**.

karyokinetic, of or pertaining to karyokinesis.

karyolymph, the transparent substance that surrounds the nucleus of a cell.

karyoplasm, the substance of the nucleus of a cell.

karyosome, a chromatin mass in the nucleus of a cell.

karyotype, the total characteristics of a cell's nucleus, esp. its size, form, and chromosome number.

katabolism, see **catabolism**.

katharsis, see **catharsis**.

katzenjammer, 1. indisposition following intoxication. 2. a feeling of worry, uneasiness, or nervousness.

keloid, a fibrous growth originating in the connective skin tissue.

Kenny method, a procedure for the treatment of poliomyelitis involving both hot applications and exercise.

kenophobia, pathological fear of empty spaces.

keratalgia, neuralgic pain in the cornea.

keratectasia, protrusion of the cornea of the eye.

keratectomy, surgical excision of part of the cornea.

keratiasis, multiple horny wart formation on the skin.

keratin, an insoluble albumoid, containing sulfur, present in horns, hair, and nails.

keratinous, relating to keratin.

keratitic, pertaining to keratitis.

keratitis, inflammation of the cornea.

keratoconjunctivitis, inflammation of the cornea and the conjuctival membrane.

keratoderma, the horny layer of the skin.

keratodermatitis, inflammation of the horny layer of the skin.

keratodermatosis, any skin disease characterized by thickening of the skin.

keratodermia, a thickening of the horny layer of the epidermis, esp. on the palms and soles of the feet.

keratoma, a horny tumor; a callosity.

keratome, a surgical knife used to make an incision into the cornea.

keratometer, an instrument to measure the curvature of the cornea.

keratoplasty, the operation by which damaged corneal tissue is replaced by healthy tissue.

keratosis, a growth of horny tissue on the skin.

keratotomy, a surgical incision of the cornea.

kernicterus, a form of jaundice occurring in infants. It is the most dangerous form of childhood jaundice, as it can cause degeneration of parts of the brain.

keto-, pertaining to or containing a ketone.

ketogenesis, the production within the body of ketone bodies, esp. in diabetes.

ketogenetic, pertaining to ketogenesis.

ketol, an organic compound including both an alcohol and a ketone group.

ketone, any of a class of organic compounds, as acetone, each consisting of a carbonyl group united to one bivalent or two monovalent hydrocarbon radicals, and often used as solvents.

ketone body, 1. an acetone body. 2. any acetone, beta-hydroxybutyric acid, or acetoacetic acid present in the blood or urine, esp. of the diabetic.

ketose, a monosaccharide having a ketone group.

ketosis, an abnormal accumulation of ketones in the body.

kidney, either of a pair of glandular organs, about four inches in length, in the back part of the abdominal cavity, which excrete urine.

kinaesthesia, see **kinesthesia.**

kinase, a substance capable of changing a zymogen into an enzyme.

kinesia, motion sickness, as seasickness, car sickness, etc.

kinesialgia, discomfort or pain caused by muscular movement.

kinesics, a study of the relationship between nonverbal body motion, as a shrug, and communication.

kinesiology, the science that investigates anatomy and organic processes in reference to human motion.

kinesioneurosis, a functional disorder characterized by tics and spasms.

king's evil, see **scrofula.**

kleptomania, an irresistible impulse to steal, usually

for no economic reason.

kleptomaniac, one affected with kleptomania.

klieg eyes, watering and inflammation of the eyes caused by immoderate exposure to very bright lights.

knee, the joint or region between the thigh and the lower part of the leg.

kneecap, the movable bone covering the knee joint in front; the patella.

knee jerk, a sudden reflex or involuntary kick of the knee caused by a blow on the patellar tendon.

knock-knee, 1. inward curvature of the legs, causing the knees to knock together in walking. 2. knees that knock together in this way.

knucklebone, 1. a bone forming the knuckle of the finger. 2. the rounded end of the fingerbone at a joint.

knuckle joint, a joint forming a knuckle.

knuckles, 1. joints of the fingers, esp. the joints at the roots of the fingers. 2. the rounded prominences of such joints when the fingers are bent.

kraurosis, a dry, atrophied condition of the skin and mucous membranes.

kraurosis vulvae, a dry condition of the membranes of the vulva.

kymograph, an instrument for graphically recording variations in motion or pressure, esp. blood pressure.

kyphoscoliosis, a curva-

ture of the spine sideways and backwards.

kyphosis, an abnormal backward curving of the spine; hunchback.

kyphotic, hunchbacked.

kysthitis, inflammation of the vagina.

labdanum, a resin obtained from rockroses and used in medicine, perfumes, and fumigants.

labia, the lips or liplike parts.

labial, pertaining to the lips.

labia majora, the two folds of hair-bearing tissue situated on each side of the opening of the vagina.

labia minora, the two thin folds of mucous membrane lying within the labia majora on each side of the opening of the vagina.

labiate, having a labium or labia; lipped.

labile, 1. apt to lapse or change; unstable. 2. pertaining to a mode of application in electrotherapy in which the active electrode is moved over the part to be acted upon.

labium, see **lip.**

labor, the process of childbirth.

labyrinth, the inner ear, including the bony and fluid-filled structures.

labyrinthectomy, surgical excision of the labyrinth.

labyrinthine, pertaining to or like a labyrinth; winding; intricate.

labyrinthine vertigo, dizziness associated with

disorders of the labyrinth.

labyrinthitis, inflammation of the labyrinth.

lacerate, to make a ragged wound or gash by tearing.

laceration, 1. an act of tearing. 2. a jagged wound or tear caused by lacerating.

lacrima, see **tear.**

lacrimal, 1. pertaining to or characterized by tears, as a lacrimal mood. 2. of, relating to, or near organs that produce tears, as, the lacrimal bone.

lacrimal abscess, an abscess in a tear duct or gland.

lacrimal gland, a gland that secretes and produces tears.

lacrimation, secretion and discharge of tears.

lacrimator, an irritant that causes the secretion of tears.

lacrimose, given to crying; tearful; tending to provoke tears.

lactagogue, a substance that stimulates the secretion of milk from the breasts.

lactalbumin, a protein belonging to the albumin class, found in milk.

lactate, to produce or secrete milk.

lactation, 1. the production of milk. 2. the time period of milk production. 3. the act of nursing or suckling young.

lactational, relating to lactation.

lacteal, relating to, producing, or resembling milk; milky.

lactean, one of numerous minute lymphatic vessels that absorb or take up lymph from the alimentary canal and convey it to the thoracic duct.

lactescent, 1. becoming or being milky. 2. producing milk. 3. concerned with the secretion of milk.

lactic, pertaining to or produced from milk.

lactic acid, a syruplike acid, present naturally in sour milk, produced commercially by synthesis or bacterial fermentation of carbohydrates, and utilized in food processing, medicine, and industry.

lactiferous, producing or conveying milk or a milky liquid.

lactiferous ducts, the ducts of the mammary glands that lead to the tip of the nipple.

lactifuge, any agent used to stop milk secretion in the mammary glands.

lactin, see **lactose.**

lactobacillus, any of the rod-shaped bacteria that produce lactic acid in the fermentation of milk and carbohydrates.

lactogenic, causing lactation.

lactose, a sugar obtained from milk, a white, odorless, disaccharide used as a sweetening agent in baby foods and other foods.

lactosuria, the presence of milk sugar in the urine.

lacuna, one of the numerous minute cavities in the substance of bone.

lacus lacrimalis, the inner

corner of the eye where tears collect.

ladanum, see **labdanum.**

lagnesis, see **nymphomania.**

lagophthalmos, inability to close the eyelids completely.

lallation, 1. a babbling form of speech. 2. the use of the letter "l" instead of "r."

lallopathology, the branch of science concerned with speech defects and their treatment.

lallopathy, any disorder affecting the speech.

lamina, a flat, thin plate, or sheet, as of bone, or a thin membrane.

laminectomy, surgical excision of the posterior arch of a vertebra.

laminitis, inflammation of a lamina.

lance, to make an incision with a lancet.

lancet, a small surgical instrument used in opening veins, tumors, or abscesses.

Langerhans's islets, see **islets of Langerhans.**

lanolin, an oily or greasy substance obtained from unwashed wool, said to be beneficial in skin ointments or lotions.

lanuginose, downy; covered with down or fine soft hair.

lanugo, woolly or downy growth, as the coat of delicate hairs covering the human fetus.

laparoenterostomy, surgical creation of an opening into the intestine through the abdominal wall.

laparotomy, surgical incision of the abdominal wall.

large intestine, the shorter and wider portion of the intestine, which prepares the feces for discharge by dehydrating the digestive residues, and which includes the cecum, colon, and rectum.

laryngalgia, neuralgic pain of the larynx.

laryngeal, pertaining to the larynx.

laryngectomy, surgical excision of the larynx.

laryngismus, spasm of the larynx.

laryngitic, pertaining to or resulting from laryngitis.

laryngitis, an inflammation of the larynx.

laryngograph, an apparatus for making a record of laryngeal movements.

laryngological, of or pertaining to laryngology.

laryngologist, one who specializes in laryngology.

laryngology, the study of the larynx and its diseases.

laryngoparalysis, paralysis of the muscles of the larynx.

laryngopharyngeal, pertaining to the larynx and the pharynx.

laryngopharyngitis, inflammation of the larynx and the pharynx.

laryngopharynx, the lower portion of the pharynx, which opens into the larynx and esophagus.

laryngoplasty, a surgical operation to repair a defect of the larynx.

laryngoscope, a reflecting instrument for examining the larynx.

laryngoscopy, the examination of the interior of the larynx with a laryngoscope.

laryngostomy, surgical operation to make a permanent opening through the throat into the larynx.

laryngotomy, surgical incision of the larynx.

laryngotracheotomy, surgical incision through both the upper portion of the trachea and the larynx to make an artificial airway through which the patient can breathe instead of through the mouth.

larynx, the cartilaginous structure at the upper end of the trachea that contains and supports the vocal cords and associated structures.

laser, a device for amplifying light radiation, in which a beam of light is shot through a crystal, causing it to emit an intense, direct light beam that is useful in micromachining and surgery.

lassitude, a feeling of weariness or weakness; listlessness of body or mind.

latent, present in a concealed form, but capable of becoming manifest, as, a latent homosexual.

latent content, the real or unconscious meaning of a dream.

latent period, the period in a disease between the moment of infection and appearance of symptoms. 2. the time between stimulation and reaction.

lateral, 1. of or pertaining to the side. 2. situated at, proceeding from, or directed toward a side, as a lateral move.

lateroflexion, bending to or curvature toward one side.

lateropulsion, the tendency to fall involuntarily to one side in cases of cerebellar and labyrinthine diseases.

lateroversion, a tendency to or a turning toward one side.

laudanum, tincture of opium.

laughing gas, see **nitrous oxide.**

lavage, the process of cleansing, as by injection, esp. the washing out of the stomach.

laxation, 1. a loosening or relaxation, or the state of being loosened or relaxed. 2. defecation.

laxative, a medicine that acts as a gentle purgative.

lead colic, severe abdominal pain caused by lead poisoning.

lead poisoning, 1. an acute, toxic condition found among persons, esp. children, whose tissues have absorbed lead. 2. a chronic condition among workers who are in contact with paint or other lead products.

lecithin, a fatty substance consisting of fatty acids, choline, phosphoric acid, and glycerol, found in the cells of plants and animals, and utilized in the drug, food, and cosmetic industries.

leech, 1. any of the blood-sucking or carnivorous, usually aquatic, worms, certain freshwater species of which were formerly used by physicians for bloodletting. 2. an instrument used for drawing blood.

leg, one of the members or limbs that support and move the body; specifically that part of the limb between the knee and the ankle.

leiomyoma, a tumor made up of nonstriated muscular tissue.

leiomyosarcoma, a malignant tumor containing smooth muscle tissue.

lenitive, 1. having the quality of softening or mitigating, as medicines; assuasive; emollient. 2. a soothing medicine or application.

lens, 1. a piece of transparent substance, usually glass, having two opposite surfaces, either both curved or one curved and one plane, used for changing the direction of light rays, as in magnifying or in correcting errors in vision. 2. a combination of such pieces. 3. the part of the eye that focuses light rays on the retina. See also **contact lens,** and **crystalline lens.**

lenticular, 1. having the form of a double-convex lens. 2. of or relating to a lens.

lentigo, 1. a freckle. 2. a

freckly condition.

leper, a person affected with leprosy.

leprosarium, a hospital or asylum for lepers.

leprose, pertaining to or resembling leprosy.

leprosy, an infectious, chronic disease caused by a microorganism and variously characterized by ulcerations, tubercular nodules, loss of fingers and toes, and anesthesia in certain nerve regions.

leprous, 1. affected with leprosy. 2. of or like leprosy.

leptomeninges, the two membranes that envelop the brain and spinal cord.

Leptospira, any of the thin-coiled, aerobic bacteria, some of which infect man.

leptospirosis, a condition resulting from Leptospira infection.

lesbian, a female homosexual.

lesbianism, female homosexuality.

lesion, an abnormal, localized change in the structure of an organ or tissue, resulting from disease or injury.

lethal, causing or able to cause death; deadly; mortal; fatal.

lethargic, 1. affected with lethargy. 2. inclined to sleep; dull; sluggish. 3. pertaining to lethargy.

lethargy, 1. unnatural sleepiness. 2. dullness; inaction; inattention; drowsiness. 3. profound sleep from which a person can scarcely be awakened.

leucaemia, see **leukemia.**

leucemia, see **leukemia.**

leucine, a white crystalline amino acid, formed in various ways, esp. by pancreatic digestion of proteins in the body.

leucocyte, see **leukocyte.**

leucocythaemia, see **leukemia.**

leucocytic, see **leukocytic.**

leucocytogenesis, see **leukocytogenesis.**

leucocytolysis, see **leukocytolysis.**

leucocytopenia, see **leukopenia.**

leucocytosis, see **leukocytosis.**

leucoderma, see **leukoderma.**

leucoma, see **leukoma.**

leucopenia, see **leukopenia.**

leucoplakia, see **leukoplakia.**

leucorrhoea, see **leukorrhea.**

leukemia, a fatal disease of the blood, in which there is a pronounced increase in the number of leukocytes; cancer of the blood.

leukemic, pertaining to leukemia.

leukocyte, a white blood corpuscle; a colorless blood cell active in the defense against infection and bacteria and occasionally found in the body tissues.

leukocythemia, see **leukemia.**

leukocytic, of or pertaining to leukocytes.

leukocytogenesis, leukocyte formation.

leukocytolysis, destruction of leukocytes.

leukocytopenia, see **leukopenia.**

leukocytosis, a temporary increase in the number of leukocytes in the blood, usually caused by an infection, and not indicative of leukemia.

leukoderma, a pigmentation deficiency of the skin, usually occurring in patches.

leukoma, a white opacity of the cornea of the eye.

leukopenia, an acute decrease of leukocytes in the blood.

leukopenic, pertaining to leukopenia.

leukoplakia, formation of white, smooth spots or patches, irregular in size and shape, on the mucous membrane of the cheek. The lesions are usually benign, but may become malignant.

leukorrhea, a whitish discharge from the vagina, usually resulting from congestion.

leukosis, any of several diseases affecting production of leukocytes.

levator, 1. a muscle that raises a part of the body. 2. a surgical instrument used to raise a depressed part of the skull.

levulose, fructose, a natural sugar found in honey and many fruits, used in foods, medicines, and preservatives.

libidinous, having a strong sexual desire; lustful.

libido, 1. the sexual instinct. 2. the instincts and drives that activate human action.

lichen, any of various eruptive skin diseases, resembling lichen in appearance.

lid, see **eyelid.**

lie in, to be confined in childbed.

lienteric, of or pertaining to lientery.

lientery, a type of diarrhea in which the food is discharged undigested.

ligament, a band of strong fibrous tissue connecting bones at a joint, or serving to hold in place and support body organs.

ligamentous, of the nature of or being part of a ligament.

ligate, 1. to bind, as with a ligature. 2. to tie, as a bleeding artery.

ligation, 1. the act of ligating or binding. 2. a bond. 3. ligature.

ligature, a thread, wire, or the like for tying blood vessels to prevent hemorrhage, or for removing tumors by strangulation. See also **suture.**

limb, one of the jointed appendages of the body, as an arm or leg.

limbo, a suspended state of mind, usually between alternatives.

limbus, a border or an edge of a part.

limen, the threshold, as of consciousness.

liminal, referring to or located at the limen, esp. pertaining to the lowest limit of perception.

lingua, the tongue or a part

that resembles the tongue.

lingual, of or pertaining to the tongue or a tongue-like part.

liniment, a liquid preparation, usually oily, for rubbing on or applying to the skin, as for sprains or bruises.

linin, the substance forming the netlike structure that connects the chromatin granules in the nucleus of a cell.

lint, a soft substance made by scraping linen, used for dressing wounds.

lip, either of two fleshy parts or folds forming the margins of the mouth and performing an important function in speech.

lipaemia, see **lipemia.**

lipase, an enzyme, occurring in the pancreas, liver, and certain seeds, which is capable of breaking down fats into fatty acids and glycerin.

lipemia, an abnormal increase of the amount of fat in the blood.

lipid, any of a group of organic substances, including fats, sterols, and waxes, insoluble in water but able to be metabolized.

lipodystrophy, a defect or disturbance of fat metabolism.

lipoid, resembling fat.

lipoidal, a substance similar to fat, as wax.

lipolysis, the breaking down of fats into fatty acids and glycerin, as by the action of lipase.

lipolytic, of or pertaining to

lipolysis.

lipoma, a fatty tumor.

lipomatosis, the deposit of excessive amounts of fat in the tissues.

lipomatous, of or pertaining to lipoma.

lipoprotein, one of the class of proteins in combination with a lipid.

lipotropic, tending to promote the utilization of fat and thus prevent excessive fat deposits in the liver.

lipuria, fat in the urine.

liquefacient, a liquefying agent, as a drug that causes the liquefaction of solid deposits.

liquefaction, 1. the act of making liquid or the process of becoming liquid. 2. the state of being liquid or melted.

liquescent, 1. melting. 2. to become liquid or fluid.

liquor amnii, the amniotic fluid in which the fetus floats surrounded by the amniotic sac.

lithiasis, the formation of stony solids in any part of the body, as in the bladder.

lythic, of or pertaining to lithiasis or lithium.

lithium, a metallic element, soft and silver-white, the lightest metal known. Its various salts are used in the treatment of gout, rheumatism, and urinary disorders.

lithology, the science dealing with the treatment of calculi in the body.

lithotomy, the surgical operation of removing stones from the bladder.

lithotripsy, see **lithotrity.**

lithotrity, the surgical operation of crushing stones in the bladder into particles that can be voided.

lithuresis, passage of crushed calculi by urination.

liver, a large reddish-brown, glandular organ situated in the right-hand side of the abdominal cavity, divided by fissures into several lobes, which secretes bile and performs various metabolic functions.

livid, 1. black and blue, as bruised flesh. 2. discolored by contusion.

lividity, the condition of being livid.

lobar, of or pertaining to a lobe, as of the lungs.

lobate, having a lobe or lobes; lobed; sometimes, having the form of a lobe.

lobe, 1. a roundish projection or division, as of an organ. 2. the soft pendulous lower part of the external ear.

lobectomy, surgical excision of a lobe of any organ or gland.

lobitis, inflammation of a lobe.

lobotomy, a treatment for some psychotic disorders involving the severing of certain nerve fibers in the brain.

lobular, of, pertaining to, or resembling lobules.

lobule, 1. a small lobe, 2. a subdivision of a lobe.

lockjaw, a form of tetanus that causes the jaws to become locked together.

locomotor, 1. one who or

that which has locomotive power. 2. of or pertaining to locomotion.

locomotor ataxia, a disease of the spinal cord caused by syphilis, marked by intense pain, difficulty in coordination and walking, and eventually paralysis.

loculate, having, composed of, or divided into loculi or cells.

loculus, a small chamber, cavity, or cell.

logagnosia, a type of aphasia.

logaphasia, see **aphasia.**

logomania, abnormal, excessive talkativeness, occurring in certain psychotic states.

logorrhea, a condition marked by excessive and incoherent talkativeness.

loin, the part or parts of the body on either side of the vertebral column between the false ribs and the hipbone.

longsightedness, see **hypermetropia.**

lordosis, abnormal inward curvature of the spine.

lordotic, of or pertaining to lordosis.

loss of memory, see **amnesia.**

lucid, rational; sane; clear to the perception.

lues, see **syphilis.**

lumbago, rheumatism or rheumatic pains affecting the lumbar region of the back.

lumbar, 1. of or pertaining to the loin or loins. 2. a lumbar vertebra, artery, or the like.

lumbricalis, one of the

wormlike muscles of the hand or foot.

lumen, 1. a duct or canal in a tubular organ, as an artery. 2. the bore of a tube, as a catheter.

lunacy, see **insanity.**

lunar caustic, silver nitrate, a compound used in medicine, esp. as a cauterizing agent.

lunatic, 1. an insane person. 2. a zany character.

lung, either of the two saclike respiratory organs.

lunula, something in the shape of a crescent, as the white crescent at the base of a fingernail.

lupulin, a fine, yellow powder obtained from the fruits of hops, used in medicine as a sedative.

lupus, any of various diseases caused by the tubercle bacillus and resulting in lesions of the skin and mucous membranes.

luteal, of or concerning the corpus luteum.

lutein, 1. a yellowish or orange compound occurring in many plants and in egg yolk, animal fat, and corpora lutea, used in certain biochemical studies. 2. a hormone preparation from corpora lutea.

luteinize, 1. to cause the formation of corpora lutea. 2. to become changed into corpora lutea.

luteinizing hormone, a secretion of the pituitary gland that stimulates the activity of the reproductive organs.

luteoma, a tumor in the

ovaries containing lutein cells.

luxate, to put out of joint, as a limb; to dislocate.

luxation, a dislocation.

lying-in, confinement during and following childbirth.

lymph, 1. a clear, coagulable bodily fluid composed of plasma and white corpuscles and carried in the lymphatic system. 2. any of similar fluids emitted from inflamed areas.

lymphadenitis, inflammation of lymph nodes or glands.

lymphatic, pertaining to, containing, or conveying lymph.

lymph cell, a cell found in lymph; lymphocyte.

lymph gland, one of the numerous glandular masses of lymphatic tissue, scattered through the lymph system, which produces lymphocytes.

lymph node, see **lymph gland.**

lymphoblast, an immature cell that becomes a lymphocyte.

lymphocyte, a leukocyte, one of the white blood corpuscles that develops in the lymphatic tissues.

lymphocytic, of or pertaining to a lymphocyte.

lymphocytoma, a malignant tumor composed of lymphocytes.

lymphocytosis, a condition of the blood involving an excessive number of lymphocytes.

lymphogranulomata, 1. inflammation of a lymph node. 2. a venereal dis-

ease marked by swollen lymphatic tissue.

lymphoid, resembling lymph, lymphatic cells, or lymphatic tissue.

lymphoma, a tumor found in lymphoid tissue.

lymphopoiesis, the formation of lymphoid tissue.

lymphosarcoma, a malignant tumor of lymphatic tissue.

lyse, to cause the dissolution of cells by lysins.

lysergic acid, an acidic crystalline solid, an ergot derivative and the base of LSD.

lysin, any of a class of substances acting as antibodies and capable of causing the dissolution or destruction of bacteria, blood corpuscles, and other cellular elements.

lysine, a basic amino acid, necessary to nutrition.

lysis, 1. the gradual recession of a disease. 2. the dissolution or destruction of cells by lysins.

Lysol, a disinfectant and antiseptic containing phenol derivatives saponified for solubility in water (trademark).

lysozyme, an enzyme capable of disintegrating bacteria, found in the latex of some plants, in tears and mucus, and in leukocytes.

-lytic, pertaining to or producing lysis.

macerate, 1. to soften or separate the parts of, as a substance, by steeping in a liquid, with or without heat. 2. to steep in order to extract soluble constituents. 3. to soften or break up, as food, by the digestive process. 4. to cause to grow lean or to waste away.

maceration, the process of macerating.

macrocardius, abnormal enlargement of the heart.

macrocephalic, having a abnormally large head or cranial capacity.

macrocephaly, the condition of having an abnormally large head.

macrocyte, a red blood cell that is abnormally large.

macrocytic, of or pertaining to a macrocyte.

macrocytosis, the condition of having macrocytes.

macrogamete, the larger of two gametes in conjugation, usually the female reproductive cell.

macroscopic, visible to the naked eye, as opposed to **microscopic,**

macroscopy, the examination of objects with the naked eye.

macula, a spot or stain, esp. a discolored spot on the skin.

macular, of or pertaining to macula.

maculate, 1. to mark with a spot or spots. 2. to stain. 3. to pollute.

maculation, 1. a spotting or spotted condition. 2. a marking of spots, as on an animal or plant. 3. a disfiguring spot or stain.

macule, see **macula.**

mad, 1. insane; mentally deranged. 2. foolish or imprudent. 3. affected with or characterized by wild excitement.

maidenhead, see **hymen.**

mal, a disease, an evil, a sickness.

mala, see **cheek** and **cheekbone.**

malacia, abnormal softening of tissues.

maladjustment, a lack of harmony between a person's desires or capacities and his external situation.

malady, any disease or ailment of the human body.

malaise, 1. a condition of unlocalized bodily uneasiness, debility, or discomfort, often a preliminary symptom of disease. 2. an indefinite feeling of morbid discontent and ill-being.

malar, pertaining to the cheek or cheekbone.

malar bone, see **cheekbone.**

malaria, a febrile disease, usually intermittent or remittent, and characterized by attacks of chills, fever, and sweating, caused by parasitic protozoans, transferred to the blood by mosquitoes.

malarial, of or pertaining to malaria.

mal de Cayenne, see **elephantiasis.**

mal de mer, see **seasickness.**

malformation, abnormal structure, esp. of a bodily part.

malignancy, the quality or condition of being malignant, as, a tumor that is malignant.

malignant, 1. increasing in danger and size, as a tumor. 2. not benign. 3. virulent, 4. tending to cause death.

malinger, to feign illness in order to avoid duty or work.

malingerer, a person who malingers.

malleal, of or pertaining to the malleus.

malleolar, pertaining to a malleolus.

malleolus, the protuberance on each side of the ankle joint.

malleus, the outermost of three small bones in the middle ear, so called from its hammerlike shape.

malnutrition, insufficient or otherwise faulty nutrition.

malocclusion, 1. faulty occlusion. 2. imperfect closing or meeting, as of the opposing teeth of the upper and lower jaws.

malodor, an offensive odor; stench.

malodorous, having an offensive odor; foul-smelling.

Malpighian body, a nodule of lymphoid tissue in the spleen.

Malpighian corpuscle, a small round body in the cortical substance of the kidney.

Malpighian layer, a layer of cells lying deep within the epidermis, which provides replacements for the outer cells of the epidermis.

malposition, faulty or wrong position, esp. of a

part or organ of the body or of a fetus in the uterus.

malpractice, improper, neglectful, or illegal performance of duty by one in a public or professional position, as a physician, lawyer, or public servant, esp. when resulting in injury or loss.

malpresentation, abnormal position of the baby during childbirth that makes delivery difficult or impossible.

Malta fever, see **brucellosis.**

maltase, an enzyme that transforms maltose into glucose by hydrolysis.

maltose, a white crystalline sugar, formed by the action of diastase, as in malt, on starch and used primarily as a sweetener.

mamma, the breast; the organ that secretes milk.

mammalgia, pain in the mamma.

mammary, referring to or resembling a mamma or the mammae.

mammectomy, see **mastectomy.**

mammilla, 1. the nipple of the breast. 2. any nipplelike process or protuberance.

mammillary, 1. pertaining to or resembling a nipple. 2. studded with nipplelike protuberances.

mammillate, 1. formed like a nipple. 2. having small nipplelike protuberances.

mammogram, an X-ray photograph of the breast or mammary glands.

mammography, study of the breast or mammary

glands by X-ray photography to diagnose cancer.

mammotomy, surgery on a breast.

mandible, the lower jawbone.

mandibular, noting or pertaining to a mandible.

mandragora, see **mandrake.**

mandrake, a plant of the European nightshade family that has strong sedative and narcotic properties.

mange, any of various skin diseases affecting animals and sometimes man, characterized by loss of hair and by scabby eruptions, and usually caused by parasitic mites.

mania, 1. intense excitement or enthusiasm. 2. a vehement passion or desire. 3. a rage or craze. 4. a form of insanity characterized by great excitement, with or without delusions, and by violence in its acute stage.

maniac, 1. a raving or wildly insane person. 2. a lunatic. 3. raving with insanity. 4. mad.

manic, of or pertaining to mania.

manic-depressive, 1. pertaining to a mental disorder characterized by marked emotional shifts from great excitement and high spirits to deep depression. 2. one afflicted with this disorder.

manifestation, the appearance of signs or symptoms of a disorder

or disease that make diagnosis possible.

manifest content, the happenings or images taking place within a dream.

manubrium, 1. a handle-shaped cell or bone. 2. the upper segment of the sternum or the handle-shaped section of the malleus.

manus, see **hand.**

marasmus, a wasting of flesh without fever or apparent disease, esp. in infants.

marijuana, see **cannabis.**

marrow, the tissue, of soft and vascular structure, present in bone cavities.

marsh fever, see **malaria.**

masculinize, to cause male secondary sex characteristics to develop, as in a female.

masochism, 1. a form of sexual perversion in which the victim takes pleasure in physical abuse. 2. propensity to derive pleasure from emotional or physical pain. 3. pathological self-destruction.

masochist, a person practicing masochism.

masochistic, of or pertaining to masochism.

massage, the act or art of treating the body by rubbing or kneading to stimulate circulation or increase suppleness.

massaging, to treat by massage.

masseter, the thick muscle that raises the lower jaw, thus assisting chewing.

masseur, a man who practices massage.

masseuse, a woman who practices massage.

mastadenitis, inflammation of breast tissue or a mammary gland.

mastadenoma, a benign tumor of the breast.

mastalgia, pain in the breast.

mastectomy, the surgical removal of a breast.

masticate, 1. to grind with the teeth in preparation for swallowing. 2. to chew.

mastication, the act of chewing.

masticatory, 1. of, pertaining to, or used in mastication. 2. a medicinal substance chewed to promote the secretion of saliva.

mastitis, inflammation of the breast.

mastodynia, pain in the breast.

mastoid, of or denoting the process or projection of the temporal bone behind the ear and parts connected with it.

mastoidal, of or pertaining to the mastoid.

mastoidalgia, pain in the mastoid region.

mastoidectomy, the surgical removal of mastoid cells or part of the mastoid process.

mastoiditis, inflammation of any of the various parts of the mastoid process.

mastopexy, surgical correction of sagging breasts.

mastoptosis, a sagging of the breast.

masturbate, to engage in

the act of masturbation.

masturbation, the handling or stimulating, usually by oneself, of the genital organs; onanism.

mater, see **mother.**

materia medica, 1. the branch of medical science that treats of the drugs employed in medicine. 2. collectively, all the curative substances employed in medicine.

maternal, of, pertaining to, befitting, having the qualities of, or being a mother.

maternity, the state or character of being a mother; motherhood.

matter, to form or exude pus.

maxilla, the upper jawbone.

maxillary, of or pertaining to the upper jawbone.

M.D., abbreviation for Doctor of Medicine.

measles, an infectious disease occurring principally in children and characterized by a widespread red rash. See also **German measles.**

meatal, of or pertaining to a meatus.

meatus, a foramen, passage, or duct of the body, as the opening of the nose or ear.

meconium, 1. the feces discharged from the bowels of a newborn infant. 2. see **opium.**

media, the intermediate layer in the wall of an artery or lymphatic vessel.

mediad, in the direction of the central line or plane.

medial, situated in or pertaining to the middle.

median, see **medial.**

mediastinal, of or pertaining to the mediastinum.

mediastinitis, inflammation of the tissue of the mediastinum.

medastinum, the division of the chest cavity from the sternum backward, dividing the cavity into two parts and enclosing all the thoracic organs but the lungs.

medic, a medical practitioner, medical corpsman, or medical student.

medicable, susceptible of medical treatment; curable.

Medicaid, a medical aid program sponsored jointly by federal, state, and local governments for the disabled or needy of any age who are not eligible for social security benefits; distinguished from **Medicare.**

medical, 1. pertaining to or connected with medicine or physicians. 2. medicinal. 3. tending to cure.

medical examiner, a medically trained public official appointed to make postmortem examinations of the bodies of victims of suicide, homicide, or other unnatural death.

medicament, 1. any substance used for healing wounds or treating diseases. 2. a healing application.

Medicare, a U.S. government insurance program, financed by social security, that provides hospital and medical care for certain persons, esp. the aged.

medicate, 1. to treat with medicine or medicaments. 2. to impregnate with a medicinal substance.

medication, 1. the act or process of medicating. 2. a medicinal preparation used to treat or cure an ailment.

medicinal, 1. pertaining to or having the properties of a medicine. 2. curative. 3. remedial, as, medicinal substances.

medicine, 1. any substance used in treating disease or relieving pain. 2. the medical profession. 3. the art or science of restoring or preserving health.

medulla, 1. the marrow of bones. 2. the medulla oblongata. 3. the soft inner substance of an organ or part, as of a kidney.

medulla oblongata, the lowest or hindmost part of the brain, continuous with the spinal cord.

medullar, of or pertaining to marrow or the medulla.

megacardia, abnormal enlargement of the heart.

megacecum, abnormally large cecum.

megacephalic, 1. largeheaded. 2. having a skull with a cranial capacity exceeding the mean.

megacephaly, the condition of being megacephalic.

megacolon, extreme distention of the colon.

megagamete, see **macrogamete.**

megalomania, a form of mental disorder characterized by extreme over-estimation of one's abilities or importance; an obsession for grandiose action.

meiosis, the process resulting in the formation of the mature reproductive cells and consisting of the reduction of the chromosome number by one-half, from the diploid to the haploid.

melancholia, a mental disease characterized by great depression, brooding, gloomy forebodings without apparent reason, a marked inaccessibility to most external stimuli, and, often, real or imagined physical ailments.

melancholy, a state of despondency, esp. frequent or lengthy despondency; somber contemplation.

melanemia, presence of free dark pigment in the blood.

melanin, any of various dark pigments in the hair, epidermis, or eyes, produced in excess by certain diseases.

melanism, an excessive development of black or dark pigment in the skin, hair, and eyes.

melanoma, a tumor, usually malignant, composed of cells containing dark pigment.

melanomatosis, the presence of many melanomas on or beneath the skin.

melanosis, 1. the deposition or development of black or dark pigment in the tissues, sometimes leading to the production of malignant pigmented tumors. 2. a discoloration caused by this.

melanotic, of or pertaining to melanosis.

melanous, black-haired and dark-complexioned.

melanuria, presence of dark pigment in the urine.

melissophobia, pathological fear of bee or wasp stings.

membrane, a thin tissue that covers organs, lines cavities or canals, or joins adjacent parts.

membrane bone, a bone that originates in membranous tissue rather than cartilage.

membranoid, resembling a membrane.

membranous, relating to or having the nature of a membrane.

membranous labyrinth, the part of the inner ear composed of membranous structures, as the cochlea.

menarche, the beginning of the menses.

Mendelism, a theory or doctrine of heredity.

Ménière's disease, a disorder of the labyrinth of the ear marked by dizziness, ringing in the ears, and more or less complete deafness.

meningeal, of or pertaining to the meninges.

meninges, three membranes, the dura mater, pia mater, and arachnoid, that envelop the brain and spinal cord.

meningioma, a tumor originating in the arachnoidal membrane of the brain.

meningism, symptoms stimulating meningitis, but without inflammation; irritation of the brain.

meningitis, inflammation of the membranes of the brain or spinal cord, esp. inflammation of the pia mater and arachnoid.

meningococcus, a microorganism that causes cerebral meningitis.

meningoencephalitis, inflammation of the brain and its membranes.

meningoencephalomyelitis, inflammation of the spinal cord, the brain, and their membranes.

meningomyelitis, inflammation of the spinal cord and its membranes.

meniscectomy, surgical excision of a meniscus, usually one from the knee.

meniscus, 1. a crescent or crescent-shaped body. 2. a lens with a crescent-shaped section. 3. a disk of cartilage located in a joint between the surfaces of the articulating bones.

menopausal, of or pertaining to the menopause.

menopause, 1. the natural and permanent cessation of menstruation, normally between the ages of 45 and 50. 2. woman's change of life.

menorrhagia, 1. profuse or prolonged menstrual discharge. 2. hemorrhage from the uterus.

mensal, occurring once a month; monthly.

menses, the monthly discharge of blood; menstruation.

menstrual, of, or pertaining to the menses of females.

menstruation, 1. the uterine discharge of blood and mucus occurring on an average every 28 days from puberty to menopause. 2. the act or time of menstruation.

menstruum, 1. any fluid that dissolves a solid. 2. a solvent.

mensuration, the act or process of measuring.

mental, of, or pertaining to the mind.

mental age, the age that corresponds to the level of a person's ability.

mental deficiency, failure in the development of intelligence, as in moronism, imbecility, and idiocy, characterized by inability to function adequately in society.

mentality, mental capacity or endowment; intellectuality; mind.

mentum, the lower extremity of the face, below the mouth; the point of the under jaw; the chin.

meperidine, a man-made narcotic, employed as an analgesic and sedative.

meprobamate, a drug used as a tranquilizer and antispasmodic.

merbromin, a compound, having the form of a green powder, which, when mixed with water, produces a red solution employed as an antiseptic and a germicide; Mercurochrome (trademark).

mercury chloride, an acid, crystalline, highly poisonous compound, used as an antiseptic, fungicide, disinfectant, and preservative.

Merthiolate, thimerosal, a germicidal and antiseptic mercurial compound (trademark).

mesarteritis, inflammation of the middle coat of an artery.

mescal, an intoxicating spirit distilled from the fermented juice of a species of agave and used as a stimulant, esp. by the Mexican Indians.

mescaline, a white, crystalline alkaloid, produced from mescal buttons, which can cause hallucinations.

mesencephalic, of or pertaining to the mesencephalon.

mesencephalon, the middle or central portion of the brain.

mesenchyme, the cells of the mesodermal layer of tissue that develop into certain structures such as the heart, blood, and lymphatic vessels, cartilage and bone.

mesenteric, of or pertaining to a mesentery.

mesenteritis, inflammation of a mesentery.

mesenterium, see **mesentery.**

mesenteron, the early stages in the development of the intestinal cavity of the embryo, bounded by endoderm.

mesentery, a fold or duplicate of peritoneum investing and attaching to the posterior wall of the abdomen, a part or parts of the intestines, or other abdominal viscera.

mesial, of or pertaining to the middle.

mesial plane, an imaginary plane dividing the body longitudinally into symmetrical parts.

mesic, having a medium amount of moisture.

mesmeric, of or pertaining to mesmerism.

mesmerism, 1. the doctrine of the induction of a hypnotic state through an influence or emanation transmitted from the operator to the subject. 2. the induction, influence, or state concerned. 3. in general, hypnotism.

mesmerize, to hypnotize; to subject to spellbinding influence.

mesoblast, the middle layer of the primitive embryo that later becomes the mesoderm.

mesoblastic, of or pertaining to the mesoblast.

mesocolic, of or pertaining to the mesocolon.

mesocolon, the peritoneal fold connecting the colon with the posterior abdominal wall.

mesoderm, the middle layer of tissue between the ectoderm and the endoderm of the embryo.

mesodermic, of or pertaining to mesoderm.

mesomorph, 1. a muscular type of body structure developed by the relative dominance of tissues derived from the mesoderm, the middle of the three cell layers of the embryo. 2. a person having this type of body structure.

mesomorphic, of or pertaining to, or characteristic of mesomorphs.

mesonephros, the central part of the embryonic renal organ.

mesothelium, the portion of the mesoderm that lines the primitive coelon of the embryo.

metabolic, of or pertaining to metabolism.

metabolism, the sum of the chemical changes in living organisms and cells by which food is converted into living protoplasm, **anabolism,** and by which protoplasm is used and broken down into simpler compounds and waste by liberation of energy, **catabolism.**

metabolite, anything produced by metabolic activity.

metabolize, to subject to or alter by metabolism.

metacarpal, 1. of or pertaining to the metacarpus. 2. a metacarpal bone.

metacarpus, the part of a hand, esp. its bony structure, included between the wrist or carpus and the fingers or phalanges.

metaplasia, the change of one kind of tissue into another kind.

metapsychology, the speculative study concentrating on the nature and function of the mind and the relation between the mental and physical processes.

metastasis, the transfer, as through the blood or lymphatics, of disease or disease-producing cells from one part of the body to another, and the condition resulting from such transfer.

metastatic, of or pertaining to metastasis.

metatarsal, a bone of the metatarsus.

metatarsus, the part of a foot, esp. of its bony structure, included between the tarsus and the toes or phalanges.

metencephalon, the posterior segment of the brain, practically coextensive with the medulla oblongata; the afterbrain; the encephalon.

meteorism, see **tympanites.**

methadone, a synthetic, habit-forming drug used to induce sleep and dull pain; also used in treatment of addiction to opium derivatives.

methemoglobin, a brownish compound, a combination of oxygen and hemoglobin, formed in the blood, occurring in the use of certain drugs.

methenamine, see **hexamethylenetetramine.**

methionine, a natural or synthetic amino acid, used in warding off or treating certain diseases of the liver.

metopic, of or pertaining to the forehead; frontal.

metra, see **uterus.**

metralgia, pain in the uterus.

Metrazol, a stimulant, pentylenetetrazol, used in treating certain heart conditions and mental disorders (trademark).

metrectomy, see **hysterectomy.**

metritis, inflammation of the uterus.

metrocarcinoma, uterine cancer.

metrocystosis, the condition of having uterine cysts.

metropathy, any disease of the uterus.

metroptosis, dropping of the uterus.

metrorrhagia, bleeding from the uterus, unconnected with the menses.

microbe, a microscopic organism, esp. a pathogenic species.

microbic, of or pertaining to a microbe.

microbiologist, one who specializes in microbiology.

microbiology, the science and study of microscopic organisms.

microcephalic, pertaining to microcephaly.

microcephaly, the condition of having an abnormally small head, often seen in idiocy.

micrococcus, any species of the genus **Micrococcus,** comprising globular or oval bacterial organisms of which certain species cause disease and others produce fermentation.

microcyte, one of the dwarf or abnormally small red corpuscles of the blood occurring in certain forms of anemia.

micron, a unit of length equal to one millionth of a meter or one thousandth of a millimeter.

microorganism, a microscopic organism, as a protozoan or bacterium.

microscope, an optical instrument consisting of a lens or combination of lenses that render minute objects distinctly visible.

microscopic, 1. visible only by the aid of a microscope. 2. minute or tiny. 3. pertaining to or resembling a microscope. 4. made by, or as by, the aid of a microscope, as, microscopic observations.

microscopy, 1. the use of the microscope. 2. investigation by means of the microscope.

microsome, one of the minute granules in the protoplasm of cells.

microtome, an instrument for cutting very fine sections of organic tissue for microscopic study.

microtomic, of or pertaining to a microtome.

micturate, see **urinate.**

midbrain, see **mesencephalon.**

middle ear, the area between the outer ear and the inner ear made up of the tympanic membrane and a cavity containing the malleus, stapes, and incus.

midriff, 1. the diaphragm. 2.the area of the body between the chest and the waist.

midwife, a woman who assists a mother in childbirth.

midwifery, the art or practice of a midwife.

migraine, a recurring headache marked by severe pain, usually limited to a single side of the head and often with attendant nausea.

miliaria, an inflammatory disease of the skin, located about the sweat glands, marked by the formation of vesicles and papules resembling millet seeds.

miliaria rubra, see **prickly heat.**

miliary, characterized by spots or vesicles resembling millet seeds, as in miliaria.

milieu, see **environment.**

milium, a small white or yellowish nodule resembling a millet seed, produced in the skin by the retention of a fatty secretion.

milk, an opaque white or bluish-white liquid secreted by the mammary glands of the female for the nourishment of the young.

milk fever, a fever caused by infection, appearing with the onset of lactation following childbirth.

milk leg, an inflammation of the veins in the leg that causes pain and swelling, often occurring in women after childbirth. See also **phlebitis.**

milk sickness, a disease brought about by the consumption of dairy products or of the meat of cattle that have grazed on certain poisonous plants.

milksop, 1. an effeminate man or boy. 2. one devoid of manliness. 3. a sissy.

milk tooth, one of the first, or temporary, teeth in children.

milligram, a thousandth part of a gram.

millimeter, a thousandth part of a meter.

millimicron, a millionth part of a millimeter, or a thousandth part of a micron.

mind, the unconscious and conscious processes that perceive, conceive, comprehend, evaluate, and reason.

miosis, 1. abnormal constriction of the pupil of the eye. 2. see also **meiosis.**

misanthrope, 1. a hater of mankind. 2. one who harbors distrust of human character in general.

misanthropist, see **misanthrope.**

miscarriage, the premature expulsion of a nonviable fetus; abortion.

miscarry, see **abort.**

miscegenation, 1. mixture of races by sexual union. 2. interbreeding between races.

miscible, capable of being mixed.

misogamist, a hater of marriage.

misogamy, hatred of marriage.

misogynist, a hater of women.

misogyny, hatred of women.

misology, hatred of reason or reasoning.

mithridate, a substance that was believed to be a universal antidote against poison.

mithridatism, the production of immunity against a poison by taking the poison in gradually increased doses.

mitosis, the usual method of cell division, characterized typically by the resolving of the chromatin of the nucleus into a threadlike form, which separates into segments of chromosomes, each of which in turn separates longitudinally into two parts, one part of each chromosome being retained in each of two new cells resulting from the original cell. Compare **amitosis.**

mitotic, of or pertaining to mitosis.

mitral, noting or pertaining to a valve in the heart that prevents the blood in the left ventricle from returning to the left auricle.

mittelschmerz, abdominal pain occurring more or less regularly midway between menstrual periods.

molar, a tooth with a broad surface for grinding, located behind the canines and incisors.

mole, 1. see **nevus.** 2. a mass of fleshy matter occurring in the uterus, usually as the result of an abortive conception.

molluscum, a skin disease characterized by tumor-like formation of nodules.

monaural, of or pertaining to sound that is perceived through only one ear.

mongolism, a congenital mental deficiency in a child characterized by slanting eyes and broad skull, face, and hands. See also **Down's syndrome.**

mongoloid, 1. of or relating to mongolism. 2. a person afflicted with mongolism.

moniliasis, an infection of the skin or a mucous membrane caused by yeastlike fungi.

moniliform, resembling the shape of a string of beads.

monocular, 1. pertaining to or intended for one eye. 2. having only a single eyepiece, as a monocular microscope.

monocyte, a large leukocyte, the nucleus of which is horseshoe-shaped.

monocytosis, an abnormal increase in the number of monocytes in the blood.

monodactylous, having only one finger or toe on a hand or foot.

monogenesis, the theoretical descent of all living things from a single cell; the theoretical descent of the whole human race from a single pair.

monomania, 1. a mental disorder in which the patient is obsessed by one idea, or is irrational on one subject only. 2. excessive enthusiasm for one idea, object, or project.

monomaniac, a person suffering from monomania.

monomaniacal, of or relating to monomania.

mononuclear, having a single nucleus.

mononucleosis, a viral

disease of the blood, characterized by the existence of too many monocytes. See also **infectious mononucleosis.**

monoparesis, paralysis of a single part of the body.

monophobia, pathological dread of being alone.

monoplegia, paralysis of a single limb or one group of muscles.

mons pubis, the rounded pubic eminence.

morbid, 1. affected by or characteristic of disease, as, morbid tissues, discharges, or symptoms. 2. pertaining to diseased parts, as, morbid anatomy. 3. being in or suggesting an unhealthy mental state. 4. unwholesomely gloomy, sensitive, or extreme.

morbidity, 1. a morbid state or quality. 2. the proportion of death, sickness, or disease in a given locality.

morgue, a place where the bodies of dead people, particularly accident victims, are kept until identified or buried.

moribund, dying; deathlike; nearing extinction.

morning sickness, nausea occurring in the early part of the day, characteristic of the first months of pregnancy.

moron, an adult with retarded intellectual development whose mentality corresponds to that of a normal child from 8 to 12 years of age.

morose, of a sullen disposition; gloomy.

morphia, see **morphine.**

morphine, a bitter crystalline alkaloid, the most important narcotic principle of opium, used in medicine, usually in the form of a sulfate or other salt, to dull pain or induce sleep.

morphinism, a morbid condition induced by the habitual use of morphine.

morphinomania, uncontrollable craving for morphine.

morphinomaniac, a person who suffers from morphinomania.

morphogenesis, the changes in form or structure in the development of an organism or part of an organism.

morphology, the study of the form and structure of organisms, without regard to function.

mortal, subject to death; causing death; fatal; pertaining to death.

mortality, the state of being mortal.

mortician, see **undertaker.**

mortuary, a funeral home.

morula, in embryology, the mass of cells resulting from the division of a cell or ovum during the cleavage state.

mother, 1. the female who gives birth to a child. 2. a female parent.

motile, 1. moving, or capable of moving, spontaneously, as, motile cells. 2. one in whose mind motor images are predominant , or esp. distinct.

motility, 1. spontaneous movements. 2. the ability

to perform voluntary movements.

motion sickness, discomfort, often including dizziness and nausea, which some people suffer in moving vehicles.

motor, 1. conveying an impulse that results or tends to result in motion, as a nerve. **2.** of or pertaining to such nerves. **3.** pertaining to or involving consciousness of action, as, motor images.

mountain sickness, an illness caused by air rarefaction, usually at altitudes above 10,000 feet, characterized by nausea, difficulty in breathing, and weakness.

mouth, 1. the opening through which man or animals take in food. **2.** the cavity containing the parts used in chewing and tasting food.

mouth-to-mouth resuscitation, a type of artificial respiration consisting of air being blown directly into the mouth and lungs of the patient by another person at short, regular intervals.

movement, 1. the act of moving. **2.** the course, process, or result of change, esp. change involving location or position. **3.** motion. **4.** the voiding of the bowels.

mucilage, any preparation of glue or gummy substance used as an adhesive.

mucin, any of a group of nitrogenous substances found in mucous secre-

tions, varying in composition according to its source; the principal constituent of mucus.

mucocutaneous, pertaining to an area where mucous membrane and skin come together, as in the nose, mouth, vagina and anus.

mucoid, any of a group of substances resembling the mucins, occurring in connective tissue and in cysts.

mucoprotein, any of various proteins containing polysaccharides, found in the body's fluids and in connective tissues.

mucosa, a mucous membrane.

mucoserous, pertaining to a fluid that contains serum or plasma with a considerable amount of mucus.

mucous, pertaining to or resembling mucus; slimy; ropy.

mucous membrane, a membrane that lines all the cavities of the body that open externally, such as the mouth, nose, or intestines, and which secretes mucus.

mucus, a viscid fluid secreted by the mucous membranes.

multicellular, having or made up of a number of cells.

multipara, a woman who has borne two or more children, or who is delivering or near to giving birth the second time.

multiparous, producing many, or more than one,

at a birth.

multiple sclerosis, a serious disease in which parts of the brain and spinal cord harden, causing tremors, muscular weakness, and other debilitating symptoms.

mumps, a disease consisting of an inflammation of the salivary glands, with swelling along the neck; see also **parotiditis.**

mural, of or pertaining to the wall of any cavity of the body.

mural pregnancy, a pregnancy occurring in the fallopian tube.

murmur, a sound emitted by the heart that is a sign of an abnormality.

muscle, 1. a tissue consisting of elongated fibers that contract on stimulation and produce bodily motion. 2. a contractive organ, consisting of muscle tissue.

musclebound, having the muscles enlarged, overstrained, and inelastic, as by overexercise.

muscular, pertaining to or consisting of muscles; performed by or dependent on muscles, as, muscular exertion.

muscular dystrophy, a disease that results in progressive deterioration and atrophy of muscle tissue.

musculature, 1. the system of muscles. 2. the muscle arrangement in an organ.

mutant, a form that is undergoing mutation or has resulted from mutation.

mutate, to change; to alter;

to undergo mutation.

mutation, 1. the act or process of changing. 2. a change or alteration, as in form, quality, or nature. 3. a sudden inheritable change appearing in the offspring of a parent organism because of an alteration in a gene or chromosome or an increase in the number of chromosomes. 4. the process by which this change occurs.

mute, 1. silent, or refraining from speech or utterance. 2. not emitting or having sound of any kind. 3. incapable of speech. 4. a person without the power of speech.

myalgia, 1. pain in the muscles. 2. muscular rheumatism.

myalgic, of or pertaining to myalgia.

myasthenia, muscular debility.

myatrophy, the wasting away of muscles.

myctes, see **fungus.**

mycetes, see **fungus.** poisoning.

mycology, the study of fungi and the diseases they cause.

mycosis, 1. the presence of parasitic fungi in or on the body. 2. a disease caused by such a fungus.

mycotic, of or pertaining to mycosis.

mycotoxin, a poison or poisonous substance produced by fungi growing in food.

mydriasis, excessive dilatation of the pupil of the eye, as a result of disease or drugs.

mydriatic, 1. pertaining to or producing mydriasis. 2. a mydriatic drug.

myelencephalitis, inflammation of the brain and the spinal cord.

myelencephalon, the posterior area of the embryonic hindbrain from which the medulla oblongata develops.

myelin, a soft, white, fatty substance encasing the axis cylinder of certain nerve fibers.

myelinic, of or pertaining to myelin.

myelinization, the process by which the myelin sheath is formed.

myelin sheath, the medullary case enclosing certain nerve fibers.

myelitis, inflammation of the spinal cord or the bone marrow.

myelocyte, a type of large cell in the red bone marrow from which leukocytes are developed.

myeloencephalitis, inflammation of the spinal cord and the brain.

myelography, X-ray inspection of the spinal cord after introduction by lumbar puncture of a substance opaque to X rays.

myeloid, 1. resembling marrow. 2. having to do with the spinal cord.

myocardiograph, an instrument that records the action of the muscles of the heart.

myocarditis, inflammation of the myocardium.

myocardium, the muscular

substance of the heart.

myogenic, having its origin in muscle.

myoglobin, hemoglobin in the muscles, similar to blood hemoglobin, but carrying less carbon monoxide and more oxygen.

myograph, an instrument used to measure muscular activity.

myology, the branch of anatomy concerned with the science of muscles and their parts.

myoma, a tumor composed of muscle tissue.

myomatous, resembling a myoma.

myoneural, of or concerning both muscle and nerves.

myopia, a condition of the eye in which images are focused in front of the retina, objects being seen distinctly only when near to the eye; nearsightedness.

myopic, of or pertaining to myopia.

myositis, inflammation of, esp. voluntary, muscle tissue.

myringa, see **tympanum.**

myringitis, inflammation of the eardrum.

myringoscope, an instrument used for examination of the tympanum.

myxedema, a disease characterized by thickening of the skin and blunting of the senses and intellect, because of diminished functioning of the thyroid gland.

myxoma, a tumor consisting of mucous and connective tissue.

naevocarcinoma, see **ne-vocarcinoma.**

naevoid, see **nevoid.**

naevous, see **nevous.**

naevus, see **nevus.**

nail, a thin, horny plate, consisting of modified epidermis, growing on the upper side of the end of a finger or toe.

nanism, abnormally small size or stature; dwarfism.

nape, the back part of the neck.

naprapath, one who practices naprapathy.

naprapathy, a system of treatment of disease based on the belief that illness is caused by disordered connective or ligamental tissues, and using massage, manipulation, and adjustment of joints and muscles as therapy.

narcissism, 1. self-love. 2. excessive admiration of or fascination with oneself. 3. an early stage in psychosexual development in which the self is the focus of erotic interest. 4. the arrest of psychosexual development at this stage.

narcolepsy, an illness characterized by the frequent, sudden, uncontrollable need for deep, but brief sleep.

narcoleptic, 1. of or pertaining to narcolepsy. 2. one who suffers from narcolepsy.

narcosis, 1. the production of stupor or insensibility by a narcotic drug. 2. a state of drowsiness or insensibility.

narcotic, 1. a substance that relieves pain, induces sleep, and in large doses brings on stupor, coma, and even death, as opium or morphine. 2. an addict. 3. something that soothes or numbs. 4. having the properties of a narcotic. 5. relating to or induced by narcotics.

narcotize, 1. to bring under the influence of a narcotic. 2. to numb the awareness of.

naris, see **nostril.**

nasal, of or pertaining to the nose.

nascent, beginning to exist or to grow; coming into being.

nasolabial, pertaining to both the nose and the lips.

nasolacrimal, pertaining to the nose and the tear glands, ducts, etc.

nasology, the study of the nose and its diseases.

nasopalatine, pertaining to both the nose and the palate.

nasopharyngeal, pertaining to both the nose and the pharynx.

nasopharyngitis, inflammation of the nasopharynx.

nasopharynx, the part of the pharynx situated above the soft palate and behind the nose (the postnasal space).

natal, of or pertaining to birth.

natality, see **birthrate.**

nates, either of the two

fleshy protuberances forming the lower and back part of the human trunk; the buttocks.

natural selection, the theory that nature tends to maintain and perpetuate those species having particular characteristics of genetic origin that best fit them for survival in their environment.

naturopath, one who practices naturopathy.

naturopathy, a method of treating illness or disease without drugs or surgery, using proper foods, heat, exercise, and massage to aid natural healing.

nausea, stomach sickness or upset, often with an inclination to vomit.

nauseate, 1. to feel nausea or disgust. 2. to affect with nausea.

nauseous, 1. causing a feeling of nausea. 2. affected with nausea.

navel, see **umbilicus.**

navicular, 1. shaped like a boat. 2. the bone of the wrist or ankle, so named for its boat shape.

near point, the shortest distance at which the eye can distinctly see a small object.

nearsighted, see **myopic.**

nearsightedness, see **myopia.**

nearthrosis, a false joint, created because of the nonunion of a broken bone.

nebula, 1. visual opacity. 2. a small cloudy spot on the cornea. 3. cloudy urine. 4. an oily medication prepared by atomization.

nebulize, 1. to reduce to fine spray; atomize. 2. to become unclear or nebulous.

nebulizer, an instrument used for spraying in a fine mist.

neck, the part of the body connecting the head and the trunk.

necrobiosis, gradual degeneration and death of a cell, cell groups, or tissue.

necrobiotic, of or pertaining to or affected by necrobiosis.

necrophobia, 1. pathological aversion to dead bodies. 2. pathological fear of dying.

necropsy, the examination of a body after death; a postmortem examination, or autopsy.

necrosis, see **necrobiosis.**

necrotic, see **necrobiotic.**

necrotize, to produce necrosis, as in an organ or tissue.

negative, not showing signs of the presence of a particular disease or organism.

negativism, an attitude or behavior disorder marked by contrariness.

negativist, one who is negativistic.

negativistic, of or pertaining to negativism.

nematode, belonging to the phylum Nematoda, of thin, unsegmented, cylindrical, parasitic worms, whose hosts may be man, domestic plants, or animals.

nematology, the branch of zoology that treats of

nematodes.

nematosis, infestation by a parasite that belongs to the phylum Nematoda.

neoarsphenamine, a yellow medicinal powder, made from arsphenamine, but not so toxic.

neo-Darwinism, Darwin's theory as developed by later students who believed that natural selection is the basis for evolution and therefore rejected that part of his theory concerned with the inheritance of acquired characteristics as an evolutionary force.

neomycin, an antibiotic, developed from the microorganism **Streptomyces fradiae,** which inhibits or destroys a broad range of bacteria, used esp. in treating skin infections.

neonatal, affecting or pertaining to a newborn infant.

neonate, a newborn infant.

neophobia, pathological fear of everything that is new.

neoplasia, the development of a neoplasm.

neoplasm, any new and abnormal growth of body tissue; a tumor.

neoplastic, of or pertaining to neoplasm.

neoplasty, surgical restoration of tissue or parts.

nephralgia, pain in the kidney region.

nephralgic, pertaining to renal pain.

nephrectomy, surgical excision of a kidney.

nepric, pertaining to the kidney or kidneys.

nephritic, of or pertaining to nephritis.

nephritis, inflammation of the kidneys.

nephrolith, a kidney stone.

nephrolithotomy, surgical incision for removal of a kidney stone.

nephroma, a kidney tumor or a tumor of renal tissue.

nephropathy, any kind of kidney disease.

nephrosclerosis, sclerosis of the kidneys.

nephrosis, a condition of the kidneys that shows degeneration without inflammation.

nervation, the arrangement or distribution of nerves.

nerve, one of the whitish fibers that proceeds from the brain and spinal cord and spreads through all parts of the body, and whose function is to convey sensation and originate motion.

nerve cell, any of the cells constituting the cellular element of nervous tissue, esp. one of the essential cells of a nerve center.

nerve center, a group of nerve cells closely connected with one another and acting together in the performance of some function.

nerve fiber, one of the primary threadlike fibers or processes known as axons or dendrites of a neuron or nerve cell.

nerve gas, a gas, used in chemical warfare, that damages or impairs the central nervous system, resulting in extreme weakness or paralysis.

nerve impulse, transmission of a wave of sensation along a nerve fiber that activates or inhibits a nerve cell, gland, or muscle.

nervous, 1. pertaining to or having nerves. 2. originating from or affecting the nerves. 3. easily agitated. 4. tense or anxious.

nervous breakdown, see **neurasthenia.**

nervousness, the state of being nervous.

nervous system, the elaborate network of nerve cells making up the ganglia, spinal cord, nerves, and brain, whose function is to receive and transmit impulses from the brain and sense organs.

nettle rash, see **urticaria.**

neural, pertaining to the nerves or nervous system.

neuralgia, pain, usually sharp and paroxysmal, along the course of a nerve.

neuralgic, of or pertaining to neuralgia.

neural tube, a hollow tubular formation of nerve tissue in the embryo made of joined ectodermal folds on each side of the neural plate and developing at one end into the brain.

neurasthenia, a condition, as from prolonged emotional tension or overwork, characterized by excessive mental and physical fatigue and sometimes by obscure physical complaints or phobias.

neurasthenic, pertaining to neurasthenia.

neuraxitis, see **encephalitis.**

neurectomy, surgical excision of a nerve or part of a nerve.

neurectopia, abnormal position or displacement of a nerve.

neurilemma, the delicate membranous sheath of a nerve fiber.

neurinoma, a tumor arising from the sheath of a nerve.

neuritis, inflammation of a nerve causing impaired reflexes or paralysis.

neuroblastoma, a malignant hemorrhagic tumor of nerve ganglia.

neurocirculatory, pertaining to the nervous and circulatory systems of the body.

neurocrine, pertaining or related to a hormone that influences nerve activity.

neurodermatitis, a severe itching irritation of the skin caused by a nervous disorder.

neurodermatosis, see **neurodermatitis.**

neurodynia, see **neuralgia**

neurofibril, any of the minute fibrils in the nerve cells, regarded as conducting elements.

neurofibroma, a tumor arising from nerve tissue or connective tissue of a nerve.

neurofibromatosis, a condition in which there

are variously sized tumors on peripheral nerves.

neurogenic, beginning in nerve tissue or in a nerve.

neurogenous, arising from some part of the nervous system.

neuroglia, the delicate connective tissue that supports and binds together the essential elements of nervous tissue, esp. in the central nervous system.

neuroglial, of or pertaining to neuroglia.

neuroglioma, a tumor of neuroglial tissue.

neurologist, a physician specializing in diagnosis and treatment of diseases of the nerves or nervous system.

neurology, the science of the nerves or the nervous system and their diseases or disorders.

neurolysin, an agent that destroys nerve cells.

neurolysis, 1. to relieve tension by stretching of a nerve. 2. disintegration of nerve tissue.

neuroma, a tumor composed of nerve tissue.

neuromalacia, abnormal softening of nerve tissue.

neuromuscular, pertaining to both nerves and muscles.

neuron, the basic functional and structural element of the nervous system, consisting of a nerve cell with all its processes.

neuronal, relating to one or more neurons.

neurone, see **neuron.**

neuropathic, relating to

neuropathy.

neuropathology, the science of the diseases of the nervous system and their causes.

neuropathy, any disease of the nervous system.

neuropharmacology, the science concerned with the study of the effects of drugs on the nervous system.

neurophysiology, the science dealing with the functions of the nervous system.

neuroplasty, surgery to repair nerves as, for instance, nerve grafting.

neuropsychiatry, the branch of medicine dealing with diseases involving the mind and the nervous system.

neurosis, a functional nervous or emotional disorder, less serious than a psychosis, marked by severe anxiety, depression, and the like, without any apparent physical origin. See also **psychoneurosis.**

neurosurgery, surgery performed on the brain, spinal cord, or nervous system.

neurosyphilis, a syphilitic stage that involves the central nervous system.

neurotic, 1. affected by or relating to a neurosis. 2. of or relating to the nerves. 3. one who has a neurosis, or whose behavior suggests one.

neurotomy, surgical severing of a nerve, as to relieve neuralgia.

neurotoxic, poisonous to

nerves or to nerve tissue such as the brain. See also **nerve gas.**

neurotripsy, the surgical crushing of a nerve.

neurovascular, pertaining to both the nervous and vascular systems.

nevocarcinoma, a cancer developing from a mole.

nevoid, resembling a nevus.

nevose, marked with moles.

nevus, 1. a congenital mark, blemish, or mole on the skin. 2. a birthmark.

newborn, 1. a recently born infant. 2. recently or just born.

Niacin (trademark), see **nicotinic acid.**

nicotine, a highly poisonous volatile alkaloid, derived from tobacco.

nicotinic acid, one of the vitamins in the B complex, consisting of a crystalline compound formed from the oxidation of nicotine, and used esp. in the prevention of pellagra.

nictitate, to wink; to blink the eyelids.

nidus, a spot in an organism that is a center of infection.

night-blind, of or pertaining to night blindness.

night blindness, a condition of the eyes in which one can see well by daylight but poorly or not at all by night or dim light.

nightmare, a fearful or terrifying dream causing intense anxiety and feelings of oppression and helplessness.

night terrors, a form of nightmare, esp. in children, causing them to wake up in terror.

nightwalking, see **somnambulism.**

nipple, 1. a protuberance on the female breast with an opening through which the milk ducts discharge. 2. anything resembling a nipple in shape or function, as the mouthpiece of a nursing bottle.

nit, the egg of a louse or similar parasitic insect.

niter, potassium nitrate or sodim nitrate. See also **saltpeter.**

nitric acid, a corrosive liquid, with powerful oxidizing properties, used in the manufacture of medicine, dyes, explosives, and metal products.

nitrogen mustard, any of a class of toxic, blistering compounds, important in the treatment of some diseases.

nitroglycerin, a highly flammable, explosive liquid produced by the action of nitric and sulfuric acids on glycerol, used primarily in making dynamite or rocket propellants, and in medicine for relaxing or dilating blood vessels.

nitroglycerine, see **nitroglycerin.**

nitrous oxide, a combination of nitrogen and oxygen that sometimes produces an exhilarating effect upon being inhaled, used as an anesthetic during dental work and surgery. Also called **laughing gas.**

noctambulation, see **somnambulism.**

nocturia, excessive urination during the night; bed-wetting.

nocuous, see **noxious.**

node, 1. a swelling. 2. a constricted region. 3. a small rounded organ. 4. a lymph gland.

nodose, knotted; knobby.

nodosity, the condition of having nodes.

nodular, characterized by or resembling nodules.

nodule, a small knot or lump.

nodulose, having small knots or nodules; knotty.

nodulus, see **nodule.**

nodus, see **node.**

noetic, 1. of or pertaining to the mind or intellect. 2. originating in the mind independent of the senses.

noma, a gangrenous ulceration of the mouth and cheeks; occurring mainly in undernourished children.

nonfattening, 1. not fattening. 2. not high in calories, as, proteins that are generally nonfattening.

nonunion, an imperfect healing of a broken bone.

nonviable, inadequately fitted to live, develop, or perform.

normal, sane; average, as, of normal intelligence.

normalcy, normality; the state or condition of being normal.

nose, 1. the human facial feature that contains the nostrils. 2. the organ that includes the nasal cavity,

the nostrils, and olfactory nerve endings, and which functions in speech, respiration, and smelling. 3. the sense of smell. 4. the organ of smell.

nosebleed, see **epistaxis.**

nosology, 1. a systematic classification or description of diseases. 2. the branch of medical science concerned with the classification of diseases.

nosomania, the delusion of being diseased.

nosomycosis, any disease caused by a parasitic fungus.

nosophobia, pathological fear of illness.

nostril, one of the two apertures of the nose that gives passage to air.

nostrum, a quack medicine; a cure-all.

notifiable disease, any disease that is required by law to be reported to the Board of Health, as for instance, scarlet fever, typhoid fever, puerperal fever.

notochord, the rodlike embryonic structure that becomes the vertebral column.

Novocaine, a local anesthetic, procaine hydrochloride (trademark).

noxious, 1. harmful or injurious to health or physical well-being, as, noxious vapors. 2. deleterious; unwholesome; morally harmful or pernicious.

nubile, of an age or stage of physical maturity suitable for marriage (said of a girl or young woman).

nubility, the state of being

marriageable (said of a girl or young woman at puberty, the final stage of sex development).

nucleic acid, a complex organic compound important in heredity and the control of the metabolism of living cells, composed of phosphoric acids, bases from purines or pyrimidines, and carbohydrates, esp. sugar.

nucleolus, an organized, conspicuous, round body in the nucleus of a cell, other than a chromosome.

nullipara, a woman who has never borne a child.

nulliparity, the condition of being nulliparous.

nulliparous, never having borne a child.

numb, without physical sensation or feeling; not able to move.

numbness, the state of being numb.

nutation, a nodding of the head, usually involuntary.

nutriment, that which nourishes; food; any matter that, taken into a living organism, serves to sustain its existence, promoting growth and replacing worn-out tissues.

nutrition, 1. the act or process by which organisms absorb proper food. 2. the process of assimilating and converting food into tissue.

nutritionist, a person who specializes in the science of nutrition.

nutritious, 1. containing or serving as nutriment. 2. promoting growth, replacing worn out tissues, and supplying energy; nourishing.

nutritive, 1. pertaining to nutrition. 2. having the quality of nourishing.

nux vomica, the strychnine-containing seed of an Asiatic tree, used in medicine.

nyctalgia, pain occurring mainly during the night.

nyctalope, a person who suffers from nyctalopia.

nyctalopia, see **night blindness.**

nyctophilia, abnormal preference of night to day.

nyctophobia, pathological fear of the dark or the night.

nympha, see **labia minora.**

nymphomania, abnormal, uncontrollable sexual desire in females.

nymphomaniac, a woman who is affected by nymphomania.

nystagmiform, resembling nystagmus.

nystagmus, an involuntary oscillation of the eyeball, usually lateral but sometimes rotary or vertical, occurring in certain diseases.

obese, excessively corpulent; fat; overweight.

obesity, the state of excessive corpulence; abnormal amount of fat on the body.

oblique, of certain muscles of the eye and the abdomen, running at an angle and not laterally.

obsess 1. to occupy a person's thoughts to an unusual degree. 2. to preoccupy the mind. 3. to harass or vex through a persistent, usually undesirable or unwanted thought or emotion.

obsession, 1. an act of obsessing. 2. a thought or emotion that comes strongly to mind with unwanted persistence. 3. the thought itself.

obsessive, of or pertaining to obsession.

obstetric, pertaining to obstetrics or to the care of a woman in pregnancy, labor, birth, and the postnatal period.

obstetrician, a physician specializing in obstetrics.

obstetrics, the branch of medical science that includes prenatal care and childbirth.

obstipation, extreme constipation, usually caused by an obstruction.

obturate, to stop up; to close.

obturator, something that closes an opening, as a surgical plate for closing an abdominal opening.

occipital, of or pertaining to the occiput; of the posterior part of the head or skull.

occipital bone, a compound bone that forms the posterior part of the skull.

occipitocervical, relating to both the occiput and the neck.

occipitofacial, pertaining to both the occiput and the face.

occipitomental, pertaining to both the occiput and the chin.

occipitoparietal, pertaining to both the occiput and the parietal bones.

occipitotemporal, pertaining to both the occiput and the temporal bones.

occiput, the back part of the head or skull.

occlude, 1. to close, shut, or stop up, as a passage. 2. to meet closely or fit into each other, as opposing teeth in the upper and lower jaw.

occlusion, the act of occluding, or the state of being occluded.

occlusive, closing or shutting up.

occult, concealed, as a hemorrhage; obscure.

occult blood, blood that occurs in such minute quantities that it can be recognized only with a microscope.

occupational disease, a disease caused by a person's occupation.

occupational therapy, a method of treatment of convalescents using light work for diversion, physical exercise, or vocational training.

ochlophobia, pathological fear of crowds or mobs.

ocular, 1. of or pertaining to the eye, ocular movements. 2. of the nature of an eye, as, an ocular organ. 3. performed by the eye or eyesight, as, ocular inspection. 4. perceived by the eye or eyesight, as, ocular demonstration. 5. derived from actual sight, as, ocular proof. 6. the eyepiece of an optical instrument.

oculist, 1. one trained and skilled in the examination and treatment of the eye. 2. an opthalmologist.

oculomotor, 1. moving the eyeball. 2. connected to or pertaining to eyeball movement.

oculomotor nerve, either of the pair of cranial nerves supplying most of the muscles moving the eyeball.

oculomycosis, any disease of the eye or parts of the eye caused by a fungus.

oculus, see **eye.**

odontalgia, see **toothache.**

odontectomy, surgical excision of a tooth.

odontitis, inflammation of a tooth.

odontoblast, one of a layer of cells that line the pulp chamber of a tooth and form dentin.

odontoid, 1. resembling a tooth. 2. related to the odontoid process. 3. the odontoid process.

odontoid process, a prominent toothlike process of the axis, or second cervical vertebra, upon which the atlas rotates.

odontologist, a dentist or dental surgeon.

odontology, the branch of anatomical science that relates to the teeth, their health, growth, structure, and diseases.

odontoma, a tumor arising from a tooth or dental tissue.

odontonecrosis, massive decay of a tooth.

odontopathy, any disease of the teeth.

odontorrhagia, bleeding from the socket of a tooth after its extraction.

odontotherapy, care of decayed or diseased teeth.

oedipal, of or pertaining to Oedipus complex.

Oedipus complex, the desire, most readily expressed in sexual terms, of a son for his mother with a consequent rivalry between the son and his father, a complex that may appear later in life as seeking a mother image in relations with other women.

officinal, stocked by a pharmacy; securable without a prescription, opposed to magistral, sanctioned by a pharmacopoeia.

ointment, any soft, unctuous substance, usually medicated, applied to the skin for medicinal and cosmetic purposes; an unguent; a salve.

olecranal, of or pertaining to the olecranon.

olecranoid, resembling the olecranon.

olecranon, the part of the ulna beyond the elbow joint and forming the bony prominence of the elbow.

olfaction, 1. the act of smelling. 2. the sense of smell.

olfactory, of or pertaining to the sense of smell.

olfactory nerve, either of two nerves that consist of sensory fibers and conduct impulses from the olfactory organ in the nose to the brain.

olfactory organ, an organ composed of membranes in the nasal cavity, sensitive to the stimuli of odors.

oligemia, a deficiency of blood in the body.

oligocholia, a deficiency of bile.

oligocythemia, a deficiency in the number of red blood corpuscles.

oligogalactia, deficient secretion of milk.

oligohemia, see **oligemia.**

oligohydramnios, abnormally low amount of amniotic fluid.

oligospermia, a deficient number of spermatozoa in the seminal fluid.

omental, of, or pertaining to the omentum.

omentectomy, surgical excision of part of the omentum.

omentitis, inflammation of the omentum.

omentum, a fold or duplication of the peritoneum passing between certain of the viscera.

omphalic, of, or pertaining to the umbilicus.

omphalitis, inflammation of the umbilicus.

omphalocele, hernia of the umbilicus.

omphalos, see **umbilicus.**

omphalotomy, the severing of the umbilical cord at birth.

onanism, 1. withdrawal during intercourse before ejaculation. 2. masturbation.

oncogenesis, the formation and development of a tumor.

oncology, the part of medical science that treats and studies tumors.

onychectomy, surgical removal of the nail of a finger or toe.

onychia, inflammation of the nailbed.

onychitis, see **onychia.**

onychoma, tumor of the nailbed.

onyx, a fingernail or toenail.

onyxis, the ingrowing of the nails.

oocyte, an ovarian egg prior to maturation.

oogenesis, a series of cell divisions starting with the primordial germ cells in the ovary, which results in the production of the ovum.

oogenetic, of, or pertaining to oogenesis.

oophorectomy, see **ovariectomy.**

oophoritis, see **ovaritis.**

oophoron, see **ovary.**

operable, capable of being treated by surgery.

operation, a process or method of operating on the body of a patient, usually with instruments.

ophidiophobia, pathological fear of snakes.

ophidism, poisoning from a snakebite.

ophthalmalgia, pain in the eye.

ophthalmia, inflammation of the eyelid, the eye, or its membranes.

ophthalmic, belonging or pertaining to the eye.

ophthalmitis, see **ophthalmia.**

ophthalmologic, of, or pertaining to ophthalmology.

ophthalmologist, a medical doctor whose specialty is ophthalmology.

ophthalmology, the science that deals with the anatomy, functions, and diseases of the eye.

ophthalmopathy, any disorder of the eye.

ophthalmoplasty, plastic surgery on the eye.

ophthalmoplegia, paralysis of the muscles of the eye.

ophthalmoscope, an instrument for viewing the interior of the eye or examining the retina.

ophthalmoscopy, viewing the interior of the eye with an ophthalmoscope.

opiate, 1. any medicine that contains opium or one of its derivatives and has the quality of inducing sleep or alleviating pain. 2. to administer an opiate to.

opium, the dried juice of the unripe fruit of the opium poppy, a poisonous, narcotic, addictive alkaloid from which morphine and codeine are derived.

opsonin, a constituent of blood serum that causes invading cells or bacteria to become more susceptible to the destructive action of the phagocytes.

optic, 1. pertaining to sight or vision. 2. pertaining to or connected with the eye as the organ of sight, or sight as a function of the brain. 3. constructed to assist sight. 4. acting by means of sight or light.

optical illusion, 1. a deceptive or misleading image or impression presented to the vision. 2. something that deceives by presenting a false impression to the eyes.

optic disc, the small area in the retina where the blood vessels and the optic nerve enter. It is insensible to light and is therefore called the **blind spot.**

optician, one who makes eyeglasses for correcting defects of vision in accordance with the prescriptions of oculists.

optic nerve, one of a pair of cranial nerves of sight.

optics, the branch of physical science that deals with vision, and the properties and phenomena of light, its origins and effects, and its role as a medium of sight.

optic thalamus, see **thalamus.**

optometric, of or pertaining to optometry.

optometrist, one who is skilled in optometry.

optometry, 1. the measurement and examination of the visual powers. 2. the practice or art of testing the eyes by means of suitable instruments or appliances for defects of vision in order to correct them with eyeglasses.

oral, 1. pertaining to the mouth, as, the oral cavity. 2. done, taken, or administered by mouth, as an oral contraceptive. 3. uttered by the mouth, or spoken, as, oral testimony.

orbit, the bony cavity in

which the eye is situated.

orchectomy, surgical excision of a testicle.

orchialgia, neuralgic pain in the testicles.

orchidalgia, see **orchialgia.**

orchidectomy, see **orchectomy.**

orchioplasty, plastic surgery of the testicle.

orchis, see **testicle.**

orchitis, inflammation of a testicle.

organ, a part or member of living organisms, as the heart, having a specific function.

organ bank, a place where human organs or tissues are stored for future surgical use as transplants.

organic disease, a disease in which there is a structural alteration in the organ involved, as opposed to functional disease.

organicism, the doctrine that symptoms and disease are caused by diseased organs only.

organotherapy, the use of extracts from animal organs, such as kidneys or thyroid glands, for therapeutic purposes.

orgasm, the ultimate emotional and physical excitement of a sexual act.

orgastic, of or pertaining to orgasm.

ornithosis, a disease related to psittacosis found in both wild and domestic fowl, milder in form when contracted by man.

oropharynx, 1. the space immediately beneath the mouth cavity. 2. the

pharynx as distinguished from the nasopharynx.

orthocephalic, having a medium or intermediate relationship between the height of the skull and the breadth or length.

orthodontia, the branch of dentistry concerned with the straightening of irregular teeth.

othodontic, of or pertaining to orthodontia.

orthodontics, see **orthodontia.**

orthodontist, a dentist who is skilled in orthodontia.

orthogenetic, see **orthogenic.**

orthogenic, pertaining to or concerned with treatment of mentally retarded or seriously maladjusted children.

orthognathism, a condition in which the jaws have little or no forward projection.

orthognathous, having a nearly vertical facial profile; having jaws that do not protrude.

orthopaedic, see **orthopedic.**

orthopaedics, see **orthopedics.**

orthopaedist, see **orthopedist.**

orthopedic, of or pertaining to orthopedics.

orthopedics, the branch of surgery dealing with the correction of skeletal deformities and with the treatment of chronic diseases of bones and muscles, esp. of the joints and spine.

orthopedist, a physician who specializes in orthopedic surgery.

orthopnea, a condition in which breathing is uncomfortable in any but an erect sitting or standing position.

orthopsychiatric, of or pertaining to orthopsychiatry.

orthopsychiatrist, one who specializes in orthopsychiatry.

orthopsychiatry, a branch of psychiatry concerned with behavioral problems and the prevention and early treatment of emotional disorders, esp. among young people.

orthoptic, pertaining to or producing normal binocular vision, as, orthoptic exercises of the eye muscles to cure certain abnormal conditions, esp. strabismus.

orthoscopic, pertaining to, characterized, by or giving correct vision.

orthotonos, a form of muscular spasm marked by rigidity of the body, which is forced to be stretched out in a straight line.

os, 1. see **bone.** 2. a mouth; an opening or entrance.

oscillogram, the tracing or record made by an oscilloscope or oscillograph.

oscillograph, an instrument for measuring and recording alternating-current wave forms.

oscillographic, pertaining to an oscillograph.

oscillography, the process of recording alternating-current wave forms.

oscilloscope, an electronic optical device that pictures changes in electric current by means of a cathode ray tube.

osmics, the science of odors.

osmidrosis, a condition in which perspiration has an abnormally strong odor.

osmose, to subject to osmosis; to go through or be subjected to osmosis.

osmosis, 1. the tendency, when two solutions of differing concentrations are separated by a semipermeable membrane, for the solution of higher density to pass through the membrane until the two solutions are equalized in pressure. 2. an instance of this passage or diffusion.

ossa, bones.

ossein, the soft gluelike protein substance of bone left after the removal of the mineral matter.

osseous, bony.

ossicle, a small bone.

ossicula auditus, the three small bones in the middle ear.

ossiculectomy, surgical excision of one of the auditory ossicles.

ossiferous, forming, composed of, or containing bone or bony tissue.

ossification, 1. the act of ossifying. 2. the change or process of changing into a bony substance. 3. bone or bonelike tissue.

ossify, 1. to form into bone. 2. to change from a soft substance into bone or a substance of the hardness of bone. 3. to become bone or like bone in hardness or rigidity.

osteal, consisting of or pertaining to bone; osseous; bonelike.

ostectomy, surgical excision of a bone or part of a bone.

ostectopy, displacement of a bone.

osteitis, inflammation of the bone tissues or bone.

osteoarthritis, a deteriorative disease of the joints, most often afflicting older persons.

osteoarthropathy, any disease of the bones or the joints, usually accompanied by great pain.

osteoblast, a bone-forming cell.

osteoblastic, of or pertaining to an osteoblast.

osteoclasis, 1. the breaking down or absorption of osseous tissue. 2. the fracturing of a bone to correct deformity.

osteoclast, 1. one of the large multinuclear cells found in growing bone and involved in absorption of osseous tissue, as in the formation of canals. 2. an instrument for effecting osteoclasis.

osteodermia, the formation of bony tissue in the skin.

osteodystrophia, see **osteodystrophy.**

osteodystrophy, defective bone development or bone formation.

osteoectomy, see ostectomy.

osteoectopy, see **ostectopy.**

osteoid, bonelike; bony.

osteologist, a physician who specializes in osteology.

osteology, the branch of anatomy that deals with bones and their structure.

osteoma, a tumor composed of bony tissue.

osteomalacia, a condition marked by softening of the bones, caused by a lack of certain vitamins and minerals.

osteomyelitic, of or pertaining to osteomyelitis.

osteomyelitis, an inflammatory, suppurative disease of bones, resulting from an infection.

osteopath, one skilled in osteopathy.

osteopathic, of or pertaining to osteopathy.

osteopathy, a method of treament resting upon the supposition that most diseases are due to deformation of some part of the body and can be relieved or cured by manipulation of bones and muscles.

osteophyte, a small bony excrescence or outgrowth.

osteophytic, of or pertaining to an osteophyte.

osteoplastic, pertaining to bone formation or to osteoplasty.

osteoplasty, the transplanting, rebuilding, or inserting of bone to correct a defect or loss.

osteoporosis, excessive porosity of bone.

osteosclerosis, abnormal hardening of bone with increasing weight.

osteoseptum, the bony part of the septum of the

nose.

osteotome, a surgical instrument for cutting or dividing bone.

osteotomy, the dividing of a bone, or the excision of part of it.

ostiole, a small orifice, opening, or pore.

otalgia, see **earache.**

otectomy, surgical removal of the three small bones in the middle ear.

otic, belonging or relating to the ear.

otitis, inflammation of the ear.

otolaryngologist, a physician who specializes in otolaryngology.

otolaryngology, the branch of medicine concerned with the ear, nose, and throat.

otolith, a small calcareous body in the internal ear.

otologist, a physician who specializes in otology.

otology, the area of medicine that deals with the ear and its diseases.

otopharyngeal, of or pertaining to both the ear and the pharynx.

otopharyngeal tube, see **eustachian tube.**

otosalpinx, see **eustachian tube.**

otoscope, 1. an instrument for examining the internal parts of the ear. 2. an instrument for auscultation of the ear.

otoscopy, examination or auscultation of the ear with an otoscope.

ovarian, pertaining to or resembling the ovary.

ovariectomy, surgical removal of one or both ovaries.

ovariohysterectomy, surgical removal of the ovaries and the uterus.

ovariotomy, surgical incision or removal of an ovary.

ovaritis, inflammation of an ovary.

ovary, one of the pair of female reproductive glands in which ova and sex hormones are formed and developed.

overexert, to put forth excessively vigorous action or effort.

oversexed, having or giving evidence of an overly strong sexual urge.

over-the-counter, a medication or drug legally sold without a prescription.

overweight, weight beyond the customary or healthful amount.

oviduct, see **fallopian tube.**

oviductal, resembling an oviduct.

ovular, of or pertaining to an ovum.

ovulate, to produce or release an ovum from an ovary.

ovulation, the act of ovulating.

ovule, 1. a tiny egg. 2. an ovum, esp. when small, immature, or unfertilized.

ovum, 1. an egg, in a broad biological sense. 2. the female reproductive cell, which, after fertilization, is capable of developing into a new individual.

oxygen, a colorless, odorless, gaseous element constituting about one-fifth of the volume of the atmosphere, which supports combustion and plays an essential role in the respiratory process of all living creatures.

oxygenate, to treat or combine with oxygen.

oxygen mask, a device covering the nose and mouth of a patient and supplying oxygen from a tank.

oxygen tent, a protective cover that makes possible delivering and retaining pure oxygen to aid a patient's respiration.

oxyhemoglobin, hemoglobin combined with oxygen, found in arterial blood.

oxytocic, 1. accelerating childbirth. 2. stimulating contraction of the muscle of the uterus. 3. an oxytocic medicine.

oxytocin, a hormone that promotes contraction of smooth muscle of the uterus and release of breast milk.

ozone, a form of oxygen, having three atoms to the molecule, with an odor suggesting that of weak chlorine.

pacemaker, 1. the area in the right atrium that controls the heartbeat. 2. a small electronic device used to stimulate and control heart action in certain pathological conditions.

pachycephaly, an abnormal thickness of the walls of the skull.

pachydermatous, having an abnormally thick skin.

pachydermia, 1. abnormal thickening of the skin. 2. see **elephantiasis.**

pachymeningitis, an inflammation of the dura mater.

packing, filling up a wound or cavity with cotton gauze or similar material.

paediatrician, see **pediatrician.**

paediatrics, see **pediatrics.**

pain, 1. physical ache, discomfort, or distress because of injury, strain, or illness. 2. emotional or mental affliction or suffering; grief.

painful, giving or accompanied by pain; distressing.

painter's colic, a type of lead poisoning marked by a slow pulse and acute pain in the abdomen.

palatable, agreeable to the palate or taste; savory.

palatal, of, or pertaining to the palate.

palate, the roof of the mouth, which separates the nasal and the oral cavities and consists of the anterior bony arch, the hard palate, and the soft palate, a muscular tissue at the posterior part of the upper mouth.

palatine, 1. of or pertaining to the palate. 2. either of the two bones, right and left, that form the hard palate.

palatitis, an inflamed condition of the palate.

palatognathus, see **cleft palate.**

palatoplasty, plastic surgery of the palate, usually to repair a cleft.

palatoplegia, paralysis of the muscles of the soft palate.

palatum, see **palate.**

palilalia, pathological repetition of words or phrases.

palindromia, the recurrence of a disease or a relapse.

palingenesis, the reproduction of ancestral structures during the development of an embryo.

palingenetic, of or pertaining to palingenesis.

pallial, of or pertaining to the cerebral cortex.

palliate, to soothe.

palliative, something that soothes; something that relieves pain but does not cure.

pallid, pale, wan; deficient in color.

pallium, the cerebral cortex.

pallor, paleness; wanness.

palm, the part of the inner surface of the hand from the wrist to the base of the fingers.

palmar, 1. pertaining to or situated in the palm of the hand. 2. similar to or of the breadth of the hand.

palpable, 1. perceptible to the touch. 2. capable of being felt. 3. tangible. 4. easily perceived and detected; plain; obvious.

palpate, to examine by the sense of touch.

palpation, examination by touch or feeling, as with the hand, to assist in diagnosing an illness.

palpebra, see **eyelid.**

palpebra inferior, the lower eyelid.

palpebral, pertaining to or situated near the eyelid.

palpebra superior, the upper eyelid.

palpitate, 1. to pulsate violently, applied particularly to an abnormally rapid and strong beat of the heart, as from fright or disease. 2. to throb; to tremble; to quiver.

palpitation, the act of palpitating.

palsy, paralysis, esp. a progressive form of paralysis culminating late in life, characterized by tremors of the limbs, muscular weakness and rigidity, and a peculiar gait and attitude.

paludism, see **malaria.**

paludrine, a drug used to treat malaria.

panacea, 1. a supposed remedy for all diseases. 2. a cure-all. 3. a solution for any difficulty.

pancreas, a gland situated near the stomach, secreting an important digestive fluid, pancreatic juice, into the duodenum, and producing insulin.

pancreatalgia, pain in the pancreas.

pancreatectomy, surgical removal of the pancreas or part of it.

pancreatic, of or pertaining to the pancreas.

pancreatic juice, an alkaline fluid containing a mixture of digestive enzymes, discharged by the pancreas into the duodenum.

pancreatin, a preparation

made from the pancreas of cattle or hogs, used as a digestive.

pancreatitis, inflammation of the pancreas.

pandemic, 1. of a disease, prevalent throughout an entire country or continent, or the world. 2. general. 3. universal. 4. a pandemic disease.

pangenesis, the Darwinian theory, now abandoned, that hereditary attributes are transmitted by gemmules that are thrown off into free circulation by individual cells from every part of the organism, and that collect in the productive cells or bodies. Compare **blastogenesis.**

panhidrosis, perspiration over the entire body.

panhysterectomy, surgical excision of the entire uterus including the cervix uteri.

panic, 1. acute fear or demoralizing terror, often contagious in a group situation. 2. an instance, outbreak, or period of such fear.

panic-stricken, 1. affected with panic or extreme fear. 2. overwrought from fear.

panidrosis, see **panhidrosis.**

pannus, vascular tissue growing from the conjunctiva into the cornea of the eye.

pansinusitis, inflammation of all the nasal sinuses at the same time.

pant, 1. to breathe quickly or spasmodically, as after exertion or from excitement. 2. to gasp. 3. to throb or heave rapidly or violently.

pantalgia, an aching of the entire body.

papilla, 1. a nipple, or one of certain small protuberances such as the papillae of the tongue or of the skin of the fingertips. 2. a process at the root of a hair. 3. the optic disc.

papillary, 1. resembling a papilla. 2. of or pertaining to the breast nipple.

papillectomy, surgical removal of a papilla.

papilledema, see **papillitis.**

papillitis, swelling and inflammation of the optic disc.

papilloma, a benign tumor of the skin or a mucous membrane, as a wart or corn, consisting of a hypertrophied papilla or group of papillae.

papillomatosis, the condition of having many papillomas.

papillose, full of papillae.

pappataci fever, see **sandfly fever.**

Pap smear, an examination of cells for evidence of uterine cancer or of any condition interpreted as precancerous.

Pap test, see **Pap smear.**

papular, resembling a papule.

papule, a small, solid, somewhat pointed elevation of the skin, usually inflammatory but not forming pus.

paraaminobenzoic acid, a part of the vitamin B complex.

para-anesthesia, the loss of sensation of two corresponding sides of the body, as, loss of sensation in both legs.

parablosis, the fusion of two organisms, sometimes naturally as in the case of Siamese twins, or a union involving surgery, as the fusion of physiological functions.

parablotic, of or pertaining to parabiosis.

parablepsis, irregular vision.

paracanthoma, a tumor arising from the innermost layer of the epidermis.

paracardiac, adjacent to the heart.

paracentesis, the surgical puncture of a cavity to remove fluid.

parachromatopsia, see **colorblindness.**

paracusia, a disorder or defect of the sense of hearing.

paracyesis, extrauterine pregnancy.

paracystitis, inflammation of the tissues and other structures around the urinary bladder.

paradenitis, inflammation of tissues surrounding a gland.

paraesthesia, abnormal sensation, as prickling or itching of the skin.

parageusia, disorder of the sense of taste.

parahepatic, parts adjacent to the liver.

parahepatitis, inflammation of parts close to the liver.

paralambdacism, a

speech defect in which the letter "l" cannot be pronounced and is replaced by other letters.

paraldehyde, a colorless liquid formed by the polymerization of ordinary aldehyde, used in medicine as a hypnotic.

paralexia, see **dyslexia.**

paralogism, 1. a fallacious argument. 2. an instance of false reasoning.

paralogistic, of or pertaining to paralogism.

paralysis, 1. impairment or loss of the power of voluntary motion, or of sensation, in one or more parts of the body. 2. a disease characterized by this.

paralysis agitans, see **Parkinson's disease.**

paralytic, 1. a person afflicted with paralysis. 2. of or pertaining to paralysis.

paralyze, 1. to affect with paralysis. 2. to destroy the energy and power of.

paramedian, near the middle line of the body.

paramedic, a person who supplements the work of professional medical personnel.

paramenia, see **dysmenorrhea.**

paramnesia, the sensation or illusion of remembering something that has never been experienced. See **déjà vu.**

paranephritis, inflammation of tissues near the kidneys.

paranephros, see **adrenal gland.**

paranesthesia, see **para-anesthesia.**

paranoia, a mental disorder characterized chiefly by systematic delusions, esp. of persecution or grandeur.

paranoiac, a person affected by paranoia.

paranoid, of, like, or characterized by paranoia.

paranoid schizophrenia, a mental disorder similar to paranoia, but often accompanied by hallucinations and behavioral deterioration.

paraphasia, the misuse of spoken words; a form of asphasia.

paraphobia, a mild form of any phobia.

paraphonia, weakness, partial loss, or abnormal change of the voice.

paraphrasia, see **paraphasia.**

paraplectic, see **paraplegic.**

paraplegia, paralysis of both legs and the lower trunk.

paraplegic, 1. one who is afflicted with paraplegia. 2. of or pertaining to paraplegia.

parapsoriasis, see **psoriasis.**

parasalpingitis, inflammation of the tissues around a fallopian or the eustachian tube.

parasite, an animal or plant that lives on or in a living organism, often injuring the host.

parasitic, of, pertaining to, or caused by parasites.

parasiticide, an agent or preparation that destroys parasites.

parasitism, the state of being infested by para-

sites or suffering disease as a result of infestation.

parasitize, to invade or live upon, as a parasite.

parasitology, the branch of science that treats of parasitism.

parasitosis, see **parasitism.**

parastruma, enlargement of the parathyroid gland because of a goiterlike tumor.

parasympathetic nervous system, the section of the autonomic nervous system made up of nerves arising in the sacral and cranial regions, which slows the heartbeat, contracts the pupils, dilates blood vessels, and in general functions in contrast to the sympathetic nervous system.

parathyroidal, of or pertaining to the parathyroid glands.

parathyroidectomy, surgical excision of one or more parathyroid glands.

parathyroid gland, any of four small glands, lying near or embedded in the thyroid gland, which control the calcium content of the blood.

parathyroid hormone, the hormone secreted by the parathyroid glands.

paratyphoid, an infectious bacterial disease with symptoms resembling typhoid fever.

paregoric, 1. camphorated tincture of opium, used to assuage diarrhea. 2. a drug used in cough remedies. 3. an anodyne that relieves pain.

parencephalitis, inflammation of the cerebellum.

parencephalon, see **cerebellum.**

parenteral, 1. not through or in the intestine. 2. introduced in a way other than through the digestive tract.

paresis, incomplete paralysis, affecting motion but not sensation.

paresthesia, a spontaneous abnormal sensation, such as tingling, itching, burning, or numbness.

paresthetic, of or pertaining to paresthesia.

paretic, pertaining to or affected with paresis.

paridrosis, any disordered condition of perspiration.

paries (pl., parietes), a wall, as of a hollow organ.

parietal, 1. pertaining to the pair of bones forming part of the top and sides of the skull. 2. pertaining to parietes or structural walls of hollow organs. 3. referring to attachment to the wall of the ovary.

parietal bone, either of the two bones forming the top and sides of the part of the skull enclosing the brain.

parietes, see **paries.**

parkinsonism, 1. Parkinson's disease. 2. a group of nervous disorders, including Parkinson's disease, that have similar symptoms.

Parkinson's disease, a progressive form of paralysis marked by loss of flexibility in the muscles, tremor, and a jerky gait.

parodontism, inflammation of the tissues around a tooth.

parodynia, 1. difficult or abnormal labor or birth. 2. labor pain.

paroniria ambulans, see **sleepwalking.**

paronychia, see **whitlow.**

parorexia, an abnormal craving for strange foods.

parosmia, any disorder of the sense of smell.

parotid, of or pertaining to the parotid gland.

parotidectomy, surgical excision of a salivary gland.

parotid gland, either of the two salivary glands on the sides of the face, one in front of each ear.

parotiditis, inflammation of the parotid gland. See also **mumps.**

parotis, see **parotid gland.**

paroxysm, 1. a sudden and violent access of passion or emotion. 2. a fit. 3. any sudden intensification of a disease or symptom, esp. one occurring with regularity, as chills.

paroxysmal, 1. of the nature of a paroxysm. 2. occurring in or pertaining to paroxysms.

parrot fever, see **psittacosis, ornithosis.**

parthenogenesis, the development of an egg without fertilization, uncommon and occurring usually only in lower plants and invertebrates.

parturient, bringing forth or about to bring forth young.

parturition, the act of bringing forth young; childbirth.

parulis, a gumboil; an abscess beneath a tooth socket.

passive, 1. not active. 2. pertaining to certain inactive but unhealthy symptoms.

pasteurization, the method of pasteurizing liquids.

pasteurize, to subject, as milk, wine, beer, fruit juices, or other liquids, to a temperature ranging from 140 to 155°F for one-half hour, in order to kill the bacteria that cause fermentation.

pasteurizer, an apparatus used for pasteurizing.

Pasteur treatment, a treatment for preventing certain diseases, esp. hydrophobia, by a series of inoculations with a virus of gradually increasing strength.

pastille, 1. a sweetened lozenge, usually medicated. 2. a troche. 3. a small roll of aromatic paste for burning as a fumigant or disinfectant.

patella, see **kneecap.**

patellar, of or pertaining to the kneecap.

patellar reflex, see **knee jerk.**

pathetic, 1. causing or arousing pity or sorrow. 2. typified by arousing such emotions. 3. affecting the feelings.

pathogen, an agent producing disease.

pathogenesis, 1. the production or development of disease. 2. the mode of production or development of a disease.

pathogenetic, of or pertaining to pathogenesis.

pathogenic, causing disease.

pathogenicity, the state of being pathogenic.

pathogeny, see **pathogenesis.**

pathognomonic, 1. skilled in judging diseases. 2. indicative or characteristic of a particular disease.

pathological, of or pertaining to the causes of disease.

pathologist, one versed in pathology.

pathology, 1. the science dealing with the nature of diseases, their causes, symptoms, and effects. 2. the entire set of circumstances that constitute a diseased condition.

pathometer, an instrument that records such physical indications of emotional strain as fluctuating blood pressure, and may be employed as a lie detector. See also **polygraph.**

pathophobia, pathological fear of disease.

patient, 1. a person who is under medical treatment. 2. bearing pain without complaining. 3. not hasty.

peccant, see **morbid.**

pectoral, 1. of or pertaining to the breast or chest. 2. thoracic. 3. good for diseases of the thorax, as a medicine.

pectoral arch, see **pectoral girdle.**

pectoralgia, pain in the chest.

pectoral girdle, the arch formed by the shoulder

blade and collarbone.

pectoralis, one of four muscles of the upper frontal part of the chest.

pectus, see **chest, breast, thorax.**

pedal, pertaining to the foot.

pedalgia, foot pain.

pederasty, sexual relations between males through anal intercourse, esp. between a man and a young boy.

pediatrician, a physician specializing in pediatrics.

pediatrics, the science that deals with the medical care and diseases of children.

pediatrist, see **pediatrician.**

pedicle, see **peduncle.**

pedicular, 1. see **peduncular.** 2. of or pertaining to pediculosis.

pediculation, see **pedunculation.**

pediculosis, the state of being infested with lice.

pedodontia, see **pedodontics.**

pedodontics, the field or practice of dentistry that specializes in child dental care and treatment.

peduncle, 1. the stem that attaches a new growth, esp. some types of tumors that hang free on a stalk. 2. a stalklike structure in the brain.

peduncular, of or relating to a peduncle.

pedunculation, developing peduncles.

pellagra, a disease affecting the skin, digestive system, and nervous system, caused by niacin deficiency.

pellagrin, one who is afflicted with pellagra.

pellagrous, pertaining to or affected with pellagra.

pellicle, 1. a thin skin. 2. a membrane.

pellucid, admitting the passage of light; translucent; limpid or clear.

pelvic, of or pertaining to the pelvis.

pelvic girdle, the arch formed by the two innominate bones.

pelvic inlet, the upper pelvic entrance.

pelvic outlet, the lower pelvic opening.

pelvimeter, a device for measuring the pelvis.

pelvimetry, the measurement of pelvic dimensions, either manually or with X rays. It helps the gynecologist to determine whether it is possible to deliver the fetus through the normal route.

pelvis, the basinlike cavity in the lower part of the trunk, formed by the innominate bones, sacrum, and coccyx. 2. the bones forming this cavity. 3. the basinlike cavity into which the ureter expands at the hilum of the kidney.

pemphigus, a disease consisting of an eruption of large watery blisters on the skin and mucous membranes.

pendulous, 1. hanging so as to swing freely. 2. swinging. 3. undecided; vacillating.

penetrometer, an instrument for measuring the strength of X rays or other penetrating radiations.

penicillin, an antibiotic produced from molds of the genus **Penicillium,** effective in inhibiting the growth of a number of disease-producing bacteria, esp. cocci.

penicillium, any fungus, genus **Penicillium,** often found as mold on ripening cheese or decaying fruit, certain species being the source of penicillin.

penile, pertaining to the penis.

penis, the male sex organ formed primarily by erectile tissue, also serving as the organ of urination.

penitis, inflammation of the penis.

pennyroyal, a low European or American mint, both used medicinally and yielding a pungently aromatic oil.

pentobarbital, a barbituric acid, used as a sedative and hypnotic, esp. in its calcium or sodium salt form, and usually administered prior to an operation.

pentylenetetrazol, a white, bitter, powdery compound, used as a stimulant in respiratory and circulatory disorders and to bring about a convulsive state in certain types of mental disease.

peotomy, surgical removal of the penis.

pepsin, 1. an enzyme formed in the stomach that reduces proteins to proteoses and peptides. 2. an extract of this enzyme, from the stomach of hogs, sheep, or cows, used for aiding digestion.

pepsinogen, a zymogen found in the gastric glands that is converted into pepsin in a mild solution of hydrochloric acid.

peptic, 1. promoting or relating to digestion. 2. relating to pepsin. 3. a medicine that promotes digestion.

peptic ulcer, a term used to cover duodenal ulcer, gastric ulcer, and pyloric ulcer, collectively. See **ulcer.**

peptidase, one of a group of enzymes that hydrolyze peptides or peptones into amino acids.

peptide, a compound of amino acids involving the linking of a carboxyl group from one acid to an amino group from another acid.

peptone, any of a class of diffusible and soluble substances into which proteins are converted by the action of pepsin or trypsin.

peptonic, of or pertaining to peptone.

peptonization, the process of peptonizing.

peptonize, 1. to convert into a peptone. 2. to subject, as food, to artificial partial digestion by means of pepsin or pancreatic extract as an aid to digestion.

per anum, through or by way of the anus.

percuss, to strike or tap for diagnostic purposes.

percussion, the striking or tapping of a part of the

body for diagnostic purposes.

percutaneous, performed or effected through the skin; referring to a procedure in which a medicated ointment is applied by rubbing into the skin or by injection.

perflation, the process of blowing air into or through a cavity to expand its walls or to expel its contents.

perforans, perforating or penetrating.

perfusion, passing of a fluid into an organ through the blood vessels.

periadenitis, an inflammation of tissue surrounding a gland.

perianglitis, an inflammation of tissue surrounding a blood or lymphatic vessel.

periarterial, placed around an artery.

periarteritis, an inflammation of the external sheath of an artery.

pericardiac, of or pertaining to the pericardium.

pericardial, see **pericardiac.**

pericardiectomy, surgical excision of part or all of the pericardium.

pericardiotomy, surgical incision of the pericardium.

pericarditis, an inflammation of the pericardium.

pericardium, the membranous sac that encloses the heart.

perichondral, of or relating to the perichondrium.

perichondrium, the membrane of fibrous connective tissue covering the surface of cartilages except at the joints.

periconchal, around the cavity of the ear.

pericorneal, placed around the cornea of the eye.

pericranium, the membrane that forms the external covering of the skull.

pericystitis, an inflammation of the tissues surrounding the urinary bladder.

peridental, surrounding a tooth or part of a tooth.

peridentitis, see **periodontitis.**

perihepatitis, an inflammation of the membranes covering the liver.

perimeter, a device for measuring the extent of the visual field.

perimetry, measurement of the scope of the field of vision with a perimeter.

perineal, of, concerning, or pertaining to the perineum.

perineorrhaphy, the closing of a wound in the perineum by suture. The wound is usually caused by laceration following labor.

perineotomy, surgical incision of the perineum, usually done to facilitate childbirth.

perineum, 1. the region between the anus and the genital organs. 2. the region of the body including the passageway for the rectum and genitourinary ducts.

perinurium, the sheath of

connective tissue that encloses a funiculus or bundle of nerve fibers.

period, the time of each month during which a woman menstruates.

periodic, 1. performed at intermittent intervals. 2. happening or returning regularly; recurring.

periodicity, the state or quality of being periodic.

periodontal, relating to the periodontium or to periodontics.

periodontics, the division of dentistry dealing with diseases of the periodontium and their treatment.

periodontist, a dentist who specializes in periodontics.

periodontitis, an inflammation or degeneration of the bone, gum, or connective tissue around a tooth.

periodontium, the bone, gum, and connective tissue around a tooth.

perionychia, an inflammation around a fingernail or toenail.

perionychium, the skin adjoining the sides and base of a fingernail or toenail.

periost, see **periosteum.**

periosteal, of or pertaining to the periosteum.

periosteotomy, surgical incision of the periosteum.

periosteum, a vascular membrane investing and nourishing the bones.

periostitis, an inflammation of the periosteum.

periotic, 1. surrounding the ear. 2. noting or pertaining to certain bones or bony elements that form or help to form a protective capsule for the internal ear, being usually confluent or fused, and constituting part of the temporal bone.

peripheral, relating to the external or outer surface.

periphlebitis, an inflammation of the external coat of a vein or the tissue surrounding a vein.

periprostatitis, an inflammation of the tissues surrounding the prostate gland.

perisalpingitis, an inflammation of the surrounding peritoneal coat of the oviduct.

peristaltic, of or pertaining to peristalsis.

peristalsis, the automatic constriction and relaxation of a tubelike muscular organ or system, as the intestines, which slowly propels the contents forward.

perisystole, the interval between the systoles in the cardiac rhythm.

perithelioma, a tumor originating in the perithelial layer of the blood vessels.

perithelium, the fibrous connective tissue of the smaller blood vessels and capillaries.

peritoneal, of or relating to the peritoneum.

peritoneum, a thin, smooth, serous membrane lining the whole internal surface of the abdomen and investing most of the viscera.

peritonitis, an inflammation of the peritoneum.

permanent tooth, any of the teeth that supplant the milk teeth; in man, one of the 32 teeth that supplant the 20 temporary teeth of babyhood.

permanganate, a dark purple salt containing potassium, manganese, and oxygen, and used in solution as an oxidizer and disinfectant.

pernicious, injurious; destructive; deadly; very severe.

pernicious anemia, a severe type of anemia caused by malformation of red blood cells, and resulting in lesions of the spinal cord, gastrointestinal, muscular, and nervous disturbances, and other complications.

perone, see **fibula.**

peroneal, pertaining to or positioned near the fibula.

peroral, by mouth; administered through the mouth.

per os, see **peroral.**

perspiration, 1. the process or act of perspiring. 2. the watery fluid or sweat excreted from the pores.

perspire, 1. to excrete perspiration through the pores of the skin. 2. to sweat.

pertussis, see **whooping cough.**

perversion, 1. abnormal sexual instinct, desire, or activity. 2. a change to what is unnatural or abnormal.

pervert, one who is affected with perversion.

perverted, changed to or being of an unnatural or abnormal kind.

pervious, 1. capable of being penetrated. 2. permeable. 3. allowing entrance or passage through.

pes, 1. a part resembling or serving as a foot. 2. see **foot.**

pes planus, see **flatfoot.**

pessary, 1. a device introduced into the vagina to correct uterine displacement. 2. a vaginal suppository. 3. a contraceptive device.

pest, see **plague.**

pestiferous, 1. pestilential. 2. infectious. 3. noxious or evil.

pestilence, any contagious disease that is epidemic and usually deadly, esp. bubonic plague.

pestilential, 1. producing or tending to produce infectious disease. 2. having the nature of an infectious and deadly disease. 3. destructive.

petechia, a small purplish spot occurring on the skin or in certain membranes, caused by hemorrhaging.

petechial, characterized by the presence of petechiae.

petrolatum, a purified, semisolid, unctuous substance obtained from petroleum and used in medical dressings and ointments.

petroleum jelly, see **petrolatum.**

petroprotein, a man-made edible protein obtained from bacteria fed on paraffin derived from petroleum.

petrosal, relating to the petrous portion of the temporal bone or to a homologous bone.

petrous, 1. like stone; hard; stony. 2. pertaining to the hard portion of the temporal bone in which the internal organs of hearing are situated.

phagedena, a severe destructive eroding ulcer.

phagocyte, a leukocyte that destroys and absorbs harmful bacteria, foreign matter, and inert cells in the bloodstream.

phagocytic, of or pertaining to phagocytosis.

phagocytosis, the absorption and destruction of bacteria, etc., by phagocytes.

phagomania, abnormal, uncontrollable craving for food.

phagophobia, pathological fear of eating.

phalange, see **phalanx.**

phalangeal, of or pertaining to the fingers or toes.

phalangitis, inflamed condition of one or more fingers or toes.

phalanx, any of the digital bones of the hand or foot.

phallic, of or pertaining to the phallus.

phallicism, worship of the phallus, as the symbol of creative power.

phallicist, one who belongs to the worshipers of the phallus.

phallism, see **phallicism.**

phallitis, an inflammation of the phallus.

phallus, see **penis.**

phantom limb, an illusion that an amputated limb still exists.

phantom pain, the sensation of having pain in a limb or part of a limb that was amputated.

pharmaceutical, 1. pertaining to the knowledge or art of pharmacy. 2. a medicine or drug product.

pharmaceutics, the science of preparing medicines.

pharmacist, 1. one skilled in the practice of pharmacy. 2. a druggist.

pharmacodynamics, the division of pharmacology that deals with the action of drugs and their effect upon the body.

pharmacognosy, the branch of pharmacology that deals with sources, characteristics, and possible uses of medicinal substances in their natural or unprepared state.

pharmacologic, of or pertaining to pharmacology.

pharmacologist, one skilled in or engaged in the science of pharmacology.

pharmacology, the science or knowledge of drugs, or the art of preparing medicine.

pharmacopoeia, 1. a book of directions and requirements for the preparation of medicines, generally published by an authority. 2. a collection or stock of drugs.

pharmacy, 1. the art of preparing and compounding medicines, and of dispensing them according to the prescriptions of medical practitioners. 2. the place where medicines are compounded or dispensed. 3. a drugstore.

pharyngeal, of, relating to, or produced in the pharynx.

pharyngitis, inflammation of the pharynx.

pharyngology, the science concerned with the pharynx and its ailments.

pharyngoparalysis, paralysis of the pharynx.

pharynx, the muscular tube that connects the mouth and the esophagus.

phase, a distinct stage in mitosis or meiosis.

phenacaine, a crystalline compound, usually administered in its hydrochloridic form as a local anesthetic, esp. for the eyes.

phenacetin, a compound, of coal-tar origin, used to relieve nervous headaches, neuralgia, or fever.

phenobarbital, a crystalline barbiturate, usually in white powder form, used as a hypnotic or sedative.

phenolphthalein, a white crystalline compound formed by the interaction of phenol and phthalic anhydride, used medicinally and to indicate the presence of alkalis, which turn it red, and of acids, which decolorize.

phenol red, a red crystalline acid-base indicator, also used in medical analysis.

phial, see **vial.**

phimosis, narrowness of the foreskin that prevents it from being pushed back over the glans penis.

phlebitis, inflammation of the inner membrane of a vein.

phlebotomist, one who opens a vein for letting blood.

phlebotomize, to bleed by opening a vein.

phlebotomy, the act or practice of opening a vein for letting blood.

phlegm, the thick mucus secreted in the respiratory passages.

phlegmatic, 1. sluggish in temperament. 2. apathetic. 3. self-possessed. 4. impassive.

phlyctena, a small watery pustule or blister.

phlyctenula, a small phlyctena.

phlyctenular, of or relating to a phlyctenula.

phlyctenule, see **phlyctenula.**

phobia, a morbid, abnormal, persistent, exaggerated, and usually illogical fear or dread.

phonation, the act of uttering vocal sounds.

phonatory, of or pertaining to utterance of vocal sounds.

phonetic, pertaining to sounds, their physical production, and written representation.

phonic, pertaining to voice, sound, or speech.

phosphatase, an enzyme secreted by the liver that hydrolyzes and synthesizes phosphoric acid esters.

phosphocreatine, an organic compound, found in muscle tissue, which furnishes the energy for contractions.

phospholipid, one of a group of lipoidal compounds, such as lecithin and cephalin, which are phosphoric esters and are found in living cells throughout nature.

photalgia, pain caused by intense light.

photic, pertaining to light or to organisms producing light.

photodermatitis, skin disorders caused by excessive exposure to light, for instance, sunburn.

photophobia, an intolerance or dread of light.

photopia, vision in bright lighting conditions.

photopsia, the sensation of flashes of light or sparks of light, purely subjective, occurring in certain retinal, optic, or brain disorders.

phototherapy, exposure to sun or artificial light rays for the treatment of disease.

phrenalgia, 1. pain in the diaphragm. 2. pain, depression, or melancholia caused by a mental process.

phrenasthenia, 1. mental feebleness. 2. paralysis of the diaphragm.

phrenic, 1. pertaining to the mind or activity of the mind. 2. pertaining to the diaphragm.

phrenology, the theory that mental powers consist of independent faculties, each of which has its seat in a definite brain region whose size, supposedly indicated by the shape of the skull over it, is commensurate with the development of the particular faculty. The system has no basis in fact.

phthiriasis, see **pediculosis.**

phylaxis, the active defense of the body itself against infection.

physiatrics, 1. a division of medicine that deals with the treatment of diseases or injuries by such physical or natural means as massage, manipulation, heat, and mud baths. 2. any kind of physical therapy. See **physiotherapy.**

physic, 1. any medicine. 2. a medicine that purges. 3. a purge. 4. a cathartic. 5. to purge with a cathartic. 6. to remedy.

physical, 1. pertaining to the body, bodily. 2. obvious to the senses.

physical education, a course of athletic training and hygiene to develop and care for the body.

physician, 1. one legally qualified to practice medicine. 2. a doctor engaged in general medical practice as distinguished from one specializing in a certain field of medicine. 3. one who is skilled in the art of healing.

physiognomy, 1. the face or countenance regarded as an indication or revelation of character. 2. the art of discerning character from the features of the body, esp. the face.

physiological, 1. of or pertaining to physiology. 2. agreeing or in accord with the normal or appropriate functioning of a healthy organism.

physiologist, one who studies physiology.

physiology, 1. the science dealing with the normal functions of living organisms or their organs. 2. the collective functions and vital processes of living matter.

physiotherapy, the treatment of disease, bodily weaknesses, or defects by physical remedies, such as massage and exercise.

physique, the physical or bodily structure, appearance, or constitution.

physostigmine, a poisonous alkaloid constituting the active principle of the Calabar bean, used in medicine as a myotic in glaucoma.

pial, belonging or relating to the pia mater.

pia mater, the delicate, fibrous, highly vascular membrane forming the innermost of the three coverings enveloping the brain and spinal cord. See **arachnoid** and **dura mater.**

pica, an unnatural craving for substances not normally considered food, as chalk or clay.

pigeon breast, a malformation of the chest in which there is abnormal projection of the sternum and the sternal region, often associated with rickets. Also called **chicken breast.**

pigment, any substance whose presence in the tissues or cells colors them.

pigmentary, relating to or forming pigment.

pigmentation, coloration with or deposition of pigment, esp. excessive deposition of skin pigment.

pigmented, colored by a deposit of pigment.

pilar, of, pertaining to, or covered with hair.

pilary, see **pilar.**

piles, see **hemorrhoids.**

pill, a small, usually globular or rounded mass of medicinal substance, to be swallowed whole.

pilose, covered with hair, usually soft, downy hair.

pilosis, excessive growth of hair.

pilosity, hairiness.

pimple, 1. a small elevation of the skin with an inflamed base. 2. see **pustule.**

pineal, pertaining to the pineal body.

pineal body, a small, usually cone-shaped body in the brain having no proven function but believed variously to be a vestigial sense or an endocrine organ. Also called **pineal gland.**

pinkeye, 1. contagious inflammation of the mucous membrane of the eyelids, affecting humans and certain animals. 2. acute conjunctivitis.

pinna, the auricle, or external ear.

pinnal, of or pertaining to the pinna.

pinworm, a small nematoid worm, infesting the intestine and rectum, esp. of children.

pisiform, having the form of a pea.

pisiform bone, a small bone of the wrist.

pitting, a function or process that makes pits, such as the hollows left by smallpox.

pituitary, 1. of or pertaining to the pituitary gland. 2. describing a form of giantism resulting from glandular malfunction. 3. the pituitary gland. 4. any of several hormone extracts taken from the pituitary gland.

pituitary gland, a small, oval-shaped endocrine gland situated at the base of the brain and secreting hormones with a broad range of effects on growth, metabolism, maturation, and other bodily functions.

Pituitrin, an extract of the pituitary gland, usually of cattle (trademark).

pityriasis, a skin disease occurring in humans and some domestic animals, consisting of irregular branlike scaly patches shed by the epidermis.

pivot tooth, a replacement crown connected by a pivot to the root of a tooth.

placebo, a preparation with little or no therapeutic value given merely to please the patient, or given as a control in experiments testing the effectiveness of a genuine drug.

placenta, the organ by which the fetus is attached to the wall of the uterus and through which the fetus receives nourishment and voids waste matter.

placental, of or pertaining to the placenta.

placentation, 1. the attachment or means of attachment of a fetus to the wall of the uterus. 2. the manner of the disposition or construction of a placenta.

placentitis, inflammation of the placenta.

plague, 1. a widespread disease with a high mortality rate. 2. pestilence, specifically a virulent, infectious, and febrile disease caused by the bacillus *Pasteurella pestis,* primarily a rodent disease but transmitted to men by fleas and occurring in several forms: bubonic, pneumonic, and septicemic.

planomania, an abnormal desire to wander and to have no social restraints.

planta, the sole of the foot.

plantar, relating or belonging to the sole of the foot.

plantar wart, a usually very painful wart occurring on the sole of the foot.

plaque, a small, flat, rounded, abnormal formation or area, as on the skin.

plasma, 1. a nearly colorless fluid in which the

corpuscles of the blood are suspended. 2. a human blood product used for transfusions and prepared by removing all red cells, white cells, and platelets from whole blood.

plasma membrane, see **cell membrane.**

plasmin, a proteolytic enzyme in the bloodstream causing fibrin breakdown and the dissolving of clots. Also called **fibrinolysin.**

plasmolysis, shrinkage and dissolution of the protoplasm in a living cell when excessive water loss occurs by exosmosis.

plasmolytic, of or pertaining to plasmolysis.

plastic surgeon, a surgeon who specializes in plastic surgery.

plastic surgery, surgery undertaken to restore or repair lost, malformed, or injured bones, other tissues, or organs of the body. See **anaplasty.**

platelet, 1. a minute plate or platelike body. 2. a blood platelet, see **thrombocyte.**

platycephalic, having a wide skull, excessively flattened from top to bottom.

platyhelminth, any of the Platyhelminthes, a phylum or group of worms having bilateral symmetry and a soft, usually flattened body, including tapeworms, planarians, and flukes. Also called **flatworm.**

platyrhine, having a short broad nose.

plethora, 1. congestion. 2. excess volume of blood.

plethoric, of or pertaining to plethora.

pleura, a thin membrane that covers the inside of the thorax and also invests the lungs.

pleural, of or pertaining to the pleura.

pleuralgia, pain coming from the pleura.

pleurectomy, a surgical excision of part of the pleura.

pleurisy, an inflammation of the pleura, often accompanied by fever and respiratory difficulties.

pleuritic, of or pertaining to pleurisy.

pleuropneumonia, an inflammation of the pleura and of the lungs.

plexor, a small hammer with a soft rubber head or the like, used in percussion for diagnostic purposes.

plexus, 1. a network of vessels, nerves, or fibers. 2. any complicated structure forming a network of interlacing parts.

plica, 1. a fold or folding, as of skin. 2. a matted, filthy condition of the hair caused by disease.

plicate, 1. pleated. 2. folded like a fan.

plumbism, poisoning by lead taken into the system.

pneumatogram, a tracing made by a pneumatograph.

pneumatograph, an instrument for measuring

the force or the quantity of air inhaled into the lungs at each inhalation and given out at each exhalation.

pneumatometer, see **pneumatograph.**

pneumectomy, see **pneumonectomy.**

pneumobacillus, the bacillus **Klebsiella pneumoniae,** associated with a type of pneumonia and other respiratory infections.

pneumococcal, of or pertaining to pneumococcus.

pneumococcus, a bacterium, **Diplococcus pneumoniae,** causing lobar pneumonia and other infectious diseases.

pneumoconiosis, an occupational disorder of the respiratory tract caused by inhalation of dust particles, mineral dust, or coal dust.

pneumogastric, 1. pertaining to the lungs and the stomach. 2. the pneumogastric nerve, see **vagus.**

pneumomassage, massage of the tympanum by pneumatic pressure.

pneumomyelography, X-ray examination of the spinal canal after injection of air.

pneumonectomy, surgical removal of all or part of a lung.

pneumonia, 1. an inflammation of the lungs. 2. an acute infectious disease of the lungs, either viral or bacteriological in origin.

pneumonic, 1. pertaining to the lungs. 2. pulmonary.

3. relating to or having pneumonia.

pneumonometer, an apparatus for measuring the capacity of the lungs. See **spirometer.**

pneumothorax, the presence of air or gas in the pleural cavity, sometimes used therapeutically in collapsing a lung.

pock, 1. a pustule raised on the surface of the body in an eruptive disease, as smallpox. 2. a pit or scar left on the skin by such a disease.

pockmark, a mark or scar on the skin made by smallpox or other disease.

podagra, gout, esp. in the foot or big toe.

podalgia, see **pedalgia.**

podiatrist, one who diagnoses and treats disorders of the human foot. See also **chiropodist.**

podophyllin, a resin obtained from the rhizome of the mayapple, used in medicine as a purgative.

pogoniasis, abnormally strong growth of beard, esp. on women.

poison, any agent, biological or chemical, that destroys life or health upon contact with or absorption by an organism.

polio, see **poliomyelitis.**

polioencephalitis, inflammatory lesions of the gray matter of the brain.

poliomyelitis, inflammation of the gray matter of the spinal cord, esp. an infectious form causing motor paralysis followed by atrophy of the muscles and sometimes lasting disability.

pollex, see **thumb.**

pollex pedis, the big toe.

pollinosis, see **hay fever.**

pollutant, something that pollutes, esp. chemicals or refuse material released into the atmosphere or water.

pollute, to make foul or unclean, as, soil, air, or water.

pollution, the act of polluting.

polychromatic, exhibiting many colors.

polyclinic, a general, nonspecialized clinic or hospital dealing with various diseases.

polycythemia, a condition in which red blood cells are abnormally increased in number.

polycythemic, of or pertaining to polycythemia.

polydactyl, having many fingers or toes, esp. more than the normal number.

polydipsia, abnormal thirst.

polydontia, having more than the normal number of teeth.

polyembryony, the production of two or more embryos from a single fertilized egg.

polygenesis, the doctrine that beings have their origin in many cells of different kinds, opposed to **monogenesis.**

polygraph, see **pathometer.**

polynuclear, having more than one nucleus.

polyp, a bulging or projecting mass of tissue that may be new growth, a center of infection, a malformation, or degenerative tissue.

polyphagous, eating or subsisting on many kinds of food.

polyphagia, excessive or extreme desire to eat.

polypnea, extremely heavy panting or breathing.

polyptome, a surgical instrument for removing polyps.

polyspermia, excessive secretion of seminal fluid.

polythelia, the presence of more than one nipple on a breast.

polyunsaturated, of or pertaining to animal or vegetable fats having two or more double bonds per molecule; when consumed by humans, they help to lower the cholesterol content of the blood.

polyvalent, pertaining to vaccine having several strains of antibodies.

pons, a band of nerve fibers in the brain connecting the lobes of the cerebellum, medulla, and cerebrum. Also called **pons Varolii.**

popeyed, having wide, bulging eyes.

popliteal, of or pertaining to the ham, the part of the leg in the back of the knee.

pore, a minute opening, as in the skin, through which fluids and other substances are excreted.

porosis, 1. formation of pores or cavities. 2. increased translucency to X rays.

porosity, state or property of being porous.

porous, having many pores or interstices.

porphyrin, any of a group of metal-free pyrrole derivatives, formed in protoplasm by the decomposition of hemoglobin and chlorophyll.

porphyrinemia, the presence of porphyrins in the blood.

portal, 1. noting or pertaining to the transverse fissure of the liver. 2. the portal vein.

portal vein, a large vein carrying blood from the stomach, intestine, pancreas, and spleen to the liver.

position, attitude or posture of the body, as, in a prone position.

posological, of or pertaining to posology.

posology, the branch of scientific study that deals with the dosage of medicines.

postclimacteric, occurring after the menopause.

posterior, the hinder part of the body; the buttocks.

posthumous, occurring or continuing after death.

posthumous child, 1. a child born after the death of the father. 2. a child taken by cesarean operation after the death of the mother.

posthypnotic, of or pertaining to the period of time following hypnosis.

postmortem, 1. subsequent to death, as an examination of the body. 2. a postmortem exami-

nation. See **autopsy.**

postmortem examination, see **autopsy.**

postnasal, 1. pertaining to the posterior cavities of the nose. 2. occurring behind the nose, as, postnasal drip.

postnatal, subsequent to birth.

postpartum, after childbirth.

postprandial, happening after a meal, esp. dinner.

postulate, 1. something postulated or assumed without proof as a basis for reasoning or as self-evident. 2. a fundamental principle. 3. an axiom. 4. a prerequisite.

posture, the position or carriage of the body and limbs as a whole.

potable, suitable for drinking.

potassium permanganate, a nearly black crystalline compound, used as an oxidizing agent, an astringent, and a disinfectant.

potency, the state or quality of being potent.

potent, 1. producing powerful physical or chemical effects, as a drug. 2. possessing sexual power, usually said of a male.

potion, 1. a draft or drink. 2. a liquid supposedly having magical or poisonous powers.

Pott's disease, caries of the vertebrae usually caused by a tubercular infection, often resulting in marked curvature of the spine.

pouch, 1. a baglike or

pocketlike part. 2. a sac or cyst.

poultice, 1. a soft dressing composed of meal, bread, or other mollifying substance, to be applied to sore or inflamed parts of the body. 2. a cataplasm.

pox, an eruptive disease characterized by pustules, as chicken pox.

practical nurse, a nurse, lacking a diploma as a registered nurse, but with sufficient training and skills to care for the sick professionally.

preadolescence, the years immediately preceding adolescence, usually from ages 9 to 12.

precancerous, of or pertaining to a condition of the tissues which, while not cancerous, may develop into cancer, as certain skin growths.

precipitant, a substance which, when added to a solution, induces precipitation.

precipitation, the process by which a substance is made to separate from another or others in a solution and fall to the bottom.

precipitin, an antibody formed in the blood that precipitates certain proteins when it unites with its antigen.

precocious, 1. forward in development, esp. mental development, as a child or young person. 2. prematurely developed, as the mind or faculties. 3. pertaining to or showing premature development.

preconscious, 1. pertaining to material absent from consciousness but readily recalled. 2. a portion of the mind on the borderline between consciousness and the unconscious.

precritical, pertaining to the period that precedes the crucial stage of disease.

predigest, to treat, as food, by an artificial process, to make it more digestible.

predisposition, a tendency, acquired or hereditary, to develop a certain disease.

pregnable, 1. capable of being taken or won by force. 2. vulnerable.

pregnancy, the state, period, or quality of being pregnant.

pregnant, 1. carrying a fetus in the womb. 2. being with child. 3. showing fertility.

prehensile, capable of or adapted to seizing or grasping.

prehension, a taking hold of or seizing.

premature, happening, arriving, existing, or done before the proper time.

premaxilla, one of a pair of bones in front of the upper jaw, situated between the maxillary bones.

premaxillary, situated in front of the maxilla.

premedical, pertaining to or engaged in studies preparatory to the professional study of medicine. Also called colloq. **premed.**

premedication, induction of a state of unconsciousness by internal drugs prior to giving general anesthesia.

premenstrual, pertaining to the period just prior to menstruation.

premolar, 1. noting or pertaining to the teeth situated in front of the molars. 2. a premolar tooth. Also **bicuspid.**

premonition, 1. a sense of foreboding concerning the future without factual substantiation. 2. previous warning, notice, or information.

premonitory, giving previous warning or notice.

prenatal, previous to birth.

preoperative, prior to an operation.

prepuce, see **foreskin.**

preputial, relating to the prepuce.

presbyatrics, see **geriatrics.**

presbyopia, an imperfection of vision in which near objects are seen less distinctly than those at a distance, common in old age.

presbyopic, of or pertaining to presbyopia.

prescribe, to designate or order for use, as a remedy or treatment.

prescriptible, 1. suitable for or subject to being prescribed. 2. depending upon or derived from prescription.

prescription, 1. a physician's direction, usually written, for the prepara-

tion and use of a medicine or remedy. 2. the medicine prescribed. 3. the act of prescribing.

presentation, the part of the unborn baby that is felt first when an examination is made through the opening of the uterus or rectum after labor has begun.

pressor, stimulating, as, a pressor nerve, a nerve whose stimulation causes an increase of blood pressure.

pressure sore, see **bedsore.**

presystole, the period of time before the systole of the heart.

preventive, 1. pertaining to a vaccine or medication for preventing disease. 2. a precautionary agent or measure. 3. a drug or other substance for preventing disease. Also **preventative.**

prickly heat, a cutaneous eruption accompanied by a prickly and itching sensation, resulting from an inflammation of the sweat glands.

primary atypical pneumonia, a typically mild form of pneumonia, probably of viral origin.

primary lesion, an original lesion from which a second one develops.

primary sore, 1. the initial sore of syphilis or chancre. 2. hardsore.

primipara, a woman who has borne but one child, or who is parturient for the first time.

primiparity, the state of

being a primipara.

privates, the external organs of sex; also called **private parts.**

probang, a long, slender, elastic rod with a sponge, ball, or the like at the end, used for removing foreign bodies from the esophagus or the larynx, or for applying medicine in those areas.

probe, an instrument for examining the depth or other circumstances of a wound, ulcer, or cavity.

procaine, a compound used in the form procaine hydrochloride as a local anesthetic.

process, a bony prominence, or other projecting outgrowth or protuberance, as of tissue, in an organism.

procreant, 1. procreating or generating. **2.** pertaining to procreation.

procreate, 1. to beget. **2.** to generate and produce. **3.** to reproduce.

procreation, the act of begetting or producing offspring.

proctalgia, pain in the anus or rectum.

proctectomy, surgical excision of the rectum or anus.

proctology, the branch of medical science dealing with the anal region and the rectum.

proctoplasty, plastic surgery for repair of the rectum or anus.

proctoscope, an instrument for interior examination of the rectum.

proctoscopy, examination of the rectum with a proctoscope.

proctostomy, a surgical operation to create a permanent opening into the rectum.

prodromal, of or relating to a prodrome.

prodrome, a premonitory symptom.

progeria, premature senility, usually occurring in childhood.

progestational, relating to certain alterations in the uterus requisite for the fertilization and growth of the ovum; receptive to pregnancy.

progesterone, 1. a female sex hormone produced in the ovaries that prepares the uterus for reception and development of the fertilized ovum. **2.** a form of this hormone obtained from pregnant cows or by synthesis.

prognathous, characterized by forward-projecting jaws, contrasted with **opithognathous.**

prognosis, a forecast of the probable course of a disease and the probability of recovery.

prognostic, of or pertaining to prognosis.

prognosticate, to foretell by means of present signs.

prognostication, the act of prognosticating.

progressive, of a disease, continuously increasing in extent or severity.

prolactin, a hormone of the pituitary gland that stimulates production of milk in the nursing female.

prolamin, one of a group of simple proteins obtained from gluten of grain, as wheat or oats, and insoluble in pure water, absolute alcohol, and neutral solvents.

prolamine, see **prolamin.**

prolan, a hormone similar to the pituitary sex hormones and present in the urine of pregnant women, permitting early diagnosis of pregnancy.

prolapse, 1. to fall or slip down or out of place. 2. a falling of an organ or part, as the uterus, from its normal position.

proliferation, growth and production by multiplication.

proline, an amino acid found in proteins.

promontory, a bodily protuberance.

pronation, 1. the motion of the arm whereby the palm of the hand is turned downward. 2. the position of the hand with the thumb toward the body and the palm downward.

pronator, a muscle of the forearm that turns the palm downward.

prone, 1. lying with face downward. 2. the position of the hand with the palm turned downward. 3. inclined, as to sickness, by disposition or natural tendency.

propagate, 1. to breed. 2. to continue or multiply by sexual reproduction.

propagation, 1. the act of propagating. 2. multiplication of the kind or species by generation or reproduction.

prophage, an intracellular bacterial virus that protects its host from active viruses.

prophase, the initial stage of cell division in which the chromosomes become distinct in the nucleus and divide longitudinally.

prophasic, of or pertaining to prophase.

prophylactic, 1. a medicine that protects or defends against disease. 2. a preventive device, as a contraceptive.

prophylaxis, preventive or protective treatment against disease.

proprioceptive, having the ability to receive stimuli originating within such body tissues as muscles and tendons.

proprioceptor, the peripheral end organ of nerves in organs that are responsive to internal stimuli.

proptosis, an outward displacement or protuberance of any organ, specifically bulging of the eyeballs.

prosector, one who dissects cadavers for the illustration of anatomical lectures or the like.

prosencephalon, the forebrain; the anterior part of the brain.

prosencephalic, of or pertaining to the forebrain.

prosoponeuralgia, facial neuralgia.

prosopoplegia, facial paralysis.

prostatalgia, pain in the prostate gland.

prostate, designating or pertaining to the prostate gland.

prostate gland, an organ, part muscle and part gland, that surrounds the male urethra at the base of the bladder and secretes a milky fluid ejected with the sperm.

prostatic, of or pertaining to the prostate gland.

prostatism, a condition resulting from a chronically diseased or enlarged prostate gland.

prostatitis, inflammation of the prostate gland.

prostatovesiculectomy, surgical removal of the prostate gland and the seminal vesicles.

prosthesis, an artificial part to supply a defect of the body.

prosthetics, the branch of surgery specializing in artificial replacements, as of limbs or teeth.

prosthodontics, the branch of dentistry dealing with the making of artificial teeth and other oral structures needed to replace missing or injured parts of the chewing apparatus; prosthetic dentistry. Also called **prosthodontia.**

prosthodontist, one who specializes in prosthodontics.

prostrate, 1. exhausted. 2. lying with body extended.

prostration, extreme physical weakness or exhaustion, as, heat prostration.

protamine, any of a class of simple, basic proteins, soluble in ammonia, uncoagulable by heat, and forming amino acids upon hydrolysis.

protease, any enzyme that exerts a digestive action on proteins.

protein, one of a class of complex chemical compounds that contain carbon, hydrogen, nitrogen, oxygen, and sulfur, are essential constituents of living matter, and on decomposition yield various amino acids.

proteinase, any of several enzymes, as pepsin and rennin, that hydrolyze proteins.

proteinic, of or pertaining to protein.

proteolysis, the hydrolysis or breaking down of proteins into simpler compounds, as in digestion.

proteolytic, of or pertaining to proteolysis.

proteose, any of a class of compounds produced in digestion and derived from proteins by hydrolysis.

prothrombin, a proenzyme in the blood that, when activated, becomes thrombin, a substance that then changes fibrogen into fibrin and brings about blood coagulation. Also called **thrombogen.**

protodiastole, the first of four phases of ventricular diastole.

protopathic, responding solely and undiscriminatingly to gross stimuli, as extreme pain, opposed to **epicritic.**

protoplasm, a complex substance, typically colorless and of viscid semifluid consistency, regarded as the physical basis of life, having the powers of spontaneous motion and reproduction; the living matter of all vegetable and animal cells and tissues.

protoplasmic, of or pertaining to protoplasm.

protozoan, any of the animals in the first or lowest zoological division or phylum, Protozoa, comprising single-celled, microscopic organisms.

protozoology, the science or study of protozoans, a division of zoology.

proud flesh, a colloquial term for an excessive development of granulations in wounds and ulcers.

provitamin, that which can become a vitamin when acted upon by certain substances in the body, as carotene, which is changed by liver action into vitamin A.

proximal, nearest the point of attachment or insertion, as the extremity of a bone or limb, opposed to **distal.**

prurient, 1. inclined or inclining to lascivious thoughts. 2. bringing about lasciviousness or lust. 3. eagerly desirous.

pseudesthesia, the sensation of itching or pain that is felt in a limb after amputation.

pseudocyesis, see **pseudopregnancy.**

pseudoplegia, hysterical paralysis.

pseudopregnancy, a condition in which all symptoms of pregnancy are present but no actual pregnancy exists.

psilocybin, an alkaloid of the fungus **Psilocybe mexicana,** used as a hallucinogen.

psittacosis, a serious, rickettsial, infectious disease that involves the lungs and is accompanied by high fever; found to be transmissible to man from parrots, and now known to occur in other birds. Also **parrot fever, ornithosis.**

psoriasis, a chronic skin disease characterized by red scaly patches.

psychasthenia, an emotional disorder manifested by morbid anxieties, fears, and phobias.

psyche, the mind, both conscious and subconscious, and all its processes.

psychedelic, 1. of, pertaining to, or causing extraordinary changes in consciousness, as the intensification of sense perception and awareness, hallucination, and delusion. 2. of or pertaining to any of a group of drugs that produce this effect, as LSD, psilocybin, and mescaline.

psychiatric, pertaining to psychiatry.

psychiatrics, see psychiatry.

psychiatrist, a physician specializing in psychiatry.

psychiatry, the field of medicine that deals with the diagnosis and treatment of emotional and mental disorders.

psychic, of or pertaining to the mind.

psycho, (slang) a mentally sick or neurotic person.

psychoanalysis, a method of studying and analyzing the subconscious thoughts of a person, as disclosed by free association or dreams, in order to detect hidden mental conflicts that may produce disorders of mind and body.

psychoanalyst, one who is qualified to practice psychoanalysis.

psychoanalytic, of or pertaining to psychoanalysis.

psychoanalyze, to examine and treat a patient by psychoanalysis.

psychobiology, 1. the study of the interaction or relationship between mind and body, esp. as shown in the nervous system. 2. the biological aspects of psychology.

psychodrama, a type of group psychotherapy that seeks to aid in the rehabilitation of patients by enabling them to dramatize roles likely to shed light on their problems.

psychodramatic, of or pertaining to psychodrama.

psychodynamic, 1. pertaining to the study of behavior in relation to motivation. 2. pertaining to the development and effect of mental processes.

psychodynamics, the study of behavior in relation to motivation.

psychogenesis, 1. the origin and development of the soul or mind. 2. origin or development due to psychic or mental, as opposed to bodily, activity.

psychogenetic, of or relating to psychogenesis.

psychogenic, of psychic or mental origin, or dependent on mental conditions or processes, as a disorder.

psychognosis, the study of the mind, esp. in relation to character.

psychological, 1. of or pertaining to psychology. 2. pertaining to the mind or mental phenomena as the subject matter of psychology.

psychological hedonism, the theory that behavior is primarily motivated by the desire to avoid pain or to experience pleasure.

psychologist, a person versed in psychology.

psychologize, to make psychological investigations or speculations.

psychology, 1. the branch of knowledge that deals with the human mind; the knowledge of the mind that is derived from a careful examination of the facts of consciousness and of behavior. 2. the aggregate of mental and behavioral qualities typical of a group or one of its members. 3. a written exposition on psychology.

psychometrics, see **psy-**

chometry.

psychometry, the measurement of the relative strength of mental facilities.

psychomotor, pertaining to movement induced by mental action.

psychoneurosis, a neurosis in which the patient's anxieties, fears, and physical complaints are emotional and without physical cause.

psychoneurotic, 1. a person who suffers from psychoneurosis. 2. of or pertaining to psychoneurosis.

psychoparesis, weakness of the mind; feeblemindedness.

psychopath, 1. a person with a psychopathic personality. 2. a mentally unstable person.

psychopathic, pertaining to a disease of the mind.

psychopathic personality, 1. a personality disorder evidenced by antisocial, nonconforming, amoral, and sometimes criminal behavior, by the inability to form deep attachments for others or to learn from experience, and by extreme personal indulgence. 2. one having this personality disorder.

psychopathology, mental pathology.

psychopathy, abnormal mental condition.

psychophysical parallelism, the theory that there is a strict correspondence between physical and mental processes but no interaction.

psychophysics, the experimental study of the connection between stimuli and sensation in its functional and quantitative aspects.

psychosis, a major mental disorder characterized by a disintegration of personality.

psychosomatic, having bodily symptoms of mental or emotional origin.

psychosomatics, a branch of medicine dealing with the interrelationship of physical disease and mental and emotional causes.

psychosurgery, surgery of the brain to relieve the symptoms of certain mental diseases.

psychotherapeutic, relating to psychotherapy.

psychotherapist, one who specializes in psychotherapy.

psychotherapy, psychological methods of treatment to correct maladjustments and mental disorders.

psychotic, of or pertaining to psychosis.

psychrophobia, abnormal fear of or sensitivity to cold.

psychrotherapy, treatment of diseases by administering cold.

ptarmic, 1. an agent that causes sneezing. 2. causing sneezing.

ptarmus, spasmodic sneezing.

pterygoid, 1. wing-shaped. 2. of or pertaining to anatomical features situated near the sphenoid bone at the base of the skull.

pterygoid process, 1. either of two processes, one on each side of the sphenoid bone, consisting of two plates separated by a notch. 2. either of these two plates.

ptilosis, loss of the eyelashes.

ptomain, see ptomaine.

ptomaine, any of a class of basic organic compounds, some of them very poisonous, produced in animal and vegetable matter during putrefaction.

ptomaine poisoning, poisoning caused by a ptomaine (applied in error to other types of food poisoning).

ptosis, 1. a falling or drooping of the upper eyelid, caused by paralysis of its levator muscle. 2. the drooping or prolapsed state of any organ.

ptotic, of or relating to ptosis.

ptyalin, an enzyme in the saliva of man, having the property of converting starch into dextrin and maltose.

ptyalism, excessive secretion of saliva; salivation.

pubertal, of or relating to puberty.

puberty, 1. the period in both male and female marked by the functional development of the generative system. 2. the age at which persons become capable of reproduction.

pubes, 1. the middle part of the lower abdominal region, covered with hair at puberty. 2. the hair growing in this region.

pubescence, the state of one who is arriving at puberty.

pubescent, arriving at puberty.

pubic, of or pertaining to the pubes.

pubis, that part of either innominate bone which, with the corresponding part of the other, forms the front of the pelvis.

pudendal, of or pertaining to the pudendum.

pudendum, the external genital organs, esp. of the female.

puerilism, immature, childish behavior by an adult, indicating an abnormal mental condition.

puerperal, pertaining to childbirth.

puerperal fever, see **childbed fever.**

puerperium, the state of a woman at and immediately following childbirth.

puffiness, swelling of tissues.

puke, see **retch, vomit.**

pulmometer, see **spirometer.**

pulmometry, determination of the capacity of the lungs.

pulmonary, of or pertaining to the lungs.

pulmonary artery, an artery conveying venous blood directly from the heart to the lungs.

pulmonary vein, any of four veins conveying oxygenated blood directly from the lungs to the heart.

pulmonectomy, see **pneumonectomy.**

pulmonic, pertaining to the lungs.

pulmotor, a mechanical device for inducing artificial respiration where respiration has ceased entirely or in part through asphyxiation or drowning.

pulp, 1. the soft part of an organ. 2. the soft vascular substance in the interior of a tooth.

pulpy, pulplike.

pulsant, throbbing, pulsating.

pulsate, 1. to beat or throb rhythmically. 2. to vibrate.

pulsatile, 1. throbbing, as the heart. 2. vibrating or sounding, as a percussion instrument.

pulsation, 1. the process of beating or throbbing. 2. a beat of the pulse. 3. a throb.

pulse, 1. the beating or throbbing of the arteries caused by contractions of the heart. 2. the pulsation of the radial artery at the wrist. 3. a pulsation. 4. any rhythmic, regular throbbing or beat.

pulsimeter, an instrument for measuring the strength and rate of the pulse.

pulverize, 1. to reduce to fine powder, as by beating, grinding, or the like. 2. to crush or demolish.

pulverulent, 1. consisting of fine powder. 2. reducible to powder. 3. powdery. 4. dusty.

pulvis, a powder.

pump, an apparatus for drawing up fluids or gases by pressure or suction, as, a breast pump to remove milk from the breast, a dental pump to remove saliva during dental procedures, a stomach pump for removing the content of the stomach.

pupil, the round, contractile aperture in the middle of the iris of the eye through which the rays of light pass to the retina.

pupillary, of or relating to the pupil.

purblind, 1. dim-sighted; almost blind. 2. deficient or lacking in understanding or insight.

purblindness, the condition of being purblind.

purgative, a medicine that evacuates the bowels; a cathartic.

purge, to evacuate the bowels by means of a cathartic.

purpura, a disease characterized by purple or livid spots on the skin or mucous membrane, caused by the estravasation of blood.

purpuric, of or pertaining to purpura.

purulent, 1. consisting of pus or matter. 2. full of or resembling pus. 3. discharging pus.

pus, a yellowish-white, more or less viscid substance produced by suppuration and found in abscesses and healing sores, consisting of a liquid plasma in which leukocytes are suspended.

pustulant, 1. causing the formation of pustules. 2. a pustulant medicine or agent.

pustular, 1. having the character of or proceeding from a pustule or pustules. 2. covered with pustules.

pustulate, 1. to form or cause to form pustules or blisters. 2. covered with glandular excrescences such as pustules.

pustulation, the act of forming pustules.

pustule, 1. an elevation of the skin having an inflamed base and containing pus. 2. any small protuberance similar to a pimple or blister.

putrefaction, 1. the act or process of putrefying. 2. the decomposition of animal and vegetable substances, producing a malodorous compound. 3. that which is putrefied.

putrefy, 1. to render putrid. 2. to cause to rot. 3. to make gangrenous.

putrescent, 1. becoming putrid. 2. growing rotten. 3. pertaining to the process of putrefaction.

putrescible, 1. capable of being putrefied. 2. liable to become putrid.

putrescine, a crystalline ptomaine, produced by putrid animal tissue.

putrid, in a state of decay or putrefaction; rotten; proceeding from or pertaining to putrefaction.

putrid fever, see **typhus.**

pyelitis, an inflammation of

the pelvis of the kidney.

pyelocystitis, inflammation of the pelvis of the kidney and the bladder.

pyelogram, see **pyelograph.**

pyelograph, a photograph produced by pyelography.

pyelography, the process of making photographs of the kidneys and other internal organs by means of X rays after the injection of a dye.

pyelonephritis, an inflammation of the kidney and the pelvis of the kidney.

pyemia, 1. a form of blood poisoning caused by pyogenic bacteria. 2. general septicemia marked by the development of abscesses.

pyemic, of or pertaining to pyemia.

pyknic, 1. characteristically short, broad, and rounded in body type. 2. endomorphic.

pylephlebitis, an inflamed condition of the portal vein.

pylic, of or pertaining to the portal vein.

pyloric, pertaining to the pylorus.

pylorus, the outlet between the stomach and the duodenum through which food passes to the intestines.

pyodermatitis, a bacterial infection and inflammation of the skin characterized by the presence of pus.

pyogenic, 1. producing or generating pus. 2. attended by or pertaining to the formation of pus.

pyorrhea, a bacterial infection of the gums in and about the sockets of the teeth, with discharge of pus and loosening of the teeth.

pyothorax, pus in the pleural cavity. See **empyema.**

pyrethrum, any of several species of the genus *Chrysanthemum,* the dried and powdered flower heads of which are used as an insecticide and for certain skin ailments.

pyretic, of or concerning fever.

pyrexia, see **fever.**

pyridoxine, vitamin B_6, a phenolic alcohol.

pyriform, having the shape of a pear.

pyrogen, a toxin that causes fever.

pyrogenic, producing fever.

pyromania, an uncontrollable impulse to set fires.

pyrometer, an instrument that measures extremely high temperatures above the range of the mercurial thermometer.

pyrometric, of or relating to pyrometer.

pyrophobia, pathological fear of fire.

pyrosis, see **heartburn.**

pyuria, the presence of pus in the urine.

Q-fever, a fever accompanied by muscular pains and chills, caused by a rickettsia, and transmitted through contact with cattle and sheep or by drinking raw milk. Also called **Queensland fever.**

quacksalver, a quack doctor.

quadriceps, a large muscle in the front of the thigh that controls the extension of the leg.

quadripara, a woman who has had four children.

quadripartite, 1. divided into four parts. 2. having four participants.

quadriplegia, a paralysis affecting all four limbs.

quadroon, the offspring of a mulatto and a white person. 2. a person having one Negro grandparent.

quadruplet, one of four children born of one birth.

quarantine, detention or isolation to prevent the spread of disease.

quartan, 1. intermitting so as to occur every fourth day, as, a quartan fever. 2. a form of malarial fever marked by paroxysms that occur every fourth day, counting inclusively.

queasy, 1. sick to the stomach. 2. affected with nausea. 3. apt to cause nausea.

Queensland fever, see **Q-fever.**

quick, living flesh, esp. sensitive areas beneath fingernails or toenails, as, nails trimmed to the quick.

quicken, to arrive at that state of pregnancy in which the fetus gives indications of life.

quinacrine, a bright yellow,

crystalline compound used in treating malaria.

quinidine, a clear crystalline alkaloid isomeric with quinine, used in its sulfate form in the regulation of the heart rhythm and the treatment of malaria.

quinine, 1. a bitter crystalline alkaloid, obtained from the bark of several species of cinchona trees, and used, esp. in the form of a salt, as a remedy for malaria. 2. a salt of this alkaloid, esp. the sulfate.

quinoidine, a brownish-black, resinous substance consisting of a mixture of alkaloids, obtained as a by-product in the manufacture of quinine and used as a cheap substitute for it.

quinsy, an inflammation of the tonsils, esp. a suppurating inflammation.

quintuplet, one of five offspring born of one birth.

quotidian, 1. anything that returns every day. 2. a fever whose paroxysms return every day.

Q wave, the wave in an electrocardiogram that is associated with the contraction of the ventricles of the heart.

rabbit fever, see **tularemia.**

rabic, of or pertaining to rabies.

rabid, affected with rabies; pertaining to rabies.

rabies, see **hydrophobia.**

racemose, arranged in the form of a raceme, as a gland.

rachialgia, a pain in the spine.

rachianesthesia, spinal anesthesia.

rachidial, of or pertaining to the spinal column.

rachidian, see **rachidial.**

rachigraph, an apparatus for outlining the curves of the spine.

rachiometer, an instrument for measuring the curvature of the spine.

rachiopathy, any spinal disease.

rachioplegia, spinal paralysis.

rachiotome, a surgical instrument for cutting and dividing the vertebrae.

rachiotomy, surgical operation of cutting into or through the vertebral column.

rachis, see **spinal column.**

rachitic, pertaining to or affected with rachitis.

rachitis, see **rickets.**

radial, pertaining to the radius bone.

radiate, to diverge from a common center.

radiation, 1. treatment for certain diseases with a radioactive substance. 2. in neurology, any group of nerve fibers that diverge from a common origin.

radiation sickness, an illness caused by exposure of body tissue to deep X rays or radioactive substances.

radical, 1. going to the root or origin in attacking the cause of a disease. 2. a form of treatment, esp. surgery, that aims at the total eradication of diseased organs or tissues.

radicle, a small rootlike part, as the beginning of a nerve fiber.

radicular, of or concerning a root or radicle.

radiculitis, an inflammation of spinal nerve roots.

radioactive, pertaining to or caused by radioactivity.

radioactivity, the emission of alpha rays, beta rays, or gamma rays in elements, as uranium, that undergo spontaneous atomic disintegration.

radiobiologic, of or pertaining to radiobiology.

radiobiologist, a scientist who specializes in radiobiology.

radiobiology, the division of biology concerned with the effects of radiant energy or radioactive material on living matter.

radiocarbon, radioactive carbon with the mass number 14, used as an analytical research tool, esp. in the dating of geological and archeological material.

radiodermatitis, inflammation of the skin caused by exposure to X rays or other radioactive elements.

radiodiagnosis, diagnosis arrived at by means of X rays.

radioelement, an element displaying radioactivity.

radiogenic, resulting from radioactive disintegration.

radiograph, an image or picture produced by the action of X rays or other rays from radioactive substances.

radiographer, a person skilled in making X-ray photographs.

radiographic, of or relating to radiography.

radiography, the production of radiographs.

radioisotope, an isotope exhibiting radioactivity, usually one created artificially from a nonradioactive element, used in research and in the diagnosis and treatment of disease. Also called **radioactive isotope.**

radiological, of or relating to radiology.

radiologist, a specialist in radiology.

radiology, 1. the science dealing with X rays or rays from radioactive substances, esp. for medical uses. 2. the process of examining or photographing organs or bones with such rays. 3. the reading of medical X rays.

radiolucency, the quality of being permeable to X rays and other kinds of radiation.

radionecrosis, the disintegration of tissues caused by exposure to radium or X rays.

radio pill, a small transmitter in a capsule which, when swallowed, sends out information on physiological, esp. gastrointestinal, conditions.

radioresistant, resistant to the action of treatment by X rays, or radium, or any other radiation, esp. of a tumor or tissues that cannot be destroyed by radiation.

radiosensitive, capable of being reduced or destroyed by certain forms of radiant energy, as, a radiosensitive tumor.

radiosurgery, the use of high-energy radioactive particles in the form of beams as an atomic knife, in treating cancers or other diseased tissues.

radiotherapeutic, of or pertaining to radiotherapy.

radiotherapeutist, see **radiotherapist.**

radiotherapist, one trained in use of radiant energy for therapeutic purposes.

radiotherapy, treatment of diseases by radioactivity, as by X rays or radioactive elements such as radium or thorium.

radium, a radioactive metallic element found in certain minerals, as pitchblende, in the uranium series, used in radiography, in medicine for treating cancer, and in luminous materials, as paints.

radius, the one of the two bones of the forearm that is on the thumb side.

radix, a root, esp. of a spinal or cranial nerve.

ragweed fever, see **hay fever.**

rale, an abnormal sound accompanying the normal respiratory murmur, as in a pulmonary disease.

ramiform, having the form of a branch; branchlike; branched. Also called **ramal.**

ramose, having many branches; branching. See also **ramiform.**

ramulose, having many small branches.

ramus, a branch, usually of a nerve, vein, or bone.

ranula, a cyst occurring beneath the tongue, caused by obstruction and subsequent swelling of a glandular duct.

ranular, of or pertaining to a ranula.

rape, the offense of sexual intercourse with a woman forcibly and against her will.

raphe, a seamlike union between two parts or halves of an organ or the like.

rarefaction, the process of decreasing density.

rarefy, to make less dense, or to increase the porosity of.

rash, an eruption on the skin, usually in the form of red spots or patches.

raspberry mark, see **nevus.**

ratbite fever, a disease transmitted through the bite of a rat carrying the bacterium **Spirillum minus,** and marked by recurring fever, skin sores, and muscular aches.

ration, a fixed allowance of food and drink for a certain period.

rauwolfia, any shrub or tree of the genus **Rauwolfia,** of the dogbane family, a source of the drug reserpine.

rave, to speak irrationally;

to be delirious; to be wild, furious, or raging.

reaction, 1. the specific effect in an organism or its systems of introduction of a foreign element. 2. depression or exhaustion as a consequence of excessive excitement or stimulation. 3. increase of activity succeeding depression. 4. abnormal behavior resulting from a personal experience or situation.

reactivate, to become or cause to become effective or operative again.

reactivation, the act of rendering active again something that was inactive.

reactive, able to respond to a stimulus.

reagent, any substance that, by the reactions it produces, can be used in chemical analysis.

reagin, an antibody.

reason, 1. normal or sound powers of mind; sanity. 2. to exercise the faculty or powers of reason.

rebound, 1. an emotional reaction following frustration. 2. the act of rebounding; resilience.

receptor, the ending of an afferent neuron that receives stimuli and transmits them to other parts of the nervous system.

recess, a cavity or indentation in an otherwise smooth surface.

recession of the gums, see **pyorrhea.**

recessive, a hidden or recessive character, as opposed to a **dominant**

character.

recidivation, 1. a relapse into crime. 2. the relapse of a disease.

recidivism, repeated or habitual relapse into crime or antisocial behavior.

recidivist, 1. a criminal who, after punishment, returns to crime. 2. a patient, esp. an insane person, who has repeated relapses.

recidivistic, of or pertaining to recidivism.

recipe, a physician's prescription.

recrement, any secretion, such as saliva, which, after having fulfilled its function, is reabsorbed into the body.

recrudesce, to break out afresh, as a sore or as disease that has been quiescent.

recrudescence, the return of a dormant disease.

rectal, proximal to, involving, or pertaining to the rectum.

rectalgia, pain in the rectum.

rectectomy, surgical excision of the rectum or anus.

rectitis, an inflammation of the rectum.

rectocolitis, an inflammation of both the rectum and the colon.

rectoplasty, see **proctoplasty.**

rectoscope, see **proctoscope.**

rectum, the lower six to eight inches of the intestine, terminating in the anus.

rectus, any of several muscles that are straight, as of the abdomen, thigh, or eye.

recumbent, reclining; lying down; reposing.

recuperate, to recover from illness or fatigue.

recuperation, restoration to health.

recurrence, the return of symptoms of an illness that has been dormant.

recurrent, 1. returning from time to time, as a fever. 2. turning back in its course, as a nerve or blood vessel.

red blood cell, a cell that contains hemoglobin and gives the red color to the blood of vertebrates.

red fever, see **dengue.**

reduce, 1. to restore to its proper place or state, as a dislocated or fractured bone. 2. to lower one's weight by dieting.

reduction, the operation of restoring a dislocated or fractured bone to its former place.

reel, sway unsteadily in standing or walking from dizziness, intoxication, or faintness.

reflector, a device that reflects waves of radiant energy or sound.

reflex, noting or pertaining to an action or movement of an involuntary nature, in which a stimulus is transmitted along an afferent nerve to a nerve center, and from there reflected along an efferent nerve to produce muscular or other activity.

reflex arc, the path followed by an impulse from afferent neurons through intermediate neurons to efferent neurons, in the production of a reflex response: the basic unit of function of the nervous system.

reflexogenic, causing a reflex action.

reflexograph, an instrument for charting a reflex.

reflexophil, characterized by reflex activity.

reflux, see **regurgitation.**

refocus, to focus again.

refraction, 1. deflection from a straight path, as of light rays as they pass through one transparent medium to another of different density. 2. correction of errors of vision due to ocular refraction.

refractory, resisting ordinary treatment, as certain diseases.

regeneration, the repair, regrowth, or restoration of damaged tissues or parts of organs.

regimen, a regulated course of diet, exercise, or manner of living intended to preserve or restore health or to attain some result.

region, a place in, or a division of, the body or a part of the body.

regional, pertaining to particular regions or parts of the body.

regression, 1. a reversion to earlier or less mature patterns of behavior. 2. progressive subsidence of an ailment or disease.

regurgitate, to rush or surge back; to pour forth,

as food.

regurgitation, 1. the act of regurgitating. 2. the backward circulation of blood through a faulty heart valve.

rehabilitate, to restore to a healthy condition or useful capacity.

rehabilitation, the process of restoring to a healthy condition or useful capacity a person who was ill or handicapped.

rehydrate, to replace water removed in dehydration.

reimplantation, replacement of tissue or an organ in its original site, as an extracted tooth in its original socket.

reinfection, a second infection of the same type as one from which a person is suffering or has recovered.

reinoculation, a second inoculation with the same organsim.

relapse, to slip or slide back, esp. from recovery or convalescence to illness.

relapsing fever, any of several chiefly tropical diseases resulting from spirochetal infections spread by ticks and lice, and marked by recurrent attacks of chills and high fever.

relax, 1. to slacken, to make lax; to make less tense or rigid. 2. to make less severe or rigorous.

relaxant, a drug that relaxes tension, esp. of muscles.

relaxation, the act of relaxing or state of being re-

laxed; a lessening of tension, effort, or severity.

relief, alleviation, mitigation, or removal of pain or grief.

relieve, to provide relief.

REM, Rapid Eye Movement; a manifestation of dreaming during sleep.

remediable, capable of being remedied.

remedial, intended to correct deficiencies or improve skills.

remediless, not admitting of a remedy; incurable; irreparable.

remedy, 1. something that cures or relieves a disease or bodily disorder. 2. a healing medicine, application, or treatment. 3. to cure, heal, or relieve. 4. to put right or restore to the natural or proper condition.

remission, 1. the act of remitting. 2. abatement. 3. a temporary subsidence of the force, violence, or symptoms of a disease or of pain.

remit, to relax; to abate; to allow to slacken.

remittent, temporarily easing or abating; having remissions from time to time.

renal, pertaining to or located near the kidneys.

reniform, having the form or shape of a kidney.

renin, a proteolytic enzyme of ischemic kidneys.

renitis, see **nephritis.**

repercussion, 1. a reaction. 2. see **ballottement.**

replicate, to fold or bend back.

reposit, to replace surgically.

reposition, the surgical restoration or replacement of an organ or tissue.

repress, to reject from consciousness, as fearful ideas or impulses.

repressed, 1. characterized by repression. 2. affected by restraint.

repression, 1. the process of repressing painful ideas in the subconscious where they continue to exert influence. 2. that which is repressed.

resect, 1. to cut or trim off surgically. 2. to cut out, as a segment of an organ.

resection, the surgical removal of a section of a bone or a piece of an organ or tissue.

reserpine, a white crystalline alkaloid, derived from the root of **Rauwolfia serpentina,** an East Indian plant, and used in medicine to alleviate extreme anxiety and hypertension.

residual, pertaining to that which is left as a residue, as the residual urine left in the bladder in case of pressure of an enlarged prostate gland on the bladder.

residue, that which remains after a part is removed; remainder.

resilience, 1. the capacity to spring back to the original shape or form after being bent, stretched, or compressed; flexibility; elasticity. 2. the capacity to rebound quickly from illness.

resilient, 1. rebounding; springing back to original shape. 2. quickly regaining spirits or health after misfortune or illness.

resolution, the diminution or disappearance of a tumor or inflammation.

resolvent, a substance that diminishes or dispels inflammation.

resonance, the sound resulting from tapping the chest or upper part of the body.

resonant, of or pertaining to resonance.

respirable, capable of respiring or fit for being respired or breathed.

respiration, the act of respiring; the inhalation and exhalation of air; breathing.

respirator, 1. a machine used for providing artificial respiration, as an iron lung. 2. a masklike contrivance covering the mouth, or nose and mouth, which serves as protection against the inhalation of cold air or harmful matter.

respiratory, of or pertaining to respiration.

respiratory quotient, the ratio of the amount of carbon dioxide exhaled in respiration to the oxygen taken in.

respire, 1. to breathe; to inhale air into the lungs and exhale it for the purpose of maintaining life. 2. to breathe easily. 3. to recover after labor, worry, or suffering.

response, the reaction of the body, a muscle, or a

gland to a stimulus.

rest, 1. the refreshing quiet or repose of sleep. 2. refreshing ease or inactivity after exertion or labor.

restiform, cordlike; twisted into ropelike strands.

restiform bodies, a pair of cordlike bundles of nerve fibers lying one on each side of the medulla oblongata and connecting it with the cerebellum.

restitution, 1. restoration to the former or original state or position. 2. the turning of a fetal head to the right or left immediately after its delivery.

restless, 1. unable to rest or sleep. 2. not satisfied to be at rest.

restorative, 1. that which restores. 2. that which is efficacious in restoring consciousness or health.

restore, to bring back to a state of health, soundness, vigor.

resuscitate, 1. to revive. 2. to recover, esp. from apparent death or unconsciousness.

resuscitation, see **artificial respiration.**

resuscitator, 1. one who resuscitates. 2. a device used to initiate respiration and relieve asphyxiation.

retardation, 1. the act of retarding. 2. the condition of being delayed. 3. that which retards. 4. abnormally slow physical, intellectual, and emotional development.

retarded, 1. exhibiting retardation. 2. abnormally slow in mental and emo-

tional development. 3. abnormally slow in action, awareness, or progress.

retch, to make an effort to vomit; to strain, as in vomiting.

rete, a network, as of fibers, nerves, or blood vessels.

retention, the retaining in the body of matter, such as urine, which is normally discharged.

retial, of or pertaining to a rete.

reticula, see **rete.**

reticular, having the form of a net; netlike.

reticulation, the formation of a network.

reticulocyte, an immature red blood cell containing a network of granules or filaments.

reticulocytosis, an abnormal increase in the number of reticulocytes.

reticulum, a network of protoplasmic structures, as cells or tissues.

retiform, see **reticular.**

retina, the innermost coat of the posterior part of the eyeball, consisting of light-sensitive cells connected to the brain by the optic nerve, and serving to receive the image transmitted by the lens.

retinene, either the orange or the yellow carotenoid pigment of the retina.

retinitis, an inflammation of the retina.

retinoscope, an apparatus used for measuring the refraction of the eye.

retinoscopy, the examination of the retina to determine the degree of any faulty refraction of the eye.

retractile, capable of being drawn back or in.

retractility, the capability of retraction.

retractor, 1. a muscle that retracts an organ or a protruded part. 2. an instrument or appliance for drawing back an impeding part, as the edge of a wound or incision.

retral, 1. at the back; posterior. 2. backward; retrograde.

retrenchment, a procedure used in plastic surgery to cut away excess tissue.

retrocede, to recede.

retroflex, bent backward.

retroflexion, a bending backward of the body of the uterus.

retrogradation, 1. backward movement. 2. decline or deterioration.

retrogress, to revert.

retrogression, 1. decline or deterioration. 2. a return to a simpler from a more complex or more perfect structure; degeneration.

retrogressive, degenerating.

retroinfection, the infection of the mother by the fetus.

retrolental, situated posterior to a lens, as of the eye.

retrolingual, situated at or behind the base of the tongue.

retromammary, situated behind the mammary gland.

retromandibular, situated behind the lower jaw.

retromastoid, situated behind the mastoid process.

retronasal, situated behind the nose.

retro-ocular, situated behind the eyeball.

retroperitoneal, situated behind the peritoneum.

retroperitoneum, the space behind the peritoneum and the front of the spinal column.

retroperitonitis, an inflammation of the retroperitoneum.

retropharyngeal, situated behind the pharynx.

retropharyngitis, an inflammation of the back of the pharynx.

retropharynx, the back of the pharynx.

retrospect, 1. to look back in thought; reflect. 2. to refer back.

retrospection, the action or faculty of looking back on things past; a survey of past events or experiences.

retrosternal, situated behind the sternum.

retrovaccination, vaccination of a human with virus obtained from a cow that had been inoculated with smallpox virus obtained from a human.

retroversion, a turning or bending backward, as of a part or an organ, esp. the uterus.

reversion, 1. a reverting or returning, as to original form or condition. 2. a return toward some ancestral type or character; **atavism.**

revulsion, 1. a sudden and strong emotional reaction or change of feeling, usually in the direction of extreme displeasure. 2. a counterirritant.

revulsive, an agent causing revulsion.

rhagades, painful linear fissures appearing esp. at the corner of the mouth or anus, caused by syphilis, intertrigo, and other affections.

rhatany, a South American shrub, the roots of which are used as an astringent and in medicine.

rheum, a thin watery fluid discharged by the mucous gland, as in catarrh.

rheumatic, 1. pertaining to or characteristic of rheumatism. 2. affected with rheumatism. 3. one subject to or afflicted with rheumatism.

rheumatic fever, a severe infectious disease, usually occurring in young adults or children, characterized by painful swollen joints, fever, and often by inflamed heart lining and valves. See also **rheumatism.**

rheumatism, a painful inflammation affecting muscles and joints, attended by swelling and stiffness.

rheumatoid, resembling rheumatism.

rheumatoid arthritis, a progressive disease of the joints causing painful swelling and shortening of fibrous tissues, frequently resulting in deformities.

rheumic, of or pertaining to rheum.

rhexis, rupture of an organ, tissue, or vessel.

Rh factor, any of several inherited antigens in red blood cells of most humans, who are Rh positive, which, under certain conditions such as blood transfusion and pregnancy, are capable of destroying red corpuscles in persons whose blood is Rh negative, or deficient in these substances; also called **Rhesus factor,** so named because it was first found in the blood of rhesus monkeys.

rhinal, pertaining to the nose; nasal.

rhinalgia, pain in the nose; nasal neuralgia.

rhinencephalic, of or pertaining to the rhinencephalon.

rhinencephalon, the olfactory portion of the brain.

rhinitis, an inflammation of the nose or its mucous membrane.

rhinodynia, see **rhinalgia.**

rhinolaryngology, the science dealing with the structure and diseases of the nose and the larynx.

rhinologist, a physician who specializes in the diseases of the nose and their treatment.

rhinology, the science dealing with the structure and diseases of the nose.

rhinophonia, a nasal sound in speaking.

rhinoplasty, plastic surgery of the nose.

rhinopolyp, a polyp (innocent tumor) of the nose.

rhinopolypus, see **rhinopolyp.**

rhinoscope, an instrument

for examining the nasal passages.

rhinoscopy, examination of the nasal cavity by means of a rhinoscope.

rhizomelic, of or concerning the roots of the hip or shoulder joints.

rhizotomy, the surgical section of the posterior roots of the spinal nerves, performed as treatment for pain or spastic paralysis.

rhodogenesis, regeneration of rhodopsin that has been bleached by light.

rhodophylaxis, the ability of the retina to regenerate rhodopsin.

rhodopsin, a photosensitive red pigment in the rodlike retinal cells of the eye that is considered important for night vision, and that in light breaks down to protein components allied to vitamin A.

rhombencephalon, the rearmost part of the brain.

rhoncal, of or pertaining to a rhonchus.

rhonchial, see **ronchal.**

rhonchus, a rattling sound, esp. when produced in bronchial tubes that are partially obstructed.

rhubarb, a large garden plant, the roots of which are used in medicine for making laxatives, tonics, and astringents.

rhypophagy, the eating of filth.

rhypophobia, abnormal aversion to the act of defecation or filth.

rhythm, a regular recurrence of a function or action, as the heartbeat.

rhythmic, of or pertaining to rhythm.

rhythm method, a system of birth control through abstinence from sexual intercourse during the estimated monthly interval of female ovulation and fertility.

rhytidectomy, plastic surgery for the removal of wrinkles.

rhytidosis, 1. wrinkling of the cornea, usually occurring with approaching death. 2. wrinkling of the face without other signs of age.

rib, one of the slender curved bones that attach from each side of the vertebral column enclosing the thoracic cavity and protecting certain important organs.

riboflavin, a growth-producing crystalline compound, orange-yellow in color, belonging to the vitamin B complex, occurring naturally in milk, liver, egg yolk, and leafy vegetables; also prepared synthetically.

ribonucleic acid, (RNA) a nucleic acid containing ribose, occurring chiefly in cytoplasm.

ribose, a monosaccharide sugar, obtained from some nucleic acids.

ribosome, one of a number of minute particles containing ribonucleic acid and protein, found in the cytoplasm of cells.

ricin, a poisonous white powder derived from the castor bean, used in medicine to cause agglutination of red corpuscles.

ricinoleic acid, an organic acid, occurring in castor oil in the form of a glyceride.

ricinolein, a glyceride of ricinoleic acid, the chief constituent of castor oil.

ricinus, the castor oil plant, yielding ricin and castor oil, the latter used as a cathartic or lubricant.

rickets, a disease of children in which there is usually some softening and distortion of the bones due to faulty deposition of calcium or a vitamin D deficiency, or both.

rickettsia, any of the microorganisms of the genus **Rickettsia,** parasitic in arthropods and transmitted by them to man, causing such diseases as typhus.

rickety, 1. affected with rickets. 2. feeble or imperfect in general. 3. irregular, as in movement.

rictus, 1. the orifice of the open mouth; the gape. 2. any opening, fissure, or cleft.

rigor, 1. rigidity. 2. a sudden coldness, accompanied by shivering, that precedes certain fevers. 3. rigidity of the body tissues or organs causing lack of response to stimuli.

rigor mortis, the stiffening of the muscles of the body after death.

rima, a slit, fissure, cleft, or crack.

rimose, full of chinks, fissures, or cracks.

rimous, see **rimose.**

rimula, a small fissure, slit or cleft.

ringworm, a disease caused by fungi, appearing in the form of rings or patches on different parts of the body, esp. on the scalp.

risus sardonicus, a facial expression resembling a sardonic grin, caused by muscle spasms and seen in persons afflicted by tetanus.

RNA, see **ribonucleic acid.**

roborant, any tonic used as a remedy.

robust, possessed of or indicating great strength or health.

Rocky Mountain spotted fever, an infectious disease caused by the microorganism **Rickettsia rickettsii,** transmitted by the bite of certain wood ticks, and marked by pain in muscles and joints, fever, prostration, skin eruptions, and chills.

roentgen, 1. the unit used internationally as a measure of radiation, named for Wilhelm Konrad Röntgen, the discoverer of X rays. 2. pertaining most commonly to X rays.

roentgenize, to subject to the action of X rays.

roentgenogram, a photograph made by means of X rays.

roentgenograph, see **roentgenogram.**

roentgenography, X-ray photography. See also **radiography.**

roentgenologic, of or pertaining to roentgenology.

roentgenologist, an expert in roentgenology.

roentgenology, the study of all applications of X rays, esp. those relating to medical diagnosis and therapy.

roentgenoscope, an apparatus having a fluorescent viewing screen on which a shadow picture of an opaque object is projected by means of X rays. See **fluoroscope.**

roentgenoscopic, of or pertaining to roentgenoscopy.

roentgenoscopy, examination by means of a roentgenoscope.

roentgenotherapy, remedial medical treatment through the use of X rays.

roentgen ray, see **X ray.**

rongeur forceps, a surgical instrument for cutting and removing bone fragments.

root, that which resembles a root of a plant in position or function, as, the root of a tooth or hair.

Rorschach test, a technique for appraising personality by an analysis of the subject's interpretation of a standard series of ten ink blots of varied design.

rosacea, a chronic skin disease occurring on the face, characterized by redness of the skin tissue and pustules.

rose fever, an allergy similar to hay fever, associated with rose pollen and usually occurring in early summer.

roseola, a kind of rose-colored rash.

rotator, a muscle that rolls a body part around its axis.

roughage, rough or coarse food, as certain fruits or bran, that is proportionately high in indigestible constituents, stimulating peristalsis.

rouleau, a group of red blood corpuscles arranged like a pile of coins.

round-shouldered, having a rounded back or stooping shoulders.

roundworm, a nematode, a parasite infesting the intestines.

rubdown, a brisk massage.

rubedo, exhibiting a red or rosy color of the face; blushing.

rubefacient, 1. producing redness of the skin. 2. a substance for external application that produces redness of the skin, not followed by blistering.

rubella, see **German measles.**

rubeola, see **measles.**

rubicund, inclining to redness; reddish; ruddy, as a complexion.

rubor, redness caused by inflammation.

rudiment, an organ or part that is nonfunctional because of its stunted capacity or size.

rudimentary, incompletely developed.

ruga, a crease, fold, or wrinkle.

rugose, wrinkled; full of wrinkles; ridged.

rumination, 1. see **regurgitation.** 2. an obsessional preoccupation of the mind by a single idea.

rupia, a skin disease characterized by cutaneous eruptions, usually seen in the third stage of syphilis.

rupture, see **hernia.**

sabulous, sandy; gritty.

sac, a bag or cyst, often a receptacle for a liquid, as, the lachrymal sac.

saccate, furnished with or having the form of a sac or pouch.

saccharate, 1. a salt of a saccharic acid. 2. a compound of sucrose and a metallic acid.

saccharic, 1. pertaining to or obtained from saccharin or compounds containing saccharin. 2. relating to or from saccharic acid.

saccharic acid, a white, crystalline, water-soluble acid, made by oxidizing glucose with nitric acid.

saccharide, 1. a carbohydrate compound containing sugar. 2. a simple sugar or a combination of sugars.

saccharification, conversion into sugar.

saccharify, to convert into sugar.

saccharimeter, an optical instrument for determining the strength of sugar solutions by measuring the amount of rotation of a plane of polarized light after it passes through a sugar solution.

saccharin, a white crystalline substance, syn-

thetically produced, which in dilute form is 300 to 500 times as sweet as cane sugar and is used primarily as a calorie-free sugar substitute.

saccharine, pertaining to, of the nature of, containing, or resembling sugar; sugary.

saccharolysis, chemical dissolution of sugar.

saccharolytic, of or pertaining to saccharolysis.

saccharometer, see **saccharimeter.**

saccharomycete, any fungus of the genus **Saccharomyces,** of the yeast family, used in the fermentation of sugar.

saccharomycosis, any disease caused by the yeast fungus.

saccharose, see **sucrose.**

saccharosuria, the presence of saccharose in the urine.

sacculate, having saccules or saclike expansions.

saccule, 1. a little sac. 2. the smaller of two sacs in the membranous labyrinth of the inner ear.

sacrad, in the direction of the sacrum.

sacralgia, pain in the sacrum.

sacrectomy, surgical excision of part of the sacrum.

sacrocoxitis, an inflammation of the sacroiliac joint.

sacrodynia, pain in the region of the sacrum.

sacroiliac, 1. pertaining to the sacrum and the ilium. 2. of or relating to the joint between these two bones and the joining ligaments.

sacrolumbar, of or pertaining to the sacrum and the loins.

sacrosciatic, pertaining jointly to the sacrum and the ischium.

sacrospinal, of or relating to the sacrum and the spine.

sacrospinalis, the large muscle on either side of the spinal column extending from the sacrum to the head.

sacrotomy, surgical excision of part of the sacrum.

sacrouterine, of or pertaining to the sacrum and the uterus.

sacrum, a bone resulting from the fusion of two or more vertebrae between the lumbar and the coccygeal regions, forming the posterior wall of the pelvis.

saddle nose, a nose with a depressed bridge.

sadism, the pathological derivation of sexual pleasure from inflicting physical or mental pain upon another; the tendency to take pleasure in cruelty. Compare **masochism.**

sadist, a person who practices sadism.

sadistic, of or pertaining to sadism.

sadomasochism, a derivation of pleasure from inflicting pain upon oneself and another.

sadomasochist, a person who practices sadomasochism.

sadomasochistic, of or pertaining to sadomasochism.

sagital, 1. pertaining to or resembling an arrow. 2. relating to the suture that unites the parietal bones of the skull. 3. of a plane that divides a body into right and left halves.

Saint Vitus's dance, see **chorea.**

salacious, lustful; lecherous.

salicin, a bitter crystalline glucoside, obtained from the bark of various species of willow and poplar or produced synthetically, used medicinally in the treatment of rheumatism.

salicylate, any salt of salicylic acid.

salicylic acid, a white powder, soluble in water, used as a food preservative and in the preparation of aspirin.

salify, 1. to form into a salt by combining an acid with a base. 2. to infuse with a salt.

salimeter, see **salinometer.**

saline, 1. consisting of salt; partaking of the qualities of salt. 2. relating to or containing chemical salt, as the alkali metals. 3. a salt spring, or any place where salt water is collected in the earth. 4. a medicinal solution of salt.

salinometer, an instrument for measuring the amount of salt present in a given solution.

saliva, the watery, viscid, slightly acid fluid secreted by the glands of the mouth, serving to moisten the mouth and food, and containing the enzyme ptyalin, which starts the digesting of starches. See **spittle**.

salivant, any agent that induces the flow of saliva.

salivary, of or pertaining to saliva.

salivary calculus, a stone in a salivary duct.

salivary glands, the glands in the oral cavity whose secretions form saliva.

salivate, 1. to secrete saliva. 2. to cause to have an abnormal secretion and discharge of saliva.

salivation, 1. the process or action of salivating. 2. an excessive flow of saliva, as caused by mercury.

salivator, see **salivant**.

salivatory, producing salivation.

Salk vaccine, an injected vaccine against poliomyelitis, made from inactivated poliomyelitis virus.

salmonella, any of a number of rod-shaped bacteria, genus **Salmonella**, associated with food poisoning, intestinal inflammations, or genital-tract diseases.

salmonellosis, infestation with bacteria of the genus **Salmonella,** which cause a form of food poisoning.

salol, a white crystalline substance, prepared by the interaction of salicylic acid and phenol, used as an antipyretic and antiseptic.

salpingectomy, the removal of a fallopian tube.

salpingemphraxis, 1. obstruction of a fallopian tube. 2. obstruction of a eustachian tube.

salpingian, 1. relating to or concerning a fallopian tube. 2. relating to or concerning a eustachian tube.

salpingitis, 1. an inflammation of a fallopian tube. 2. an inflammation of a eustachian tube.

salpinx, 1. a fallopian tube. 2. a eustachian tube.

salpingocyesis, a tubal pregnancy; a fetus starting to develop in a fallopian tube.

salsoda, crystalline sodium carbonate, used as a cleansing agent.

saltation, 1. a leaping or jumping. 2. palpitation. 3. a mutation in macroevolution.

saltatorial, of or pertaining to saltation.

saltatory, see **saltatorial**.

saltpeter, potassium nitrate, a crystalline compound used as a fertilizer.

salubrious, conducive to health; healthful.

salutary, 1. promoting health. 2. producing a beneficial effect.

salutiferous, see **salutary**.

Salvarsan, an organic arsenical compound used in the treatment of syphilis and other spirochetal diseases (trademark). Since the development of penicillin, Salvarsan is rarely used in the treatment of syphilis.

salve, a soothing ointment applied to wounds or sores; a balm; anything that heals, relieves, or placates.

sanative, having healing

power; curing.

sanatorium, an establishment for the treatment of diseases, or for recuperation of invalids or convalescents.

sanatory, conducive to health; healing; curing; hygienic.

sand-blind, having imperfect eyesight.

sandfly, 1. a small biting fly of the family Psychodidae, inhabiting the seashore. 2. a bloodsucking fly of the genus **Phlebotomus,** whose bite transmits certain diseases, as sandfly fever.

sane, mentally sound; not deranged; having reason and the other mental faculties.

sanguicolous, living in the blood, as a parasite.

sanguifacient, making blood.

sanguiferous, conveying blood, as the arteries and veins.

sanguinaria, a plant of the poppy family, having a white flower, lobed leaves, and a red juice; the rhizome of this plant, used as an emetic or expectorant. Also called **bloodroot.**

sanguine, 1. having the color of blood. 2. ruddy, as a complexion. 3. characterized by vigor and confidence.

sanguineous, pertaining to or containing blood.

sanguinolent, tinged or mingled with blood; bloody.

sanies, a thin serous fluid, often greenish, discharged from ulcers or wounds.

sanious, of or pertaining to sanies.

sanitarian, 1. promoter of sanitary measures, public health, or the like. 2. clean; healthful.

sanitarium, see **sanatorium.**

sanitary, see **sanatory.**

sanitary napkin, a pad of absorbent material, usually cotton, used by women during the menstrual period.

sanitate, 1. to subject to sanitation. 2. to make sanitary by applying sanitary equipment.

sanitation, 1. the adoption of sanitary measures to eliminate unhealthy elements. 2. hygiene.

sanitize, to render sanitary; to disinfect.

sanity, 1. the state of being sane or of sound mind. 2. rationality. 3. reasonableness.

santonica, 1. a species of wormwood of the Old World. 2. a drug consisting of the dried flower heads of this plant used to expel parasitic intestinal worms.

santonin, a crystalline compound, the active principle of santonica.

saphena, either of the two large veins of the leg.

saphenous, pertaining to the large superficial veins of the leg, the long or internal saphena on the inner side of the leg, and the short, external, or posterior saphena on the outer and posterior sides.

saphenous nerves, the inner and the outer saphenous nerves, which follow the course of the saphenous veins.

sapid, having an agreeable flavor; savory.

sapiens, the specific name of modern man, **Homo sapiens.**

sapor, 1. that which affects the taste sense. 2. taste; savor; flavor.

saporific, of or pertaining to sapor.

saporous, see **saporific.**

sapphism, see **lesbianism.**

sapremia, a form of blood poisoning, esp. that due to the absorption of the toxins produced by certain microorganisms.

sapremic, of or relating to sapremia.

saprogenic, producing putrefaction or decay, as certain bacteria.

saprogenous, see **saprogenic.**

saprophilous, living on decayed substances.

saprophyte, a plant, as one of various bacteria or fungi, that grows on decaying vegetable matter.

saprophytic, of or relating to a saprophyte.

sarcitis, an inflammation of tissue, esp. muscle tissue.

sarcoid, a sarcomalike tumor.

sarcology, the branch of medicine that deals with the anatomy of soft tissue.

sarcoma, any of various malignant tumors originating in the connective tissue.

sarcomatoid, resembling a sarcoma.

sarcomatosis, a condition in which many sarcomas are present in the body.

sarcomatous, see **sarcomatoid.**

sarcous, belonging to or consisting of flesh or muscle.

sardonic grin, see **risus sardonicus.**

sartorial, pertaining to the sartorius.

sartorius, a flat, narrow muscle, the longest in man, running from the ilium to the top of the tibia and crossing the thigh obliquely in front, the chief muscle involved in rotating the leg to the cross-legged position.

sate, 1. to satisfy completely, as the appetite or desire. 2. to glut or satiate.

satiable, capable of being satiated or satisfied.

satiate, see **sate.**

saturnine, 1. morose; of a gloomy temper; sluggish; heavy. 2. pertaining to lead or the absorption of lead, as a person with lead poisoning.

saturnism, see **lead poisoning.**

satyriasis, an uncontrollable sexual appetite in males.

sauriderma, see **ichthyosis.**

scab, a crust formed over a sore in healing.

scabby, 1. covered or coated with scabs. 2. affected with scabies.

scabies, an easily transmitted skin disease, the itch caused by the itch mite, afflicting cattle and sheep as well as man.

scabious, pertaining to or of the nature of scabies.

scabrities, a roughened, scaly condition of the skin.

scabrous, rough with minute points or projections.

scald, 1. a burn caused by hot liquid or steam. 2. affected with scall or scurf.

scalene, relating to the scalenus.

scalenous, see **scalene.**

scalenus, any of a group of three muscles on either side of the cervical vertebrae that aid in respiration and in bending the neck.

scall, a scaly or scabby skin eruption, esp. on the scalp.

scalp, 1. the integument of the upper part of the head, usually including the associated subcutaneous structures. 2. a part of this integument with the accompanying hair.

scalpel, a small, sharp-bladed knife used in anatomical dissection and surgical operations.

scaly, 1. covered with or abounding in scales or scale. 2. characterized by scales. 3. consisting of scales or scale. 4. of the nature of scales.

scanner, 1. one who scans. 2. an instrument that inspects, as for accuracy or performance, a certain operation or condition.

scanning speech, slow and hesitating speech with the pronunciation of words in syllables, usually a symptom of various diseases of the nervous system.

scansion, the act of scanning.

scaphocephalic, having a deformed, boat-shaped head.

scaphoid, boat-shaped.

scaphoid bone, 1. a boat-shaped bone on the radial side of the carpus. 2. a boat-shaped bone on the inner side of the tarsus.

scaphoiditis, an inflammation of the scaphoid bone.

scapula, the shoulder blade.

scapular, of or pertaining to the scapula.

scapulectomy, surgical excision of part or the whole shoulder blade.

scar, the mark of a wound remaining on the skin after healing; a cicatrix.

scarfskin, see **epidermis.**

scarification, the making of a number of small incisions or pricks into the skin, as for vaccination.

scarificator, a medical instrument used to produce scarification.

scarify, to superficially pierce the skin.

scarlatina, a mild form of scarlet fever.

scarlatinal, pertaining to or of the nature of scarlatina.

scarlet fever, a contagious streptococcal disease, usually of children, characterized by fever, inflammation of the throat, and an extensive scarlet rash.

scar tissue, connective tissue that has contracted and replaced normal tissue destroyed by disease, surgery, or injury.

scathe, hurt, harm, or injure, esp. by scorching or searing.

scatology, the study of dung, or of savage practices in which excrement or filth is used.

Shick test, an injection of small amounts of diluted diphtheria toxin, just below the surface of the skin, used to test immunity to diphtheria, nonimmunity being indicated by reddening of the skin.

schistoprosopia, a congenital fissure of the face.

schistosis, see **silicosis.**

schistosome, any trematode worm of the genus **Schistosoma,** including some flukes that parasitize blood vessels of man and other mammals and cause schistosomiasis in man.

schistosomiasis, 1. infestation with schistosomes. 2. a disease caused by schistosomes.

schizo, (slang) a person who is schizophrenic.

schizogenesis, reproduction by fission.

schizogony, the asexual reproductive process of protozoans by multiple fission, as of many of the sporozoans.

schizoid, 1. one whose behavior suggests a tendency toward the abnormalities characteristic of schizophrenia. 2. pertaining to, resembling, or predisposed to schizophrenia.

schizomycete, any of the Schizomycetes, a class or group of plant organisms allied to the fungi.

schizomycetous, of or pertaining to schizomycetes.

schizomycosis, any disease caused by schizomycetes.

schizont, a cell found in certain sporozoans that reproduces itself by repeated asexual fission to form many small cells.

schizonychia, a split condition of the fingernails or toenails.

schizophrenia, a psychosis characterized by emotional, intellectual, and behavioral disturbances, such as withdrawal from reality, delusions, and progressive deterioration. Also called **dementia praecox.**

schizophrenic, 1. one afflicted with schizophrenia. 2. pertaining to schizophrenia.

schizothymia, a schizoid tendency characterized by introversion and withdrawal but remaining within the range of normality.

schizothymic, of or pertaining to schizothymia.

sciatic, 1. affecting or pertaining to the hip or to the sciatic nerves, either of two nerves distributed along the back part of each thigh and leg. 2. a nerve or part that is sciatic.

sciatica, 1. pain and tenderness in a sciatic nerve and its branches. 2. sciatic neuritis. 3. sciatic neuralgia

scirrhoid, pertaining to or like a scirrhus.

scirrhoma, see **scirrhus.**

scirrhosis, the process of scirrhus formation.

scirrhous, indurated; knotty.

scirrhus, a relatively hard tumor, frequently in fibrous tissue, often cancerous, or terminating in a cancer.

scission, 1. the act of cutting or dividing. 2. the state of being cut or split. 3. a division. 4. a separation. 5. a fission.

scissor leg, an abnormal condition in which the legs are crossed in walking because of disease of both hip joints or contraction of thigh abductor muscles.

scissura, see **scission.**

sclera, the fibrous white outer coating that is contiguous with the cornea. Also called **sclerotica.**

scleradenitis, an inflammation and hardening of a gland.

scleral, of or pertaining to the sclera.

sclerectoiridectomy, surgical excision of part of the sclera and the iris, necessitated for the treatment of glaucoma.

sclerencephalia, sclerosis of the brain tissues.

scleritis, an inflammation

of the sclera.

scleroderma, a disease in which the skin becomes hard and rigid.

sclerodermatitis, a skin disease characterized by inflammation of the skin, accompanied by thickening and hardening.

scleroid, having a hard texture; indurated; hardened.

sclerometer, an instrument for determining with precision the degree of hardness of a substance.

sclerose, to affect or become affected with sclerosis; to harden.

sclerosis, 1. a hardening and thickening of a tissue or a part, usually from excessive growth of fibrous or connective tissue. 2. a disease exhibiting such hardening.

sclerotic, 1. pertaining to the sclera, as the sclerotic coat of the eye. 2. hard, firm, as the sclera. 3. affected with or pertaining to sclerosis.

sclerous, hard; bony.

scolecology, see **helminthology.**

scolex, the round, headlike segment at one extremity of a tapeworm, serving as an organ of attachment. 2. the larva of a tapeworm.

scoliometer, an instrument for measuring the curvature of the spine.

scoliorachitic, of or relating to scoliosis and rickets.

scoliosis, a curvature, particularly lateral, of the spine.

scoliotic, pertaining to scoliosis.

scoop, a spoonlike instrument used in extracting the contents of cysts or cavities.

scopolamine, a crystalline alkaloid obtained from the rhizome **Scopolia carniolica** or other solanaceous plants, used as a sedative, truth serum, and mydriatic.

scopophobia, a pathological fear of being seen.

scorbutic, pertaining to or affected with scurvy.

scorbutus, see **scurvy.**

scorch, a superficial burn.

scotoma, a blind spot in the field of vision.

scotomatous, of or pertaining to scotoma.

scotometer, a medical instrument used for the detection and measuring of blind spots in the visual field.

scotophobia, a pathological fear of darkness.

scotopia, the adaptation of the eye to see in the dark.

scratch test, a test to determine allergic susceptibility by the application of allergens into scratches made in the skin, an allergic condition being indicated by subsequent inflammation of the area.

screen, in dreams, a person or object that symbolizes another, concealing the real object of the emotions of the dreamer.

screwworm, the larva of a fly, a dipterous insect that deposits its eggs in sores or in the nose. The larvae live upon the tissue of the host.

scrobiculate, furrowed or pitted.

scrobiculus, any small groove or pit.

scrofula, a constitutional disorder of a tuberculous nature, characterized chiefly by swelling and degeneration of the lymphatic glands, esp. of the neck, and by inflammation of the joints.

scrofuloderma, a skin disorder, usually of tuberculous origin.

scrofulous, of or pertaining to scrofula.

scrotal, of or pertaining to the scrotum.

scrotitis, an inflammation of the scrotum.

scrotocele, hernia in the scrotum.

scrotum, the external pouch that contains the testicles.

scruple, 1. to hesitate or be reluctant on conscientious or similar grounds. 2. a modern unit of apothecaries' weight equivalent to 20 grains or one-third of a dram.

scrupulous, 1. having or showing a strict regard for what is right. 2. minutely careful, precise, or exact.

scurf, 1. matter composed of minute scales of dry skin flaking from the body, as dandruff. 2. a crusty or scaly layer of matter adhering to a surface.

scurvy, a disease characterized in part by swollen and readily bleeding gums, livid skin patches, and generalized exhaustion, affecting persons who are deprived of vitamin C.

scutiform, shaped like a shield.

scutum, any shield-shaped bone.

scyphoid, cup-shaped.

seasickness, nausea and vomiting produced by the rolling or pitching of a vessel at sea; one of a group of motion sicknesses.

sebaceous, 1. pertaining to sebum. 2. pertaining to or containing fat. 3. made of or secreting fatty matter. 4. fatty.

sebaceous cyst, a swelling beneath the skin formed by blockage of the duct of a sebaceous gland and filled with sebaceous material.

sebaceous gland, small glands under the skin, secreting sebum.

sebiparous, producing sebaceous matter.

seborrhea, an excessive increase in the sebum secreted by the sebaceous glands.

seborrheic, of or pertaining to seborrhea.

sebum, the fatty secretion of the sebaceous gland.

secondary sex characteristic, any manifest characteristic specific to either sex but not necessary to reproduction, and due to the effect of gonadal secretions of hormones, as the development of beards or breasts in humans at puberty.

second childhood, dotage; senility.

second-degree burn, a burn characterized by blistering and redness of the affected area, without destruction of the epidermis.

secretagogue, 1. any agent that causes secretion of glands. 2. anything that stimulates secreting organs.

secrete, 1. to produce, release, or discharge by secretion. 2. causing or promoting secretion.

secretin, a hormone, produced in the lining of the small intestine, that stimulates the secretory activity of the pancreas.

secretion, 1. the process by which functionally specialized and excretory substances are separated from the blood, elaborated into different materials, such as bile, saliva, mucus, or urine, and released into or from the body. 2. a secreted substance.

secretory, 1. pertaining to secretion. 2. performing the act of secretion. 3. a secretory organ, gland, or the like.

section, 1. the act of cutting or separation by cutting, as in surgery. 2. a thin slice of material for microscopic examination.

sector, a separate part; a special area of the body.

secundines, see aftanbirth.

sedation, the practice or act of alleviating pain, distress, or tension through the use of sedatives.

sedative, 1. tending to calm

or tranquilize. 2. allaying irritation and irritation. 3. assuaging pain. 4. a medicine that allays irritability and irritation and assuages pain.

sedentary, 1. accustomed to sit; requiring such sitting; inactive; indolent. 2. staying in one locale, as contrasted with migratory. 3. permanently affixed to something.

segment, 1. one of the parts into which anything naturally separates or is divided. 2. a division or section. 3. any section of a leg or the like between joints. 4. to separate or divide into segments.

segmental, 1. pertaining to a segment or segments. 2. composed of segments. 3. of the nature of a segment. 4. having the form of a segment of a circle, as a segmental arch.

segmentation, a division into segments.

segmentation cavity, the central cavity of a blastula.

segregation, 1. the act of segregating, or the state of being segregated; isolation. 2. the separation of paired or allelic genes into different gametes in the process of meiosis.

Seidlitz powders, an aperient consisting of two powders, one tartaric acid and the other a mixture of sodium bicarbonate and Rochelle salt, which are dissolved separately and the solutions mixed and drunk while effervescing.

seismotherapy, a treatment of disease by use of mechanical vibration.

seizure, 1. a sudden attack, as of some disease. 2. a fit, as an epileptic fit, a heart attack, or a stroke.

self-abasement, degradation of oneself, esp. because of feelings of guilt, inferiority, or shame.

self-abuse, 1. the act of belittling oneself. 2. self-reproach. 3. disregard of one's own health. 4. masturbation.

self-analysis, the search for understanding of oneself, usually by methods similar to those of professionals but without the services of such trained persons.

self-centered, 1. centered in oneself; engrossed in self, selfish. 2. being itself fixed as a center.

self-conscious, 1. aware of the existence, actions, or thinking of oneself. 2. conscious of oneself or one's own thoughts or actions. 3. excessively conscious of oneself. 4. given to thinking excessively of oneself as an object of observation to others. 5. exhibiting shyness or embarrassment.

self-deception, the act or fact of fooling or deceiving oneself.

self-delusion, see **self-deception.**

self-deprecating, undervaluing or belittling oneself; overly modest.

self-destruction, the destruction of oneself or itself; suicide.

self-hypnosis, self-induced hypnosis.

semeiology, see **symptomatology.**

semeiotic, see **symptomatic.**

semen, the whitish, viscous substance that carries spermatozoa and is secreted by the male reproductive organs.

semicircular canals, three curved tubular canals in the labyrinth of the ear, responsible for maintaining equilibrium.

semilunar, resembling in form a half moon; crescent-shaped.

semilunar valve, one of two valves situated at the entrance to the aorta and to the pulmonary artery, having three crescentic cusps that prevent regurgitation of blood into the ventricles of the heart.

seminal, pertaining to or consisting of seed or semen.

seminal vesicle, one of two small saclike glands, lying behind the bladder of the male. Their ducts join the ducts that carry semen from the testicles.

semination, see **impregnation.**

seminiferous, seed-bearing; producing or bearing semen.

semipermeable, permeable only by certain substances, as a membrane that permits the passage of a solvent but not the solute.

semiprivate, somewhat but not completely private, as a hospital room containing two or three beds.

senega snakeroot, a milkwort of the Northeastern U.S., the root of which is used medicinally as an expectorant and a diuretic.

senescence, the state of growing old.

senile, 1. pertaining to old age. 2. characterized by the weakness of old age, esp. a decline in mental faculties.

senilism, old age, esp. when premature.

senility, the state of being senile; old age, esp. the infirmity of age; dotage.

senna, any of various leguminous herbs, shrubs, or trees of the genus **Cassia,** the dried leaflets of which are used as a laxative medicine.

sensate, perceived by a sense or the senses.

sensation, 1. an impression made upon the mind through the medium of one of the organs of sense. 2. the power of feeling or receiving impressions. 3. a non-localized feeling arising from intrapsychic sources and not dependent upon bodily stimulation, as a sensation of awe.

sense, any of the special faculties connected with bodily organs by which man and other animals perceive external objects and their own bodily changes, as sight, hearing, smell, taste, and touch.

sense organ, a specialized organ, such as the nose, ear, or eye, that is sensitive to or registers external stimuli; a receptor.

sensitive, 1. having the capacity to receive impressions from external influences. 2. having feelings easily excited.

sensitivity, 1. the state of being sensitive. 2. the state of being readily affected by the action of appropriate chemical or other agents. 3. readiness of muscles or nerves to respond to stimuli.

sensitization, the state of being sensitized.

sensitize, to render sensitive, particularly to agents that produce allergies.

sensitizer, any agent that produces sensitization.

sensorium, 1. the supposed seat of sensation, or sensory nerve center in the brain. 2. the whole sensory apparatus of the body.

sensory, 1. relating to the sensorium or to sensation. 2. conveying sense impulses, as sensory nerves.

sensual, 1. pertaining to the body and the physical senses as distinguished from those of the spirit. 2. pertaining to excessive gratification of physical appetites.

sensualism, a state of subjection to the sensual appetites; sensuality.

sensualize, to make sensual; to debase by carnal gratification.

sensuous, 1. pertaining to the senses. 2. appealing to the senses, esthetically as well as physically. 3. readily affected through the senses. 4. alive to the pleasure to be received through the senses.

sentience, 1. the state of being sentient. 2. the capability for perceiving or feeling. 3. consciousness not involving thought.

sentient, of or pertaining to sentience.

sepsis, a poisoned state of the system caused by a spread of infection through the blood.

septal, of or pertaining to a septum or septa.

septate, divided by a septum or septa.

septectomy, surgical excision of a septum, esp. the nasal septum or part of it.

septic, 1. pertaining to or of the nature of sepsis; putrefactive; infective; pusforming. 2. a substance that causes putrefaction or sepsis.

septicemia, the presence in the bloodstream of infectious microorganisms or their toxins; blood poisoning.

septicemic, of or pertaining to septicemia.

septic sore throat, an acute infection of the throat caused by streptococcus bacteria and characterized by inflammation of the throat and tonsils, fever, toxemia, and often prostration.

septimetritis, an inflammation of the uterus caused by sepsis.

septometer, an instrument for measuring the width of the nasal septum.

septonasal, of or pertaining to the nasal septum.

septotome, a surgical instrument used in operations on the nasal septum.

septotomy, surgical incision of a septum.

septum, a dividing wall, membrane, or the like; a dissepiment or partition of tissue.

septuplet, one of seven children born of a single pregnancy .

sequel, 1. the consequence of a disease. 2. a morbid affection that results from and follows another.

sequela, see **sequel.**

sequestral, of or pertaining to a sequestrum.

sequestration, 1. the formation of a sequestrum. 2. isolation or quarantine of a patient.

sequestrectomy, surgical excision of a sequestrum.

sequestrum, a detached dead bone fragment that adjoins sound bone.

sero-albuminuria, the presence in the urine of serum albumin (albumin derived from the blood serum).

serocolitis, an inflammation of the serous coat of the colon.

seroculture, the growing of a bacterial culture on blood serum.

serohepatitis, an inflammation of the membran-ous covering of the liver.

serologist, one specializing in serology.

serology, the scientific study of the nature and actions of blood serum.

serolysin, a bactericidal substance in the blood serum.

serosa, a serous membrane, esp. the peritoneal membrane that coats most of the viscera of the intestines.

serositis, an inflammation of a serous membrane.

serotherapy, the treatment of a disease by injecting human or animal blood serum containing antibodies.

serotonin, a crystalline substance, normally found in certain blood, brain, and intestinal cells, that causes muscle contraction and vasoconstriction.

serous, 1. resembling serum. 2. of a thin, liquid nature. 3. containing or secreting serum. 4. pertaining to serum.

serous membrane, any of various thin membranes, as the peritoneum, that line certain cavities of the body and secrete serous fluid.

serpigo, a skin disease that spreads from one area to another, as ringworm.

serum, 1. a clear, pale-yellow liquid that separates from the clot in the coagulation of blood. 2. a fluid obtained from the blood of an animal that has been rendered immune to some disease by inoculation, used as an antitoxic or therapeutic agent.

serum albumin, 1. a simple protein that is the principal one found in plasma and the body's serous fluids. 2. such a substance precipitated from animal blood and prepared for commercial use.

serum globulin, a plasma protein that may be separated by electrophoresis into three blood fractions, alpha, beta, and gamma globulin, which have been shown to serve related functions; the last named is responsible for the body's ability to resist certain infections.

serum sickness, an allergic reaction that may occur after serum injections.

serum therapy, see **serotherapy.**

sesamoid, resembling a sesame seed in form, as some nodular cartilages and bones.

setaceous, bristlelike; bristle-shaped; bristly; stiff.

seventh cranial nerve, the facial nerve.

sex, 1. the total physical and behavioral differences, properties, and characteristics by which the male and female are distinguished. 2. activities relating to or based on sexual attraction, sexual relations, or sexual reproduction. 3. sexual intercourse.

sex chromosome, a chromosome that carries sex-linked traits and acts as a determinant of the offspring.

sexed, 1. belonging to a sex or possessing sexual traits. 2. being sexually attractive or appealing.

sex hormone, a hormone affecting the growth or function of the sexual organs or the development of secondary sex characteristics.

sex hygiene, the part of hygiene concerned with sexual activity as it affects personal and community well-being.

sexless, 1. having or seeming to have no sex. 2. exciting or evidencing no sexual desires.

sex-linked, designating a gene contained in a sex chromosome, or a character controlled by such a gene.

sexological, of or pertaining to sexology.

sexologist, a scientist specializing in sexology.

sexology, the science that deals with sexual behavior, esp. of humans.

sextuplet, one of six children born of a single pregnancy.

sexual, 1. pertaining to sex or the sexes. 2. motivated by or exhibiting sex. 3. denoting reproduction by processes involving both a male and a female.

sexual intercouse, coitus; copulation.

sexuality, 1. sexual character; possession of sex. 2. the recognition or emphasizing of sexual matters.

sexual organs, the genitalia.

sexy, involving excessive sex; sexually provocative or exciting.

shaft, the long middle portion of a bone.

shake, to move with jerky vibrations to and fro, up and down, or in different directions; to quiver, tremble, shiver, or vibrate by or as if by a physical or mental cause, condition, or blow.

shaking palsy, see **Parkinson's disease.**

shaky, given to shaking; shaking; trembling; weak or feeble, or not strong in health.

shamble, to walk or go awkwardly or unsteadily; shuffle.

shank, see **shin.**

sharp-eyed, see **sharp-sighted.**

sharp-nosed, possessing an acute sense of smell.

sharp-sighted, having acute vision.

sharp-witted, having acute mental faculties.

sheath, a closely enveloping part or structure.

shell shock, combat fatigue, a kind of nervous breakdown of soldiers during or after battle.

shin, 1. the forepart of the leg between the ankle and the knee. 2. the sharp-edged front of the tibia, or shinbone.

shinbone, see **shin.**

shingles, a painful viral infection involving the central nervous system and characterized by the eruption of groups of blisters on the skin along the affected nerves. Also called **herpes zoster.**

shiver, to shake involuntarily or tremble, as with cold, fear, or excitement.

shock, a sudden debilitating effect on the bodily functions caused by a violent impression on the nervous system, as from a severe injury, a surgical operation, an emotional disturbance, or the like. 2. the resulting condition of nervous depression or prostration. 3. the effect produced on the body by the sudden passage through it of a current of electricity.

shock therapy, a treatment for mental disorders, based on the coma or other shock effects induced by injections of drugs, such as insulin, or by the application of electrical currents to the brain.

shock treatment, see **shock therapy.**

shortsightedness, see **myopia.**

short-winded, see **dyspnea.**

shoulder, the joint by which the arm is connected with the body.

shoulder blade, either of the two large, flat triangular bones in the upper back on either side, forming the dorsal part in humans. Also called **scapula.**

shoulder girdle, the bony or cartilaginous semicircular band or arch that serves for the attachment and support of the upper extremities.

show, the discharge of a small amount of blood from the vagina prior to the first stage of labor.

shudder, an agitation or convulsive shaking of the body; tremor.

sialaden, a salivary gland.

sialadenitis, an inflammation of a salivary gland.

sialagogue, a medicine that promotes the salivary flow.

sialagogic, of or relating to sialagogue.

sialaporia, deficiency in secretion of saliva.

sialic, of or pertaining to saliva.

sialine, see **sialic.**

sialism, an excessive flow of saliva.

sialoadenectomy, surgical excision of a salivary gland.

sialoadenitis, see **sialadenitis.**

sialoangitis, an inflammation of the salivary ducts.

sialolithiasis, the presence of stones in a salivary gland or duct.

sialoncus, a tumor under the tongue, usually caused by the presence of an obstruction in a salivary gland or duct.

Siamese twins, 1. Siamese male twins born joined at the chest by a cartilaginous band. 2. any twins congenitally united.

sib, 1. a relative, esp. a sister or brother; a sibling. 2. kinsmen or relatives collectively.

sibilant, hissing.

sibilus, a hissing rale.

sibling, see **sib.**

sick, affected with disease of any kind; not healthy; ill.

sick bay, the portion of a ship used as a hospital.

sickbed, a bed on which a sick person lies, often specially built for the purpose.

sick call, the time of day when sick military personnel may report for treatment.

sicken, to become sick; to feel wearied.

sick headache, headache accompanied by nausea; migraine.

sickish, nauseating or sickening; indisposed or somewhat sick.

sick leave, time away from work or duty, usually with pay, accorded to employees when ill.

sickle cell, a crescent-shaped red blood cell having abnormal hemoglobin, often causing a fatal anemic disease.

sickle-cell anemia, a hereditary chronic blood disorder, usually found only in blacks, in which the red blood cells take on a crescent shape, causing a crystallization of the cells within erythrocytes, distorting them and clogging blood vessels.

sickly, habitually ailing or indisposed; not robust.

sickness, the state of being sick; disease; ill health; any disordered state.

sickroom, a room occupied by a sick person.

side effect, an unintended,

esp. harmful, secondary reaction to a drug or chemical.

siderodromophobia, a pathological fear of trains.

sideropenia, iron deficiency in the blood.

sideropenic, pertaining to sideropenia.

sideroscope, an opthalmological instrument for detecting small particles of iron or steel in the eye.

siderosis, a disease of the lungs caused by inhaling particles of iron or other metals, occurring mainly in iron miners or welders.

siderous, of, pertaining to, or containing iron.

sigh, to emit a prolonged and audible breath, as from sorrow, weariness, relief, or yearning.

sight, 1. the power or faculty of seeing. 2. the sense whereby objects are perceived with the eyes. 3. vision. 4. the act or fact of seeing. 5. the range or field of vision.

sightless, see **blind.**

sigmoid, 1. shaped like the letter S. 2. of or pertaining to a flexure of the colon, specifically its last curve before terminating in the rectum.

sigmoidal, see **sigmoid.**

sigmoid colon, see **sigmoid flexure.**

sigmoidectomy, the surgical excision of all or part of the sigmoid flexure.

sigmoid flexure, a sharply curving final segment of the decending colon, beginning at a point opposite the crest of the ileum

and ending in juncture with the rectum.

sigmoiditis, an inflammation of the sigmoid colon.

sigmoidoscope, an illuminated tubular surgical instrument that is passed into the anus for examination of the sigmoid flexure.

sigmoidoscopy, the examination of the sigmoid colon with a sigmoidoscope.

sigmoidostomy, the surgical creation of an artificial anus in the sigmoid flexure.

sign, any objective indication of disease.

signature, that part of a prescription giving directions for the use of the prescribed medicine.

sign language, a system of manual signs or gestures used as a substitute for speech by the deaf. Also called **hand language.**

silicon, a nonmetallic element having both crystalline and amorphous forms, occurring in a combined state in rocks and minerals, and constituting more than one-fourth of the earth's crust.

silicone, a compound made by substituting silicon for carbon in substances such as oils, greases, synthetic rubber, and resins, to provide greater stability and resistance to water and to temperature extremes.

silicosis, a disease of the lungs caused by inhalation of silica dust, as by stonecutters.

silicotic, of or pertaining to silicosis.

silver protein, any of several colloidal preparations of protein and silver used in solutions as external antiseptics.

simple, 1. something not mixed or compounded. 2. formerly, a medicinal herb or a medicine obtained from a single herb.

simple fracture, a bone fracture with no complications.

simulate, to feign disease.

simulation, the act of simulating or feigning a disease or symptoms of a disease.

simulator, one who simulates.

sinapism, a mustard plaster.

sincipital, of or pertaining to the sinciput.

sinciput, the upper part of the head, esp. the front; see also **forehead.**

sinew, see **tendon.**

sinewy, 1. consisting of or resembling sinews. 2. well braced with sinews. 3. strong. 4. having prominent sinews.

singultus, see **hiccup.**

sinister, on the left hand or the left side; left.

sinistral, 1. of, pertaining to, or inclining to the left side. 2. left-handed.

sinistraural, hearing better with the left ear.

sinistrocardia, a displacement of the heart to the left side of the medial line.

sinistrocerebral, pertaining to or located in the left cerebral hemisphere.

sinistrocular, having stronger vision in the left than the right eye.

sinistromanual, left-handed.

sinistropedal, left-footed.

sinuate, bent in and out; winding.

sinuosity, a curve, bend, or turn.

sinuous, abounding in curves, bends, or turns; winding.

sinus, 1. any of various cavities, recesses, or passages, as a hollow in a bone, or a reservoir or channel for venous blood. 2. a cranial hollow, containing air, which connects with the nasal cavities. 3. a dilated part in a canal or vessel. 4. a narrow, elongated abscess with a small orifice. 5. a narrow passage leading to an abscess or the like.

sinusal, of or pertaining to a sinus.

sinusitis, an inflammation of a sinus, as of those in the bones of the face.

sinusoid, resembling a sinus.

sitiergia, a hysterical refusal to take food (probably closely related to **anorexia nervosa**).

sitiology, the branch of medicine that relates to diet and nutrition.

sitology, see **sitiology.**

sitomania, a periodic abnormal craving for food.

sitophobia, a pathological abhorrence of food, either generally or of specific dishes.

sitosterol, any of several

sterols or groups of sterols that occur widely in plants, esp. soybeans, and are used in varying forms and combinations for the synthetic production of steroid hormones.

sitotherapy, the medical use of food; treatment by dieting.

situs, the proper or original position, as of a part or organ.

sitz bath, a form of bath, usually taken for therapeutic purposes, in which only the hips and thighs are covered with water.

skeletal, of or pertaining to the skeleton.

skeleton, the total bony framework that sustains the softer body parts.

skiagram, see **skiagraph.**

skiagraph, an object shown by shadowed outline, as by X rays; a radiograph.

skiagraphy, the act or art of delineating shadows; the making of skiagraphs.

skiametry, the examination of the eye by skiascopy.

skiascope, an instrument used for detecting errors of refraction in the eye by observing the movement of light and shadow from the retina as it is illuminated from various angles. See **retinoscope.**

skiascopy, examination of the eye and testing of the vision with a skiascope.

skin, the external covering or integument of the body.

skin graft, the viable skin transplanted in skin grafting.

skin grafting, a process

whereby pieces of healthy skin are transplanted from a donor's or the patient's body to replace skin that has been destroyed, as by burns.

skinny, 1. very thin; undesirably slender; emaciated. 2. consisting of or like skin.

skin test, a test in which a particular substance, as pollen, is applied to or injected into the skin in order to determine the extent of the patient's allergic sensitivity to it. See also **Schick test, scratch test.**

skull, the cranium or bony case that forms the framework of the head and encloses the brain.

skull and crossbones, representation of a human skull, with two bones crossed beneath it, formerly the design on a pirate flag, now a generalized warning of danger to life.

slabber, to unintentionally dribble saliva; to slobber.

slaver, see **slabber.**

sleep, 1. to take the repose or rest afforded by a suspension of the voluntary exercise of the bodily functions and the natural suspension, complete or partial, of consciousness. 2. the state of a person who sleeps.

sleeper, one who or that which sleeps; a slumberer.

sleeping sickness, a disease, generally fatal, that is common in certain parts of Africa, characterized usually by fever, weight loss, and progressive lethargy and caused by a parasitic protozoan, **Trypanosoma gambiense**, transmitted through the bite of a tsetse fly.

sleepless, without sleep; wakeful; unable to sleep; watchful.

sleepwalk, see **somnambulate.**

slipped disk, an inflamed or displaced intervertebral disk causing pressure on the spinal nerve.

slobber, see **slabber.**

slouch, to sit or stand in an awkward, drooping posture; to fail to maintain an erect posture.

slough, a mass or layer of dead tissue that separates from the surrounding or underlying living tissue.

slow-witted, slow of wit, of intelligence, or understanding; dull.

slumber, to sleep, usually lightly; to drowse or doze.

small intestine, the long, narrow, upper section of the intestines, which extends from the pyloric valve of the stomach to the cecum of the large intestine, and which serves, through its secretion of enzymes, to digest and assimilate nutritive substances.

smallpox, an acute virus disease, highly contagious, and marked by fever and pustular eruptions that leave permanent scarring of the skin.

smegma, secretions of sebaceous glands, esp. the thick cheesy secretion found under the labia minora and under the foreskin.

smegmatic, of or relating to smegma.

smell, 1. to perceive through the function of the olfactory nerves in the nose; to perceive or detect the scent or odor of. 2. the sense or faculty of perceiving by smelling with the nose. 3. that which affects the olfactory organs.

smelling salts, ammonium carbonate, often scented, used for resuscitation and stimulation.

snaggletooth, a tooth growing beyond or apart from others.

snare, a looped wire instrument for excising tumors or other such growths.

sneeze, 1. to emit air or breath suddenly, forcibly, and audibly through the nose and mouth by involuntary, spasmodic action. 2. the act or sound of sneezing.

sniffle, 1. to sniff repeatedly, as from a cold in the head or from repressing tears. 2. the act or sound of sniffling.

snore, 1. to breathe during sleep through the open mouth, or the mouth and nose, making hoarse or harsh sounds. 2. the act or sound of snoring.

snow blindness, temporarily reduced vision caused by the glare of sunlight reflected by snow.

sob, to weep with convulsive catching of the breath.

soda lime, a mixture of sodium hydroxide or caustic soda and calcium hydroxide or slaked lime, used in the production of ammonia and for the absorption of moisture, esp. from certain gases.

sodium bicarbonate, a white crystalline compound used in making baking powder and as an antacid and in other medical preparations.

sodium chloride, common table salt.

sodium citrate, white granular powder, salty in taste, water soluble, and used as an anticoagulant in blood transfusions.

sodium iodide, a compound resembling potassium iodide.

sodium salicylate, a white compound powder, used as an analgesic and antipyretic.

sodium sulfate, Glauber's salts, used as a mild cathartic and diuretic.

sodomite, one who practices sodomy.

sodomy, unnatural sexual intercourse, esp. of one man with another or of a human being with an animal.

soft palate, see **palate.**

solar, of or pertaining to the sun.

solar plexus, a network of nerves situated at the upper part of the abdomen, behind the stomach and in front of the aorta.

sole, the bottom or under- surface of the foot.

soleprint, a print of the sole of the foot, esp. as used in hospitals to identify infants.

solution, 1. the crisis or termination of a disease. 2. a rupture or separation such as a laceration or fracture. 3. the homogeneous combination of a liquid, solid, or gas with another liquid or, more rarely, a gas or solid; the preparation formed by this combination.

solvent, any substance that dissolves other substances.

soma, 1. all the body cells of an organism excluding the germ cells. 2. the body as distinguished from the mind.

somatic, of or pertaining to the body.

somatic cell, any of the cells that compose the various organs, tissues, and other parts of the body, except the reproductive cells; opposed to **germ cell.**

somatogenic, having origin in or affecting somatic cells.

somatology, 1. the science dealing with the body in all its physical aspects. 2. a branch of anthropology in which the physical nature of evolving man is subjected to comparative study and evaluation.

somatopathic, of or pertaining to somatopathy.

somatopathy, any physical bodily disease, as distinguished from a mental disease.

somatoplasm, the protoplasm making up the composition of a body or soma cell of an organism, distinguished from **germ plasm.**

somatopleure. the embryonic layer formed out of the association between the ectoderm and the parietal layer of the lateral mesoderm.

somatopsychic, pertaining to both body and mind.

somatotype, 1. physique. 2. body type. 3. one of the types of body build, ectomorph, endomorph, or mesomorph, differentiated by the relative prominence of structures developed from one of the three embryonic germ layers.

somesthetic, pertaining to the sensory structures of the body.

somite, any of the embryonic segments from which various organs are derived.

somitic, of or pertaining to a somite.

somnambulate, to walk while asleep.

somnambulism, the state or practice of walking or performing other motor acts while asleep; sleepwalking.

somnambulist, a person who is subject to somnambulism.

somnifacient, producing or inducing sleep or sleepiness.

somniferous, causing or inducing sleep, as a narcotic; soporific.

somniloqui, the act of talking during sleep.

somnolence, sleepiness; drowsiness.

somnolent, sleepy; drowsy; inducing sleep; inclined to sleep.

sonorous, giving out or capable of giving out a sound, esp. a deep or resonant sound.

sonovox, an electronic device for transmitting recorded sounds to the laryngeal area to be emitted in turn as words through the mouth, as by a person whose larynx has been removed.

sopor, a deep, unnatural sleep; stupor.

soporiferous, tending to bring sleep; soporific.

soporific, see **soporiferous.**

soporose, pertaining to or resembling morbid sleep.

soporous, see **soporose.**

sorbose, a simple crystalline sugar, produced industrially by bacterial oxidation of sorbitol, a main agent in the chemical synthesis of vitamin C.

sore, 1. painful or tender, as a bruise, wound, or inflammation on the body or skin. 2. stiff and tender, as from physical exercise. 3. suffering mental anguish and grief, as, sore in mind and heart. 4. a place where the skin or flesh is bruised, cut, infected, or painful. 5. any cause of sorrow, pain, misery, or vexation.

sore throat, an inflammation of the pharynx,

fauces, or tonsils, marked by pain, esp. in swallowing.

souffle, a soft blowing sound heard through the stethoscope in auscultation, as a cardiac souffle (heart murmur), etc.

sound, 1. the sensation produced in the organs of hearing by certain vibrations or sound waves conveyed by the atmosphere, water, or other elastic medium. 2. to examine by percussion or auscultation, as a physician sounds a patient's chest. 3. to explore, as a body cavity, or to dilate, as strictures in a canal, by means of sound. 4. a long, slender, usually curved instrument for sounding or exploring cavities or canals of the body.

Spanish fly, a blister beetle, esp. **Lytta vesicatoria,** used in medicine, after drying and powdering, as a counterirritant or a diuretic. See **cantharis.**

Spanish influenza, 1. a contagious respiratory disease produced by a virus and resulting in fever, coughing, and general body pains. 2. the worldwide epidemic of such respiratory infections in 1917–18.

spargosis, 1. expansion of the female breasts with milk. 2. see **elephantiasis.**

sparteine, a bitter, poisonous liquid alkaloid obtained from the common broom, **Cytisus scopar-**

ius, used in medicine.

spasm, 1. a sudden, abnormal, involuntary muscular contraction. 2. an affection consisting of continued muscular contraction (tonic spasm). 3. a series of alternating muscular contractions and relaxations (clonic spasm).

spasmodic, pertaining to or of the nature of spasm; characterized by spasms; resembling a spasm or spasms.

spastic, 1. pertaining to, of the nature of, or characterized by spasm, esp. muscular spasm. 2. a person given to spasms or convulsions, esp. one suffering from cerebral palsy.

spastic paralysis, a paralytic condition marked by prolonged muscular contractions and increased reflexes of the tendons.

spay, to remove the ovaries, usually said of animals.

specialist, a medical practitioner who devotes his attention to a particular class of diseases.

specific, 1. produced by a special cause or infection, as a disease. 2. having special effect in the cure of a certain disease.

specimen, a sample of a body substance to be analyzed for diagnostic purposes.

spectacles, a device to aid defective vision or to protect the eyes from light, dust, or the like.

spectroscope, an optical instrument used to form

and analyze spectrums.

spectrum, a series of colors (red, orange, yellow, green, blue, indigo, and violet) produced when white light is passed through a prism.

speculum, a surgical instrument for rendering a part accessible to observation, as by enlarging an orifice.

speech, the faculty or power of expressing thoughts and emotions by articulated sounds and words.

sperm, the reproductive seminal fluid of males.

spermacrasia, lack of spermatozoa in the seminal fluid.

spermary, the organ in males in which spermatozoa are produced; testis.

spermatemphraxis, an obstruction that prevents the discharge of semen.

spermatic, 1. pertaining to, resembling, or conveying sperm; seminal. 2. relating to spermary.

spermatic cord, the cord by which the testicle is suspended within the scrotum, and which contains the vas deferens, the blood vessels, and the nerves of the testicle.

spermatid, a cell developed from a lower cell, called a spermatocyte, which will grow into a fully developed male reproductive cell.

spermatism, ejaculation, voluntary or involuntary, of semen.

spermatocele, a cystic tumor arising in or around a testicle containing spermatozoa.

spermatocyst, see **spermatocele.**

spermatocyte, a primary male germ cell that develops from the division of a spermatogonium and then itself divides to produce a spermatid and subsequent spermatozoon.

spermatogenesis, the genesis or origin and development of spermatozoa.

spermatogenic, of or pertaining to the origin and development of spermatozoa.

spermatogonium, one of the primitive germ cells that give rise to the spermatocytes.

spermatoid, resembling spermatozoa; like semen.

spermatology, the science and study of the seminal fluid.

spermatolysis, the destruction of spermatozoa.

spermatopathy, any disorder of sperm cells, their secreting ducts, or glands.

spermatorrhea, the involuntary discharge of semen, abnormally frequent, without sexual intercourse.

spermatozoic, of or pertaining to spermatozoa.

spermatozoon, 1. one of the numerous minute, usually actively mobile bodies contained in semen or sperm that fertilize the ovum of the female. 2. any mature male reproductive cell.

spermaturia, discharge of semen with the urine.

spermiogenesis, the production of male reproductive cells.

spew, to discharge the contents of the stomach through the mouth; to vomit.

sphenoid, pertaining to the sphenoid bone.

sphenoidal, see **sphenoid.**

sphenoid bone, the wedge-shaped bone at the base of the skull.

spherocyte, an erythrocyte that is nearly spherical and more fragile than normal.

sphincter, a contractile ringlike muscle surrounding and capable of closing a natural orifice or passage.

sphincteral, of or pertaining to a sphincter.

sphincteralgia, pain in the muscles of the anal sphincter.

sphincterectomy, surgical excision of any sphincter.

sphygmogram, a tracing of the pulse produced by the sphygmograph.

sphygmograph, an instrument which, when applied over an artery, graphically records the uniformity, strength, and rapidity of the pulse.

sphygmographic, of or pertaining to a sphygmograph.

sphygmography, the graphical recording of the pulse movement.

sphygmoid, resembling the pulse.

sphygmomanometer, an instrument for measuring the pressure of the blood in an artery.

sphygmomanometric, of or pertaining to the blood pressure in an artery.

sphygmometer, an instrument that measures the rate and force of the pulse. See also **sphygmograph.**

sphygmophone, an instrument for making the pulse beat audible.

sphygmoscope, an instrument for making the pulsation of arteries and veins visible.

sphygmotonometer, an instrument for determining the elasticity of the walls of an artery.

sphygmous, of or pertaining to the pulse.

sphygmus, see **pulse.**

spica, a plaster or plain bandage having a spiral and reversed form and looking like a spike of wheat.

spiloma, see **nevus.**

spina bifida, the protrusion of the spinal membranes due to a fissure in the lower part of the spine, usually congenital.

spinal, pertaining to or resembling the spine or backbone.

spinal analgesia, an anesthetic injected into the spinal cord.

spinal canal, the tube or canal that holds the spinal cord as well as its membranes and _ is formed by the vertebral arches.

spinal column, the series of small bones or vertebrae forming the axis of the skeleton and protecting the spinal cord.

spinal cord, the cord of nervous tissue extending through the spinal canal and enclosed within the spinal column.

spine, the backbone that provides the main support for the body. See **spinal column.**

spinobulbar, pertaining to the spinal cord and the medulla oblongata.

spinocerebellar, pertaining to the spinal cord and the cerebellum.

spinose, see **spinous.**

spinous, 1. of or pertaining to the spine. 2. spinelike or spiniform. 3. slender and sharp-pointed, as a bone process.

spinous process, the dorsal bony projection from the middle of the neural arch of a vertebra.

spireme, the chromatin of a cell nucleus when it assumes a continuous or segmented threadlike form during mitosis.

spirillemia, the condition of having bacteria of the genus **Spirillum** in the blood.

spirillum, a microscopic, flagellate bacterium of the genus **Spirillum.**

spirit, a solution in alcohol of an essential or volatile principle.

spirochete, any of the slender threadlike bacteria characterized by spiral or screwlike shapes that constitute the genus **Spirocheta,** some species of which cause diseases, as syphilis and yaws.

spirochetosis, any disease, infection, or condition caused by spirochetes.

spirograph, an instrument for recording the frequency and extent of respiratory movements.

spiroid, resembling a spiral.

spirometer, an instrument for determining the air capacity of the lungs.

spirometry, the measurement of the air capacity of the lungs.

spirophore, a device used for artificial respiration. See **iron lung.**

spit, 1. to eject saliva from the mouth; to expectorate. 2. saliva, esp. when ejected; spittle.

spittle, the secretion of the salivary glands.

splanchna, the intestines or viscera.

splanchnemphraxis, obstruction of the intestines or any other internal organ.

splanchnic, of or pertaining to viscera or intestines.

splanchnicectomy, the surgical removal of a part of a splanchnic nerve.

splanchnic nerves, the three nerves that control the viscera.

splanchnicotomy, the surgical operation of incising a splanchnic nerve.

splanchnology, the branch of medicine that deals with the study of the viscera.

splanchnopathy, any pathological condition of the viscera.

splayfoot, 1. a broad, flat foot, esp. one turned more or less outward. 2. the condition or deformity of having a splayfoot.

spleen, a spongy glandular organ situated in the upper part of the abdomen, being one of the ductless glands.

splenalgia, pain in the spleen.

splenectasis, an enlargement of the spleen.

splenectomy, the surgical removal of the spleen.

splenectopia, see **splenectopy**.

splenectopy, mobility or displacement of the spleen; a floating spleen.

splenetic, see **splenic**.

splenic, pertaining to the spleen; situated in or near the spleen.

splenitis, an inflammation of the spleen.

splenius, a broad, flat muscle of the upper dorsal region and the back and side of the neck, which divides into two sections in ascending the neck and serves in rotating the head and neck, as well as in drawing the head backward.

splenocele, a hernia of the spleen.

splenoid, resembling the spleen.

splenoma, a tumor of the spleen.

splenomegaly, an abnormal growth of the spleen resulting in gross enlargement.

splint, a thin piece of wood or other stiff material used to hold a fractured or dislocated bone in position when set, or to maintain any part of the body in a fixed position.

spondylalgia, a painful condition of a vertebra.

spondylitis, a disorder of the spine or vertebrae that causes inflammation, rigidity, or deformity.

spondylopathy, any disorder of the vertebrae.

spondylosyndesis, a surgical joining of vertebrae.

spontaneity, 1. the fact, state, or quality of being spontaneous. 2. activity or behavior that is spontaneous.

spontaneous, arising from one's own tendencies or impulses, without forethought, constraint, or external effort.

spontaneous fracture, a fracture caused by the state of the bone, due to defects in the bone and not to accident.

spot, a blemish or flaw, as a small scar, eruption, or birthmark. See also **macula**.

spotted fever, any of various fevers characterized by spots on the skin. See **Rocky Mountain spotted fever**.

sprain, 1. to strain or wrench, as the ankle, wrist, or other part of the body at a joint, so as to injure without producing dislocation. 2. an act of spraining; the condition of being sprained.

sprue, a tropical disease characterized by inflammation of the mucous membranes of the digestive tract. See also **thrush.**

spud, a surgical instrument with a spadelike blade to dislodge foreign substances.

spur, a sharp or pointed, usually horny or bony projection.

sputum, spittle or any matter mixed with saliva that is expectorated.

squama, a scale or scalelike part, as of epidermis or bone.

squamaceous, scaly, shaped like a scale.

squamate, provided or covered with scales.

squamosal, 1. pertaining to a thin, scalelike element of the temporal bone in the skull. 2. a squamosal bone.

squamous, see **squamaceous.**

squamulose, see **squamate.**

squint, 1. to look with partially closed eyes, as toward a brilliant light. 2. see **strabismus.**

stabile, 1. unaffected by moderate degrees of heat, as some serum components. 2. stable. 3. noting or pertaining to a mode of application of electricity in which the active electrode is kept stationary over the part to be acted upon. 4. fixed in position.

stable, firm; steady; stationary.

stage, a definite phase in the course of disease, characterized by certain symptoms.

stagger, to sway from side to side while standing or walking as a symptom of various diseases.

stain, a reagent or dye used in staining microscopic specimens.

stamina, 1. strength of physical constitution. 2. power to endure conditions of difficulty or hardship, as disease, fatigue, or privation.

staminal, of or pertaining to stamina.

stammer, 1. to pause, hesitate, or falter involuntarily while speaking. 2. a stammering manner of speaking; a defective utterance.

stanch, to stop the flow of, as a liquid, esp. blood; to stop the flow of blood from, as a wound.

stapedectomy, the surgical excision of the stapes in the ear.

stapedial, of, pertaining to, or shaped like the stapes.

stapes, the innermost of the three small bones in the middle ear.

staph, see **staphylococcus.**

staphyle, see **uvula.**

staphylectomy, the surgical removal of the staphyle.

staphyline, see **uvular.**

staphylitis, an inflammation of the staphyle.

staphylococcus, any of certain bacteria of the genus **Staphylococcus** in which the individual organisms form irregular clusters, resembling a bunch of grapes.

Staphylococcus aureus, a species of staphylococci that causes inflammation and the formation of pus, and is formed in boils and carbuncles.

staphylohemia, the presence of staphylococci in the blood.

staphylorrhaphy, the suture of a cleft palate.

stasis, the retardation or stoppage of the regular flow of fluids in the body, as of the contents of the intestines or of blood in the circulatory system, because of disease.

state, the condition of a person.

status asthmaticus, the state or condition of having persistent and intractable asthma.

status epilepticus, the state or condition of having a succession of epileptic attacks without regaining consciousness during the intervals.

statutory rape, sexual relations with a female under the legal age of consent.

staunch, see **stanch.**

steapsin, the lipase of the pancreatic juice.

stearate, a salt or ester of stearic acid.

stearic acid, a monobasic organic acid used in making lubricants, cosmetics, and medicine.

steariform, resembling fat.

stearodermia, a disease of the sebaceous glands of the skin.

steatitis, an inflammation of the adipose (fatty) tissues.

steatoma, see **lipoma.**

steatopathy, any disease of the sebaceous glands of the skin.

steatopygia, abnormal accumulation of fat on and about the buttocks.

steatorrhea, excess fat in the feces, caused by a disease of the intestine or pancreas and usually accompanied by diarrhea and weight loss.

stegnosis, see **stenosis.**

stellate, resembling the form of a star; radiated.

stenocephaly, an abnormal narrowness of the cranium.

stenosed, contracted or narrowed.

stenosis, the contraction of a passage or canal.

stenotherm, an organism capable of existing only within a narrow range of temperature.

stenotic, of or pertaining to stenosis.

stereognosis, the ability to recognize the form and nature of objects by touch.

stereotype, 1. a set image. 2. a standardized or typical image or conception held by or applied to members of a certain group.

stereotypy, maintenance of a posture or repetition of an action or a speech pattern with such frequency as to be considered abnormal, as in certain mental disorders.

sterile, 1. free of living germs or microorganisms. 2. incapable of producing offspring; barren.

sterility, the condition of being sterile.

sterilize, 1. to render sterile, esp. to free from living germs, as by heating. 2. to inhibit or destroy by surgery the reproductive capabilities of the sex organs.

sterilizer, an appliance for sterilizing, as medical instruments, by heat.

sternal, of or pertaining to the sternum.

sternalgia, pain in the sternum.

sternocostal, in the area between the sternum and the ribs or functionally related to the area.

sternoid, resembling the sternum.

sternum, a bone or series of bones extending along the middle line of the ventral portion of the body, consisting of a flat, narrow bone connected with the clavicles and the true ribs; the breastbone.

sternutation, the act of sneezing.

sternutator, a substance used in chemical warfare that causes sneezing, coughing, and other nasal and respiratory irritations.

sternutatory, causing sneezing; a substance that induces sneezing.

steroid, a class of fat-soluble organic compounds including sterols, bile acids, sex hormones, and certain digitalis compounds.

stertor, 1. see **snoring.** 2. a heavy snoring sound accompanying respiration in certain diseases.

stethoscope, an instrument used in auscultation to convey sounds in the body, esp. those in the chest, to the ear of the examiner.

stethoscopic, of or relating to a stethoscope.

stethoscopy, examination by means of a stethoscope.

sthenic, 1. attended with abnormal increase of activity in the heart and arteries. 2. extremely vigorous; strong.

stigma, 1. a mark or small spot on the skin. 2. a mental or physical mark characteristic of a specific disease or condition.

stigmasterol, a water-insoluble, plant sterol, obtained from soybeans and Calabar beans, and used in manufacturing progesterone and other steroids.

stigmata, marks like the wounds on the crucified body of Christ, said to have been supernaturally impressed upon the bodies of certain persons.

stigmatic, of or relating to a stigma.

stigmatism, 1. a condition characterized by the presence of stigmata. 2. a condition of the eye in which there is no astigmatism.

stigmatist, a person marked with stigmata resembling the wounds of Christ.

stilbestrol, a synthetic crystalline compound similar to but more powerful than estrogen.

stillbirth, 1. the birth of any fetus or offspring that is dead. 2. a stillborn fetus or offspring.

stillborn, dead at birth; abortive.

stimulant, an agent, such as caffeine, that produces a quickly diffused and transient increase of vital energy, activity, and strength in an organism or a part.

stimulate, to produce a quickly diffused and transient increase of vital energy and strength of action; to act as a stimulus.

stimulus, something that incites to action or exertion; a stimulant.

sting, 1. to prick or wound with a sharp-pointed often venom-bearing organ, as a sting or fang of bees and certain other animals. 2. to be affected painfully or irritatingly as the result of contact with certain plants, as, to be stung by nettles.

stirrup, see **stapes.**

stitch, 1. a sudden sharp pain. 2. a suture.

stoma, a minute opening, as a pore.

stomach, 1. the pouchlike enlargement of the alimentary canal, being the principal organ of digestion. 2. to be able to eat, retain, or digest.

stomachache, see **gastralgia.**

stomachic, 1. pertaining to or strengthening the stomach. 2. exciting the action of the stomach. 3. a medicine that strengthens the stomach and stimulates digestion.

stomatitis, an inflammation of the mouth.

stomatologist, a specialist in the treatment of diseases of the mouth.

stomatology, the medical science dealing with the mouth and its diseases.

stomatomycosis, any disease of the mouth caused by fungi.

stomatoschisis, see **harelip.**

stomodeum, the oral or anterior part of the alimentary canal or digestive tract, beginning as an invagination of the ectoderm in the embryo.

stone, 1. a calculous concretion in the kidneys or bladder. 2. the disease arising therefrom.

stool, the discharge from the bowels.

stoop, a stooping movement; a stooping attitude or carriage of body, as a slouch.

strabismal, pertaining to or afflicted with strabismus.

strabismic, see **strabismal.**

strabismus, a disorder of vision due to the turning of one eye or both eyes from the normal position so that both cannot be directed at the same point or object at the same time; squint; cross-eye.

strabometer, an instrument for measuring the degree of strabismus.

strain, 1. to impair, injure, or weaken by stretching or overexertion, as a muscle or tendon. 2. to filter.

strainer, 1. one who or that which strains, esp. a filter. 2. a device for stretching or tightening.

strangle, to kill by compressing the windpipe; to choke.

strangulation, 1. the act of strangling; the state of being strangled. 2. the state of a part too closely constricted, as the intestine in hernia.

strangury, a condition in which the passing of urine occurs drop by drop and is accompanied by pain.

strawberry mark, a reddish, usually raised, vascular birthmark.

strep, colloq. streptococcal.

strep throat, a communicable streptococcal infection of the throat.

streptobacillus, any of the rod-shaped anaerobic, pathogenic or parasitic bacteria of the genus **Streptobacillus,** grouped together in the form of a chain.

streptococcus, any of several spherical or oval bacteria of the genus **Streptococcus,** usually found in long chains or pairs and usually nonmotile.

streptokinase, an enzyme present in certain streptococcal cultures that is used clinically to break down blood clots and fibrinous material.

streptomyces, any of a group of soil microorganisms, genus **Streptomyces,** some of which are cultured for the antibiotic substances they form.

streptomycin, an antibiotic derived from a soil fungus, **Streptomyces griseus.**

stress, a constraining, urging, or impelling physical force; strain.

stria, a slight furrow or ridge; a narrow stripe or streak.

striae atrohicae, fine pinkish-white or gray lines that occur on the skin of the abdomen or breasts following stretching of the skin by obesity, tumor, or pregnancy.

stricken, afflicted with disease, trouble, or sorrow.

stricture, a morbid contraction of any canal or duct of the body; stenosis.

stridor, a harsh respiratory sound caused by any of various forms of obstruction.

stroke, an attack of apoplexy or paralysis.

stroma, 1. the supporting framework of an organ or part, usually consisting of connective tissue. 2. the colorless, spongelike framework of a red blood corpuscle or other cell.

stromal, of or pertaining to a stroma.

strongyl, any of certain nematode worms constituting the family Strongylidae, parasitic in the organs and tissues of man and many animals, and often giving rise to serious pathological conditions.

strongyle, see **strongyl.**

strongyloides, a species of intestinal roundworms.

strongylosis, any disease caused by strongyls.

strophanthin, a glycoside drug obtained from the seeds of an African plant of the dogbane family, used as a stimulant in the treatment of heart disease.

struma, 1. a scrofulous swelling or tumor; scrofula. 2. see **goiter.**

strychnine, a colorless, crystalline, poisonous alkaloid used as an antidote for poisoning by depressant drugs.

strychninism, a morbid condition induced by an overdose, or by excessive use, of strychnine.

stump, any basal portion remaining after the main part has been removed, as after the amputation of a limb of the body.

stunt, to hinder from normal or free growth or progress; to check in development; to dwarf.

stupe, a heated wet compress, sometimes medicated, applied to a wound or sore.

stupefactive, a drug or agent that produces stupor.

stupefy, to put into a state of stupor; to deprive of sensibility; to benumb or dull the faculties; to make stupid, as with a narcotic.

stupor, a state of suspended or deadened sensibility; mental torpor or apathy.

stuporous, affected with stupor.

stutter, 1. to utter involuntary or spasmodic repetitions of syllables or sounds in the effort to speak, esp. habitually, from a defect in the power of speech; to stammer. 2. a stuttering mode of utterance.

sty, a small inflammatory protuberance or enlargement of a sebaceous gland on the edge of the eyelid.

stye, see **sty.**

style, a slender blunt-pointed probe.

stylet, the stiffening wire or rod in a flexible catheter; a probe.

styloid, pertaining to certain stylus-shaped skeletal processes, as on the ulna, the radius, or the temporal bone.

stype, see **tampon.**

styptic, 1. having the quality of stopping the bleeding of a wound. 2. astringent.

styptic pencil, a pencil-shaped stick containing a styptic material, used to check bleeding, as from a razor nick in shaving.

subacute, between the stages or degrees of acute and chronic, as of some diseases.

subcartilaginous, 1. situated under the clavicle. 2. referring to a vein, artery, or similar part under the clavicle.

subclavian artery, the main artery of the arm,

beneath the clavicle.

subclavian vein, the main vein beneath the clavicle leading to the arm.

subclinical, referring to a disorder virtually undetectable in general clinical tests because its symptoms are so moderate.

subconscious, 1. existing or operating beneath or beyond consciousness; imperfectly or not wholly conscious. 2. the part of the mental process that is not in the realm of consciousness.

subcortex, the parts of the brain that lie directly beneath the cerebral cortex.

subculture, 1. to transfer a small portion of, as a bacterial culture, onto a new medium. 2. a bacterial culture derived from another culture.

subcutaneous, 1. situated, used, lying, or made immediately under the skin. 2. introduced beneath the skin, as an injection.

subcutis, the lowest part of the dermis.

subfebrile, a moderate rise in temperature, usually considered as less than 101°F.

sublatio, the removal or detachment of a part.

sublatio retinae, the detachment of the retina.

sublimate, 1. to transfer the energy of, as a basic drive, to a higher, nobler, or more ethical goal. 2. to vaporize and condense a solid.

subliminal, 1. below consciousness. 2. noting

stimuli that lack the intensity to produce a clear perception or sensation.

sublingual, situated under the tongue.

submaxilla, see **mandible.**

submaxillary, 1. of, pertaining to, or just beneath the lower jaw. 2. pertaining to or situated near the submaxillary gland.

submaxillary gland, one of the salivary glands.

submicroscopic, of a size smaller than is visible with an ordinary microscope.

subnormal, of less than normal intelligence.

subocular, situated below the eye.

suborbital, situated below the orbit of the eye.

subscapular, situated beneath the scapula.

subsidence, the gradual abatement of symptoms or manifestations of a disease.

substantia alba, the white substance of the brain and nerves.

substantia cinerea, the gray matter (substance) of the brain and spinal cord.

subtetanic, referring to muscle tension not yet tetanic; remittently contracted.

succedaneous, acting as or relating to a substitute.

succedaneum, a substitute, as one medicine taking the place of another of similar properties.

succussion, a shaking of the patient to determine if fluid or gas is present in a body cavity.

suckle, to nurture; to nurse from the breast.

suckling, an unweaned child or other mammal.

sucrase, see **invertase.**

sucrate, a compound of a metallic oxide with a sugar, as, calcium sucrate.

sucrose, a crystalline compound, the ordinary sugar obtained from sugarcane, sugar beets, and sorghum.

sudamina, see **prickly heat.**

sudation, the act of sweating.

sudatorium, a hot-air bath for inducing sweating.

sudor, see **perspiration, sweat.**

sudoriferous, producing sweat; secreting perspiration.

sudorific, 1. causing sweat. 2. a medicine that produces sweat.

suffocate, 1. to choke or kill by stopping respiration. 2. to stifle, as by depriving of air. 3. to smother. 4. to become choked, stifled, or smothered.

suffocation, the stoppage of breathing.

sugar, see **sucrose.**

suggestion, the insinuation of an idea, belief, or impulse into the mind of a subject, whether by words, gestures, or otherwise, but without the normal critical command, thought, or action.

suicidal, 1. pertaining to, involving, or suggesting suicide. 2. tending or leading to suicide.

suicide, 1. one who intentionally takes his own life. 2. the intentional taking of one's own life.

sulcate, furrowed or grooved.

sulcus, a fissure between two convolutions of the surface of the brain.

sulfa, 1. chemically related to sulfanilamide. 2. of or concerning sulfa drugs. 3. containing or consisting of a sulfa drug or drugs.

sulfa drug, any of a family of bacteriostatic drugs closely related in chemical structure to sulfanilamide.

sulfanilamide, a colorless, crystalline compound, a derivative of sulfanilic acid, used for its therapeutic action in numerous bacterial infections.

sulfur, a nonmetallic element existing in several forms, the common one being a yellow crystalline solid that burns with a blue flame and a suffocating odor, and is used, among others, in medicine.

sulpha, see **sulfa.**

sulphanilamide, see **sulfanilamide.**

sulphur, see **sulfur.**

sunburn, 1. an inflammation of the skin, caused by prolonged exposure to the sun's rays. 2. the discoloration so produced. 3. to affect or be affected with sunburn. Also called **actinodermatitis.**

sunstroke, see **heat stroke.**

sunstruck, 1. having sunstroke. 2. affected by the sun.

superciliary, 1. pertaining to the eyebrow. 2. situated or being above the eyelid.

supercilium, see **eyebrow.**

superego, 1. a system within the mind which, acting consciously or unconsciously, brings perceived parental, social, or moral standards to bear upon the actions and decisions of the ego. 2. the conscience plus a memory of perceived ideals.

superfecundation, fertilization of two ova during the same menstrual cycle by two different acts of coitus.

superfetation, a second conception after a prior one, by which two fetuses exist at once in the same womb.

superficial, lying on or pertaining to the surface.

superficies, 1. the surface. 2. the appearance. 3. the exterior part or face of a thing, consisting of length and breadth without thickness, and therefore forming no part of the substance or solid content of a body.

superinduce, to bring in or on as an addition to something.

supernormal, 1. above or beyond what is normal. 2. beyond average human intelligence or ability.

supernumerary, 1. a person or thing beyond what is necessary or usual. 2. exceeding a designated,

necessary, or usual number; extra; superfluous.

supersaturate, to saturate to excess or beyond normal, under known conditions of temperature and pressure as, to supersaturate a solution.

supinate, 1. to render supine. 2. to rotate or place, as the hand or forelimb, so that the palmar surface is upward when the limb is stretched forward horizontally. 3. to rotate, as a limb or joint, upward and away from the midline of the body. 4. to become supinated.

supination, 1. the position of the hand extended with the palm upward. 2. the rotating of a limb or joint upward and away from the midline of the body.

supinator, a muscle that aids in turning the palm of the hand upward.

supine, lying on the back, or with the face or front upward.

suppository, a mass of some prepared substance, usually in the form of a cone or cylinder, for introduction into the rectum, vagina, or urethra.

suppress, 1. to restrain from utterance. 2. to conceal, as one's feelings.

suppression, 1. the act of suppressing. 2. the state of being suppressed. 3. the deliberate, conscious retention of an utterance, action, impulse, or desire.

suppurant, 1. producing or

characterized by the production of pus. 2. any agent that causes formation of pus.

suppurate, 1. to generate pus. 2. to contain pus. 3. to fester.

suppuration, the formation of pus.

suppurative, something that promotes suppuration, esp. a drug.

supraliminal, above the threshold of consciousness; opposed to subliminal.

supramaxilla, the upper jawbone.

supraorbital, situated or being above the orbit of the eye.

suprarenal, 1. situated above the kidneys. 2. pertaining to an adrenal gland.

suprarenal gland, see **adrenal gland.**

suprascapular, situated above the scapula.

sura, the calf of the leg.

sural, of or pertaining to the calf of the leg.

surdity, see **deafness.**

surdomute, see **deafmute.**

surgeon, a specialist in the practice of surgery.

surgeon's knot, any of the knots used by a surgeon in tying ligatures or stitches.

surgery, 1. the practice that involves the performance of operations on the human subject to cure disease or injuries of the body. 2. the operative branch of medicine. 3. a room where surgical operations are performed.

surgical, relating to surgery.

susceptibility, 1. the state or quality of being susceptible. 2. sensitiveness. 3. capacity for feeling or emotional excitement.

susceptible, 1. capable of being acted on or affected in any way. 2. admitting any change. 3. capable of emotional impression.

susceptive, see **susceptible.**

suspend, to cease for a time; to interrupt temporarily.

suspended animation, a temporary cessation of vital bodily functions.

suspension, 1. the act of suspending or hanging up. 2. the act of delaying, interrupting, or stopping for a time. 3. a cessation of operation.

suspensory ligament, any of several fibrous tissues that support certain anatomical parts, esp. the ring-shaped tissue holding the lens of the eye.

suspire, to breathe with a long, deep breath; to sigh.

suspiration, the act of sighing.

sustentacular, supporting or sustaining.

sustentation, 1. support; sustenance. 2. support of life.

susurrus, a soft, humming, murmuring sound; a whisper; a rustling.

suture, 1. the uniting of the lips or edges of a wound

or incision by stitching. 2. one of the seams uniting the bones of the skull.

swab, a small bit of cotton or other material attached to a stick used in cleansing or as a medical applicator.

swathe, to bind or wrap with a band or bandage. 2. a bandage, band, or wrapping.

swayback, an unnatural downward curving or sagging of the back.

sweat, the watery fluid excreted through the pores of the skin. 2. to perspire, esp. profusely.

sweat gland, one of the minute, coiled, tubular glands of the skin that secrete sweat.

sweating, the act of excreting sweat.

swelling, 1. the state of being swollen. 2. that which is swollen. 3. an abnormal protuberance. 4. a tumor.

swoon, to faint; to sink into a fainting fit.

sycoma, a large soft wart.

sycosis, a disease characterized by an eruption of tubercles on the hair follicles of the beard and scalp.

symbion, an organism that lives with another organism in a state of symbiosis.

symbiont, see **symbion.**

symbiosis, the state of two different organisms living in close relationship, each benefiting from the association.

symbiotic, of or pertaining to symbiosis.

symbol, 1. an image that articulates a subconscious complex of meanings, as a dream image. 2. an action or affect that takes the place of the gratification of a repressed desire or the resolution of unconscious conflict.

symbolism, a condition in which everything that occurs is interpreted by the patient as a symbol of his own thoughts.

sympathectomy, the excision or interruption of part of the sympathetic nerve pathways.

sympathetic, relating to the part of the nervous system that, with the parasympathetic nerves, makes up the autonomic nervous system.

sympathetic nervous system, the section of the autonomic nervous system originating in the thoracic and lumbar regions, which stimulates the heartbeat, dilates the pupils, contracts the blood vessels, and, in general, functions in opposition to the parasympathetic nervous system.

sympathin, a substance produced at the nerve endings of the sympathetic nervous system, having an effect similar to adrenalin.

symphysion, the most anterior point of the lower jaw.

symphysis, 1. the growing together, or the fixed or movable union, of bones, as that of the two halves of the human lower jaw, or that of the two human pubic bones at the lower anterior point of the abdomen. 2. a line of junction or articulation of other parts so formed.

symptom, a circumstance or condition that results from or accompanies a disease, by which the nature of a disease may be diagnosed.

symptomatic, pertaining or relating to a symptom or symptoms.

symptomatology, the branch of medicine that treats of the symptoms of diseases.

synapse, the area in which contact takes place and a neuron transmits nerve impulses to another neuron.

synapsis, a stage in meiosis in which homologous chromosomes pair up.

synaptic, of or pertaining to synapsis.

synarthrosis, a union of two bones that prevents either from moving; a fixed articulation.

syncopal, relating to a syncope.

syncope, a temporary diminution or suspension of heart action, characterized chiefly by loss of consciousness.

syncytium, a mass of multinucleate protoplasm, not definitely divided into cells.

syndactyl, having certain digits partially or wholly united.

syndesis, see **synapsis.**

syndesmosis, a connection of bones by ligaments, fasciae, or membranes other than those of the joints.

syndesmotomy, a surgical section of ligaments.

syndesmus, see **ligament.**

syndrome, the combination of symptoms in a disease; a number of symptoms occurring together.

syndromic, of or pertaining to syndrome.

syneresis, the contraction of a gel causing exudation of liquid, as the separation of serum from a blood clot.

synergetic, working together; cooperative; as, synergetic muscles.

synergism, any cooperative effort of discrete agencies that produces a more effective result than the sum of the results produced by the same agencies acting independently of one another, as two drugs.

synergy, 1. combined action. 2. the cooperative action of two or more parts or organs of the body. 3. the cooperative interaction of different drugs.

synesthesia, 1. sensation produced in one part of the body when a stimulus is applied to another part. 2. the bringing about, through a sensation produced by one stimulus, of a mental image corresponding to another, as when hearing a particular sound induces the visualization of a particular color.

synesthetic, of or pertaining to synesthesia.

syngamy, the union of female and male gametes during fertilization.

syngenesis, sexual reproduction.

synostosis, union by means of ossified cartilage or bone.

synovia, a lubricating liquid resembling the white of an egg, secreted by certain membranes, as those of the joints.

synovial, of or pertaining to synovia.

synovitis, an inflammation of the synovial membrane.

syntonic, of a personality, marked by emotional responsiveness to environment.

syphilis, a chronic, infectious venereal disease caused by a microorganism, either congenital or communicated by contact and usually having three sequential degenerative stages occurring over the course of many years.

syphilitic, 1. pertaining to or affected with syphilis. 2. one affected with syphilis.

syphilology, the sum of scientific knowledge concerning syphilis.

Syrette, a disposable tube attached to a hypodermic needle for injecting medicines (trademark).

syringe, a small, portable device for drawing in a quantity of a fluid and ejecting it in a stream, used for cleansing wounds or injecting fluids into the body.

syringitis, an inflammation of the eustachian tube.

syringomyelia, a disease affecting the spinal cord in which liquid accumulates in abnormal cavities, replacing the nerve tissue and causing spasticity and muscle atrophy.

syringotome, a surgical instrument for incision of a fistula.

syssarcosis, the union or connection of bones attached by muscle.

systaltic, having alternate contraction and dilatation, as the heart; pulsating.

system, 1. an assemblage of parts or organs of the same or similar tissues or concerned with the same function, as the nervous system. 2. the entire human body as a physiological unity or anatomical whole.

systemic, 1. pertaining to a particular system of parts or organs of the body. 2. pertaining to or affecting the entire bodily system or the body as a whole.

systole, the regularly repeated contraction of the heart that forces the blood through the circulatory system; opposed to diastole.

systolic, of or pertaining to the systole.

systremma, a cramp in the calf muscles of the leg.

tabella, medicated material formed into a tablet.

tabes, a gradually progressive emaciation accompanying a disease.

tabes dorsalis, a disease of the spinal cord caused by syphilis, marked by intense pain, difficulty in coordination and walking, and eventual paralysis.

tabetic, of, pertaining to, or affected with tabes or tabes dorsalis.

tabic, see **tabetic.**

tablature, the division between two plates of cranial bones.

tablet, a small disk or lozenge of medicine.

taboparesis, a general paralysis usually associated with tabes.

tache, a colored spot on the skin, as a freckle.

tachetic, marked by taches.

tachistoscope, an apparatus for testing visual perception that exposes to view, for a selected brief period of time, an object or groups of objects, as letters or words.

tachistoscopic, pertaining to the tachistoscope.

tachycardia, excessively rapid heart action.

tachycardiac, of or pertaining to tachycardia.

tachylalia, abnormally rapid speech.

tachyphrasia, excessive volubility of speech, often a sign of a mental disorder.

tachyphrenia, abnormally rapid activity of the mental processes.

tachypnea, abnormally rapid respiration.

tactile, 1. pertaining to or possessing the sense of touch. 2. capable of being touched or felt.

tactile corpuscle, any of numerous minute oval bodies, esp. of the fingers and toes, concerned with the sense of touch.

taction, the act of touching.

tactual, see **tactile.**

tactus, see **touch.**

taedium vitae, the condition or state of feeling that life is not worth living, often leading to suicide.

taenia, 1. a ribbonlike structure, as certain bands of white nerve or muscle fibers. 2. any of the various tapeworms of the genus **Taenia.**

taeniacide, an agent that destroys tapeworms.

taeniasis, a diseased condition caused by the presence of tapeworms.

talalgia, pain in the heel or ankle.

taligrade, walking with the weight on the outer edge of the foot.

taliped, one who has a clubfoot.

talipes, see **clubfoot.**

talipomanus, see **clubhand.**

talking book, a tape recording or phonograph record of a reading of a magazine, book, or other literary piece, esp. as prepared for the blind.

talocalcanean, of or pertaining to the talus and the calcaneous.

talpa, see **mole.**

talus, the anklebone or astragalus; the ankle.

tamarind, a tropical legu- minous tree, the fruit of which, containing an acid pulp, is used in medi- cines.

tampon, 1. a plug of cotton or the like inserted into an orifice or wound, as to stop hemorrhage. 2. to fill or plug with a tampon.

tan, 1. to become tan- colored or sunburned. 2. a brown skin color result- ing from exposure to the rays of the sun.

tantalum, a rare, gray- white metallic element that is hard, ductile, and resistant to single acids, used as wire suture and to repair cranial injuries.

tantrum, an outburst of anger or rage; a violent display of temper.

tapeinocephalic, of or per- taining to tapeinocephaly.

tapeinocephaly, flattening of the top of the skull.

tapetum, any of certain membranous layers or the like, as in the retina.

tapeworm, any of various flat or tapelike cestode worms, parasitic when adult in the alimentary canal of man and other vertebrates, and usually characterized by having larval and adult stages in different hosts.

taphophobia, a pathologi- cal fear of being buried alive.

tarantism, a nervous affec- tion characterized by manic, hysterical fits of dancing, stupor, melan- choly, popularly believed to result from a bite of a tarantula.

tarantula, any of various spiders, usually large and hairy, of the family Theraphasidae, which have a painful although not very poisonous bite and are common in the southwestern U.S.

taraxacum, any of the composite plants con- stituting the genus **Tar- axacum,** as the dande- lion, the dried roots of which are used as a tonic, diuretic, and gentle laxa- tive.

tarsal, 1. of or pertaining to the tarsus of the foot or to the tarsi of the eyelids. 2. a tarsal part, as a bone or joint.

tarsalgia, pin in the tarsus.

tarsalia, the tarsal bones.

tarsectomy, 1. the surgical excision of the tarsus or a tarsal bone. 2. the re- moval of a tarsal plate in the upper eyelid.

tarsectopia, a dislocation of the tarsus of the foot.

tarsitis, 1. an inflammation of the tarsus of the foot. 2. an inflammation of the tarsal plate of the upper eyelid.

tarsometatarsal, of or per- taining to the tarsus and the metatarsus.

tarsoplasty, plastic surgery of an eyelid.

tarsotibial, of or pertaining to the tarsus of the foot and the tibia.

tarsotomy, the surgical in- cision of either the tarsal cartilage of an eyelid or the tarsus of the foot.

tarsus, 1. the proximal segment of the foot; the instep. 2. the collection of bones between the tibia and the metatarsus, entering into the construction of the ankle joint. 3. the plate of connective tissue along the border of an eyelid.

tartar, a yellowish, hard substance deposited on the teeth, consisting chiefly of calcium phosphate.

tartaremetic, potassium antimonyl tartrate, a poisonous, water-soluble salt, with a sweetish metallic taste, occurring as a white crystal or a granular powder, and used as an emetic, an expectorant, and a diaphoretic in medicine.

tartaric, of, pertaining to, or referring to tartar.

taste, 1. to perceive or distinguish flavor by the sense of taste. 2. the sense by which flavor or savor of things is perceived when they are brought into contact with the taste buds in the mouth.

taste bud, one of the many tiny end organs of the sense of taste located in the epithelium of the tongue.

tattoo, 1. the act or practice of marking the skin with indelible patterns, pictures, or legends by puncturing and inserting pigments. 2. a pattern, legend, or picture so made.

taxis, the replacing of a displaced part, or the reducing of a hernial tumor or the like, by manipulation and without incision.

TB, see **tuberculosis.**

tear, 1. a limpid, droplike liquid secretion of the lacrimal gland that moistens the surface of the eye and cleanses it of foreign particles. 2. .the liquid appearing in the eyes or flowing from them, esp. through grief or joy.

tease, to pull apart or separate the adhering fibers of, as in preparing a specimen for microscopic examination.

teat, the projecting structure through which milk is drawn from the breast of females; a nipple.

tectocephaly, having a roof-shaped cranium.

tectum, any structure resembling or serving as a roof.

teethe, to grow teeth; to cut teeth.

teething ring, a ring made of plastic, rubber, or the like, on which a teething baby may bite.

teethridge, the inner gum surface of the upper jaw between the front teeth and the hard palate.

tegmen, a cover, covering, or integument.

tegmental, of or pertaining to the tegmentum.

tegmentum, a roof or covering, as the skin, but esp. a portion of the midbrain.

tegumen, see **tegmen.**

tegument, a natural covering, as the skin covering the body.

tegumental, of or pertaining to the skin.

teichopsia, attacks of temporary blindness accompanied by subjective zig-zag lines in the visual field, sometimes accompanying migraine headaches.

tela, any weblike structure.

telaesthesia, see **telesthesia.**

telangiectasis, dilation of the capillaries and other small blood vessels, as caused by congenital defects, alcoholism, or cold weather, producing a form of angioma, usually on the face.

telangiitis, an inflammation of the capillaries.

telencephalic, of or pertaining to the telencephalon.

telencephalon, the anterior division or section of the forebrain or prosencephalon.

teleneuron, any nerve ending.

telepathist, a person who claims to have the ability to read the mind of others.

telepathy, the communication of one mind with another by means beyond normal sensory perception.

telesthesia, ability to respond to a stimulus beyond or presumed to be beyond the usual range of the senses.

telesthetic, of or pertaining to perception at a distance beyond the usual range of the senses.

telesystolic, pertaining to the end of the cardiac systole.

teletactor, a device that enables the deaf to receive vibrations through the skin and thus "hear."

telotism, the complete performance of a function, as that of one of the senses.

temper, 1. mental balance or composure, equanimity, or calmness, as, to keep one's temper. 2. a particular frame of mind, feeling, or humor. 3. heat of mind or passion, shown in outbursts of anger or resentment.

temperament, 1. the combination of elements or qualities that make up a personality. 2. the peculiarity of physical organization by which the manner of acting, feeling, and thinking of each person is permanently affected; disposition.

temperance, 1. the observance of moderation in emotions, thoughts, or acts. 2. customary moderation with regard to indulging the natural appetites and passions. 3. sobriety.

temperate, of or pertaining to temperance; moderate.

temperature, the body heat; any amount of body heat above a normal level, as above 98.4°F.

temple, the flattened region on either side of the human forehead.

temporal, 1. of or pertaining to the temple or temples of the head. 2. noting or pertaining to either of a pair of complex bones that form part of the sides and base of the skull.

temporal bone, one of the two compound bones situated on either side of the head.

temulence, intoxication; drunkenness.

tenaculum, a small, sharp-pointed hook set in a handle, used for picking up and maintaining a hold on parts, such as arteries, in operations and dissections.

tenalgia, pain in a tendon.

tender, acutely or painfully sensitive, as a tender bruise.

tendinitis, an inflammation of a tendon.

tendinous, of, relating to, or full of tendons; sinewy.

tendo Achilles, see **Achilles tendon.**

tendon, a hard, tough cord or bundle of fibers by which a muscle is attached to a bone or other part that it serves to move.

tenesmic, pertaining to or like tenesmus.

tenesmus, an urge to void the bowels or bladder, accompanied by straining, but without discharge.

tenia, see **taenia.**

teniacide, see **taeniacide.**

teniasis, see **taeniasis**

tennis elbow, a pain at the side of the elbow, usually caused by overexertion of the arm, only rarely caused by playing tennis.

tenodesis, the surgical fixation of a tendon to restore the lost function or to increase the power of the motion of a joint.

tenontitis, see **tendinitis.**

tenophyte, an osseous growth in a tendon.

tenotome, a surgical instrument for cutting a tendon.

tenotomist, a specialist in tenotomy.

tenotomy, the surgical section of a tendon.

tense, 1. stretched tight; taut or rigid. 2. in a strained nervous or emotional condition. 3. referring to an instance of high mental pressure involving strain on emotions and nerves.

tensile, pertaining to tension; capable of tension or being extended.

tension, 1. mental or emotional strain, as in worry or excitement. 2. an intense or uncomfortable feeling between people or groups of people.

tensor, a muscle that stretches or tightens some part of the body.

tent, 1. a roll of lint or linen used to dilate an opening in the flesh, or to keep open a sore from which matter is discharged. 2. to hold open with a tent or pledget; to probe.

tentative, 1. experimental. 2. in a diagnosis, meaning subject to change.

tenth nerve, see **vagus.**

tenum, see **penis.**

tenuity, the state of being thin or fine; slenderness.

tenuous, thin or slender; of little density; weak.

tephromyelitis, an inflammation of the gray matter of the spinal cord. Also called **poliomyelitis.**

teras, a badly deformed

fetus.

teratic, of, or pertaining to a badly formed fetus.

teratology, the study of monstrosities or malformations in fetuses.

teratoma, a tumor containing embryonic elements of all three primary germ layers.

teratophobia, the pathological fear of giving birth to a malformed fetus.

terebene, a terpenic mixture used in medicine.

terete, slender and smooth, with a circular traverse section.

term, see **parturition.**

terminal, pertaining to causing death, as a disease.

Terramycin, an antibiotic derived from a soil mold, effective against many disease-causing microorganisms (trademark).

tertian, 1. recurring every third day. 2. a tertian ague, esp. malaria.

tertiary syphilis, syphilis in the third stage.

testectomy, the surgical removal of a testicle or testicles; castration.

testicle, one of the two oval-shaped reproductive glands in the male, enclosed in the scrotum, which secrete the spermatozoa and several of the fluid elements of the semen.

testiculate, shaped like a testicle; ovoid.

testis, see **testicle.**

testopathy, any disease of the testicles.

testosterone, a male testicular hormone that pro-

motes male secondary sex characteristics.

tetanic, of, pertaining to, or causing tetanus.

tetaniform, see **tetanoid.**

tetanode, see **tetanoid.**

tetanoid, resembling tetanus.

tetanus, 1. an infectious, often fatal disease, caused by a specific bacterium, **Clostridium tetani,** which gains entrance to the body through wounds, characterized by more or less violent tonic spasms and rigidity of many or all of the voluntary muscles, esp. those of the neck and lower jaw; see **lockjaw.** 2. the specific bacterium that causes this disease. 3. the condition of prolonged contraction that a muscle assumes under rapidly repeated stimuli.

tetany, a disorder or condition characterized by irregularly intermittent muscular spasms and pain, esp. in the extremities, and usually occurring because of defective metabolism of calcium salts.

tetracycline, a yellow crystalline powder, produced artificially by chemical synthesis or naturally by certain soil bacilli of the genus **Streptomyces,** used as an antibiotic.

tetrad, 1. a tetravalent or quadrivalent element, atom, or radical. 2. the arrangement of four chromosomes, formed during meiosis by the splitting of paired chromosomes.

tetraplegia, see quadri-plegia.

tetter, any of several cutaneous diseases, as herpes, impetigo, etc.

texis, childbearing.

thalamencephalic, of or pertaining to the thalamencephalon.

thalamencephalon, the segment of the brain behind the prosencephalon or forebrain, containing the optic thalami and the pineal gland; the between-brain.

thalamic, of or pertaining to the thalamus.

thalamus, a part of the diencephalon composed of gray matter that relays sensory impulses to the cortex of the brain.

thalassophobia, a pathological fear of the sea.

thanatoid, resembling death.

thanatology, the science dealing with death.

thanatomania, the condition of a suicidal or homicidal craze.

thanatophobia, see **necrophobia.**

thanatopsy, see **postmortem.**

Thanatos, in Freudian theory, the death instinct.

theca, caselike tissue enclosing anatomical structures.

thecal, of or pertaining to a sheath.

thecitis, an inflammation of the sheath of a tendon.

theleplasty, a surgical operation on the nipple.

thelitis, an inflammation of the nipple.

thelium, a nipple; a papilla.

thenal, of or pertaining to the palm of the hand.

thenar, the fleshy part of the palm of the hand at the base of the thumb.

theobromine, a white, poisonous, crystalline powder found in the seeds of cacao, used primarily in medicine, as a vasodilator and diuretic.

theomania, religious insanity.

theomaniac, 1. a person afflicted with religious insanity. 2. of or pertaining to theomania.

theophobia, a pathological fear of God.

therapeutic, pertaining to therapeutics; curative.

therapeutics, the branch or part of medicine dealing with the treatment of diseases.

therapeutist, a person skilled in therapeutics.

therapist, see **therapeutist.**

therapy, 1. the treatment of disability or disease, as by some remedial or curative process, as serumtherapy. 2. any soothing or curative device, process, or activity. 3. curative or therapeutic quality or ability.

therm, a unit of heat or thermal capacity.

thermal, of, caused by, or pertaining to heat.

thermic, see **thermal.**

thermoanesthesia, the loss of the ability to distinguish between heat and cold.

thermocauterectomy, surgical excision by thermocautery.

thermocautery, cautery using heat, either with a cauterizing iron or with an electrically heated loop of platinum.

thermogenesis, heat created in the body by metabolic processes.

thermogenetic, of or pertaining to thermogenesis.

thermogenic, see **thermogenetic.**

thermogram, a record made by means of a thermograph.

thermograph, a thermometer that automatically records the temperature.

thermolabile, subject to destruction or loss of characteristic properties through the action of moderate heat.

thermolysis, 1. the dispersion of heat from the body. 2. decomposition or dissociation by heat.

thermolytic, of or pertaining to thermolysis.

thermometer, an instrument by which temperature is measured, consisting usually of a closed glass tube containing liquid, most often mercury or alcohol, which expands or contracts with variations of temperature.

thermophore, an apparatus for applying heat to parts of the body.

thermoplegia, see **heatstroke.**

thermostable, able to withstand moderate heating without loss of characteristic properties.

thermotaxic, of or pertain-

ing to thermotaxis.

thermotaxis, 1. the property in a cell or organism of movement toward or away from a heat source. 2. the regulation of the body temperature.

thermotherapy, the use of heat in treatment of disease.

thermotropic, of or pertaining to thermotropism.

thermotropism, the property in organisms of turning or bending a part of the organism either toward or away from a heat source.

thews, 1. well-developed muscles or strong sinews. 2. strength or power, esp. muscular.

thiamine, a B-complex vitamin compound of white crystals, found in both animal and plant sources but also made synthetically, necessary for proper activity of the nervous system and carbohydrate metabolism. Also called vitamin B_1.

thigh, the part of the leg between the hip and the knee.

thighbone, see **femur.**

thigh joint, see **hip joint.**

thigmesthesia, sensitivity to touch.

thimerosal, a light-colored, water-soluble crystalline powder used as a germicide and an antiseptic.

think, to form or conceive mentally, as a thought.

thinking, 1. able to think; using the faculty of reasoning; rational. 2. the act or state of thinking; thought.

thiocarbamide, see **thiourea.**

thiopental, a barbiturate, administered intravenously as a sedative and hypnotic for surgical procedures and psychotherapeutics.

thiopental sodium, see **thiopental.**

thiouracil, an antithyroid agent, used in the treatment of thyrotoxicosis to reduce the production of hormones by the thyroid gland.

thiourea, a colorless crystalline substance, with a bitter taste, regarded as urea with the oxygen replaced by sulfur, and used esp. in external medicine and organic synthesis.

third cranial nerve, the nerve that regulates eye movements.

third-degree burn, a charring burn in which the epidermis is destroyed, exposing nerve endings.

thirst, 1. the distressing sensation of dryness in the mouth and throat caused by want or need of fluids. 2. the physical condition resulting from this want.

thirsty, having thirst; craving drink.

thoracal, see **thoracic.**

thoracentesis, the surgical puncture of the chest to remove fluid.

thoracic, of or pertaining to the chest.

thoracic duct, the largest lymphatic vessel in the body, lying along the vertebral column and serving to convey lymph to the left subclavian vein, where it enters the circulatory system.

thoracostomy, the opening of the chest, usually for drainage.

thoracotomy, an incision of the chest wall.

thorascope, an instrument for visual inspection of the chest cavity.

thorascopy, diagnostic examination of the chest cavity with a thorascope.

thorax, 1. the cavity of the body formed by the spine, ribs, and breastbone, and containing the lungs and heart. 2. the chest.

thoroughwort, see **boneset.**

threadworm, any of various nematode worms, esp. a pinworm, which inhabit the intestines.

three-day fever, see **dengue.**

threonine, an amino acid, considered essential to nutrition.

threshold, the point at which a stimulus to the sensory organism is just intense enough to be felt, as, the threshold of consciousness.

thrill, 1. to affect with a keen emotion, as of delight or excitement. 2. to vibrate. 3. to produce a tingling sensation. 4. to feel a shivering sensation through the body.

throat, the passage that leads from the nose and mouth to the lungs and stomach and includes the esophagus, the fauces, and the pharynx.

throb, 1. to beat, as the heart or pulse, with more than usual force or rapidity. 2. to show, exhibit, or feel emotion. 3. to palpitate, quiver, or vibrate. 4. a beat or strong pulsation; palpitation.

throbbing, rhythmic beating movement.

throe, 1. a violent spasm or pang. 2. a paroxysm. 3. a sharp attack of emotion. 4. the pains of childbirth. 5. the agony of death. 6. any violent convulsion or struggle.

thrombin, 1. the enzyme that causes the coagulation of blood. 2. a preparation to control capillary bleeding.

thromboangiitis, an inflammation of the lining of a blood vessel with formation or existence of a blood clot.

thrombocyte, any blood platelet.

thromboembolism, an embolism that has become dislodged from the thrombus and is blocking a blood vessel.

thrombogen, see **prothrombin.**

thrombogenic, of or pertaining to thrombogenesis

thrombogenesis, the formation of a blood clot.

thrombolysis, the breaking up of a thrombus.

thrombolytic, pertaining to or causing thrombolysis.

thrombophlebitis, an inflammation of any blood vessel accompanied by a thrombus.

thromboplastic, bringing about or speeding up the formation of blood clots.

thromboplastin, a lipoprotein that promotes blood clotting and is esp. found in blood platelets.

thrombosis, 1. a coagulation of the blood in a blood vessel or in the heart during life. 2. the formation or existence of a thrombus.

thrombotic, of or pertaining to thrombosis.

thrombus, a fibrinous clot of blood that forms in and obstructs a blood vessel.

throttle, to strangle; to choke or suffocate.

throwback, a reversion to an ancestral type or character.

throw up, see **vomit.**

thrush, a disease, esp. in children, characterized by whitish spots and ulcers on the membranes of the mouth, fauces, or the like caused by parasitic fungus.

thumb, the short, thick, opposable inner digit of the human hand, next to the forefinger.

thylacitis, an inflammation of the sebaceous glands of the skin.

thymectomy, the surgical excision of the thymus gland.

thymic, of or related to the thymus gland.

thymion, see **wart.**

thymitis, an inflammation of the thymus gland.

thymolysis, the dissolution of thymus tissue.

thymolytic, destructive to thymus tissue.

thymoma, a tumor in the thymus gland.

thymus, a ductless gland of uncertain function situated in the upper thoracic cavity and attaining its maximum development at the second year, becoming vestigial in adults.

thyroadenitis, an inflammation of the thyroid gland.

thyrocele, see **goiter.**

thyrochondrotomy, an incision of the thyroid cartilage.

thyroid, 1. noting or pertaining to the principal cartilage of the larynx. 2. noting or pertaining to a ductless gland adjacent to the larynx and upper trachea.

thyroid cartilage, the principal cartilage of the larynx, forming the projection known in men as the Adam's apple.

thyroidectomy, the surgical excision of the whole or a part of the thyroid gland.

thyroid gland, a ductless two-lobed gland adjacent to the larynx and upper trachea, furnishing an important secretion for regulating body development and metabolism.

thyroptosis, a condition in which the thyroid gland is partially or completely displaced into the thorax.

thyrotome, a surgical knife for cutting into the thyroid cartilage.

thyrotomy, a surgical incision of the thyroid gland.

thyrotoxicosis, a disorder caused by an overabundant secretion of the thyroid gland resulting usually in an enlarged thyroid gland, bulging of the eyes, tremors, and rapid heart beat; hyperthyroidism.

thyroxin, see **thyroxine.**

thyroxine, 1. an active iodine compound of the thyroid gland that controls metabolism and is used in treating hypothyroidism. 2. a similar compound prepared synthetically or extracted from animals.

tibia, the large bone of the lower leg; the shinbone.

tibial, of or pertaining to the tibia.

tic, a habitual spasmodic contraction of certain muscles, esp. of the face.

tic douloureux, severe facial neuralgia accompanied by convulsive twitchings of the facial muscles.

tick, any of various parasitic mites or acarids, as those of the genus **Ixodes,** which bury the head in the skin of the host and suck the blood, and often are carriers of disease.

tick fever, any fever transmitted to man or animals by a mite or acarid of the families Ixodidae and Argasidae, as Rocky Mountain spotted fever afflicting man, and Texas fever occurring in some animals, esp. cattle.

tilmus, involuntary picking at the bedclothes by seriously ill, delirious patients.

tincture, an extract or solution of the active principle of some substance in a solvent.

tinea, ringworm or any similar fungus infection of the skin.

tinnitus, a ringing, buzzing, or other similar subjective or pathological sensation in the ears.

tired, exhausted, as by exertion; fatigued; weary.

tissue, an aggregate of cells usually of similar structure that perform the same or related functions, as, xylem or muscle tissue.

tissue culture, the growing of tissue in a culture medium outside the parent body.

tit, see **teat.**

titubation, a disturbance of body equilibrium in standing or walking, resulting in an uncertain gait and trembling, usually caused by diseases of the cerebellum.

tobacco heart, a functional disorder of the heart, characterized by a rapid and often irregular pulse, resulting from excessive use of tobacco.

tocology, see **obstetrics.**

tocopherol, any of four phenolic compounds obtained from oils of various plants, as wheat germ and cottonseed, and possessing the active principle of vitamin E.

toddle, 1. to walk with short steps in a tottering way, as a child or an old person. 2. the act of walking in this manner; an unsteady gait.

toddler, one who toddles.

toe, one of the terminal members or digits of the foot.

toilet, the cleansing of a part after an operation, esp. in the peritoneal cavity.

tolbutamide, a drug of the sulfonamide group, used to control some types of diabetes.

tokology, see **tocology.**

tolerable, capable of being borne or endured; sufferable.

tolerance, the capacity to endure or resist the action of a drug or poison.

tolerant, capable of tolerance.

tolerate, to endure or resist the action of, as a drug or poison.

toleration, see **tolerance.**

tomentum, a blood vessel network found within the cortex of the brain and the cerebral surface of the pia mater.

tomography, an X ray technique by which detailed images of a structure lying in a specific layer of tissue may be obtained, with images of structures in other layers eliminated or blurred.

tonaphasia, the loss of the ability to remember a tune because of cerebral lesions.

tone, that condition of a vital body in which the parts have tension, the organs function normally, and the tissues are firm, sound, and resilient. See also **tonus.**

tone-deaf, lacking the capability to express or to detect distinctions in musical pitch.

tongue, 1. the freely moving organ within man's mouth, having the power to shape itself for different purposes, as tasting, swallowing, articulation, or speech. 2. a receptor with taste buds and nerve endings.

tongue-tie, restricted movement of the tongue, esp. from a shortened frenum.

tongue-tied, 1. unable to articulate distinctly. 2. having an impediment in the speech or having tongue-tie.

tonic, a tonic agent or remedy; anything invigorating or bracing, physically, mentally, or morally.

tonicity, the normal elastic tension of living muscles, arteries, and other parts by which the tone of the system is maintained. See also **tonus.**

tonometer, any of various physiological instruments, as for measuring the tension of the eyeball, or for determining blood pressure within the vessels.

tonometric, of or pertaining to a tonometer or tonometry.

tonometry, the measurement of tension of the eyeball or blood pressure with a tonometer

tonsil, one of two oblong masses of lymphoid tissue, situated on each side of the throat.

tonsillar, of or pertaining to a tonsil.

tonsillectome, a surgical instrument used to excise a tonsil.

tonsillectomy, the surgical removal of enlarged or inflamed tonsils.

tonsillitis, an inflammation of the tonsils.

tonsillotomy, incision of a tonsil.

tonus, the normal condition of tension in muscles, making possible response to a stimulus.

tooth, one of the hard bodies or processes, usually attached in a row to each jaw, serving for the prehension and mastication of food, composed chiefly of dentin surrounding a sensitive pulp and covered on the crown with enamel.

toothache, pain in a tooth or teeth arising from decay; also called **adontalgia.**

toothpaste, a dentifrice in paste form.

tooth powder, a powdered dentifrice.

tophus, a uratic or calcareous deposit formed in the fibrous tissue of the body, as around or at a joint or on the roots of teeth, esp. in gout.

topical, pertaining or applied to a particular part of the body.

topology, the study of the structure of a particular region or part of the body.

toponym, the name of a particular region or part of the body, as contrasted with an organ.

toponymic, of or pertaining to a toponym.

toponymy, 1. the study of

toponyms. 2. regional nomenclature of the body.

toric, of, or pertaining to a torus, esp. noting or pertaining to a lens with a surface forming a portion of a torus, used in eyeglasses.

tormina, gripping pains accompanying intestinal colic.

torpid, having lost motion or the power of motion and feeling; numb; dull; sluggish.

torpidity, numbness; sluggishness.

torpor, a state of suspended physical powers and activities; sluggish inactivity or inertia; lethargic dullness or indifference; apathy.

torporific, causing torpor.

torrefy, to dry, roast, scorch, or parch by heat, as drugs.

torrify, see **torrefy.**

torsion, the act of twisting or the resulting state.

torso, the trunk of the human body.

torticollis, an affliction in which the neck is twisted and the head inclined to one side, caused by spasmodic muscular contraction; also called **wryneck.**

torus, a rounded ridge; a protuberant part.

touch, 1. the tactile sense. 2. to place the hand, finger, or part of the body on or in contact with something; to come into or be in contact. 3. the act of touching; the state or fact of being touched. 4. the sense by which anything material is perceived by means of the contact with it of some part of the body. 5. the sensation or effect imparted or experienced by touching something.

tourniquet, a bandage that is tightened by twisting with a stick, or a pad pressed down with an elastic, to arrest hemorrhage.

toxalbumin, a toxic albumin.

toxanemia, anemia caused by poison.

toxemia, a form of blood poisoning, esp. one in which toxins produced by certain microorganisms enter the blood.

toxic, of, pertaining to, or caused by a toxin or poison; of the nature of a poison; poisonous.

toxical, see **toxic.**

toxicant, 1. a poison; any toxic agent of a stimulating, narcotic, or anesthetic nature, as an intoxicant. 2. being toxic or poisonous.

toxicity, poisonous or toxic quality, or the degree or state of being toxic; poisonous.

toxicoderma, skin disease caused by poison.

toxicogenic, 1. generating or producing toxic products or poisons. 2. caused or produced by poisonous or toxic substances.

toxicologist, a specialist in the field of poisons, their detection and treatment.

toxicology, the science of

poisons, their effects, antidotes, etc.

toxicosis, an abnormal or diseased condition produced by the action of a toxin or poison.

toxin, 1. any of various usually unstable organic poisons produced in living or dead organisms or their products, as venom, or ptomaine. 2. any of the specific poisonous products generated by pathogenic microorganisms, and constituting the causative agents in various diseases, as tetanus or diphtheria. Compare **antitoxin**.

toxin-antitoxin, a mixture or combination of antitoxin and toxin for inducing, esp. formerly, active immunity from various diseases.

toxinic, of or pertaining to a toxin.

toxiphobia, an abnormal or morbid fear of being poisoned.

toxoid, a toxin whose toxic property has been eliminated, usually by a chemical agent, but which retains its antigenic qualities that produce immunity on injection into the body by initiating antibody production.

toxoplasmosis, a disease, esp. of the nervous system, resulting from infestation of tissue by **Toxoplasma gondii**, a parasitic protozoan, occurring sporadically in certain animals and occasionally in man.

trabecula, 1. the tissue supporting an organ. 2. a structural part resembling a small beam or crossbar.

trabecular, of or pertaining to a trabecula.

trachea, the tube extending from the larynx to the bronchi, serving as the passage for conveying air to and from the lungs.

tracheal, of or pertaining to the trachea.

tracheitis, an inflammation of the trachea.

tracheobronchial, in the region of, related to, or acting upon both the bronchi and the trachea.

tracheobronchoscopy, examination of the trachea and bronchi through a bronchoscope.

tracheoscopist, a specialist in tracheoscopy.

tracheoscopy, examination of the interior of the trachea, as with a laryngoscope.

tracheostomy, an incision of the trachea for insertion of a tube to overcome an obstruction.

tracheotome, a surgical instrument used for opening the trachea.

tracheotomy, incision of the trachea.

trachitis, see **tracheitis**.

trachoma, a contagious inflammation of the conjunctiva of the eyelids, characterized by the formation of granulations or small rounded growths.

trachomatous, of, pertaining to, or affected with trachoma.

tract, a particular area of the body, esp. a system of related organs, as, the digestive tract.

traction, the action of pulling on an organ or muscle to relieve or lessen pressure, or to repair dislocation.

tragus, a small cartilaginous eminence at the front entrance of the external ear.

trait, a distinguishing or peculiar feature or quality; a characteristic.

trance, an unconscious, cataleptic, or hypnotic condition.

tranquilize, to render tranquil; to pacify when agitated, esp. by administering drugs.

tranquilizer, that which tranquilizes or soothes; any of several drugs capable of relieving tension.

transect, to cut across; to divide by passing across; to dissect transversely.

transection, cross section.

transference, the revival and transferral of emotions, esp. those related to forgotten childhood experiences, toward a different person than that to whom they were initially directed, usually a psychoanalyst.

transfuse, to transfer, as blood, from the veins or arteries of one person to those of another.

transfusion, the act of transfusing.

transilluminate, to throw a strong light through, as an organ or part, as a means of diagnosis.

transillumination, examining a cavity or organ by throwing a strong light

through its walls.

transmigration, the act of passing across or through, as the passage of white blood cells through capillary membranes, or the passage of the egg cell from the ovary to the womb.

transmutation, the act of transmuting, or state of being transmuted; change into another substance, form, or nature.

transmute, to change from one nature, form, or substance into another; to change into another thing or body; to metamorphose; to transform.

transpiration, 1. the act or process of transpiring. 2. exhalation of moisture through the skin. See **perspiration.**

transpire, to excrete, as waste matter, in the form of perspiration, through the pores of the skin.

transplant, 1. to transfer, as an organ or a portion of tissue, from one part of the body to another or from one person to another. 2. to undergo transplanting, esp. in a manner specified. 3. the act of transplanting. 4. something that has been transplanted.

transudate, see **transudation.**

transudation, 1. the act or process of transuding. 2. a fluid or substance that has transuded.

transude, to pass or ooze through the pores of a substance, as, a membrane.

transverse, lying athwart; being in a cross direction.

transverse colon, the part of the colon that extends across the abdominal cavity from right to left, as distinguished from the ascending and descending parts.

transversectomy, the surgical excision of a transverse process of a vertebra.

transverse process, a lateral extension of a vertebra.

transvestism, the practice of wearing or the compulsion to wear clothes appropriate to the other sex.

transvestite, a person addicted to transvestism.

trapezium, a bone of the wrist, so named from its shape.

trapezius, each of a pair of large flat triangular muscles of the back of the neck and adjacent parts serving to draw the head back or to the side and move the shoulders.

trauma, 1. a wound; a bodily injury produced by violence or shock; the condition produced by this. 2. a disordered or disturbed state, either mental or behavioral, which is an effect of stress or injury, and which sometimes has a lifelong effect; a shock.

traumatic, of or pertaining to trauma.

traumatism, any morbid condition produced by a trauma.

traumatize, 1. to damage, as tissues, by force or by chemical or other agents.

2. to produce a trauma or shock in, as in a person's brain.

travail, 1. the pain and labor involved in childbirth. 2. to suffer the pangs of childbirth.

treatment, the manner of proceeding in applying medicinal remedies or surgery to cure an illness.

tremble, 1. any condition or disease characterized by continuing trembling or shaking. 2. to shake involuntarily.

trembler, one who trembles.

tremor, involuntary shaking of the body or limbs, as from fear, weakness, or fever; a fit of trembling.

tremulant, see **tremulous.**

tremulous, characterized by trembling.

trench fever, a recurrent rickettsial fever spread by body lice that occurred commonly among the troops during World War I.

trench foot, a condition of the feet resembling frostbite, frequently terminating in gangrene, and caused by exposure to wet and cold, as in trench warfare.

trench mouth, see **Vincent's angina.**

trepan, an early form of **trephine,** a surgical instrument.

trephine, 1. an improved form of a surgical trepan for removing disks of bone from the skull, having a transverse handle and a center pin that is fixed in the bone to steady the instrument during operation. 2. to operate upon with a trephine.

trepidation, trembling of the limbs, as in paralytic affections.

treponema, any spirochete of the genus **Treponema,** parasitic on man and other mammals, as the organism that causes syphilis.

triceps, a muscle having three heads or points of origin, esp. one extending along the humerus at the back of the upper arm.

trichiasis, an inversion or ingrowth of an eyelid, causing irritation of the eyeball by the eyelashes.

trichina, a parasite sometimes present as an encysted larva in the muscular tissues of man and certain animals, esp. pigs and rats.

trichiniasis, see **trichinosis.**

trichinize, to infect with trichinae.

trichinosis, a disease caused by the presence of the trichina worm, **Trichinella spiralis,** in the intestines and muscular tissues.

trichinous, 1. infected with trichinae. 2. pertaining to or of the nature of trichinosis.

trichoid, hairlike; capillary.

trichomonad, any flagellate protozoan, genus **Trichomonas,** parasitic in many animals and certain species in human beings.

trichomoniasis, 1. a trichomanadal infection. 2. vaginitis or urethritis in humans caused by **Trichomonas vaginalis** infestation, resulting in an inflammatory reaction characterized by a persistent discharge.

trichromat, a person having normal color or trichromatic vision.

trichromatic, having or pertaining to the combining or using of three colors, as in printing; characterized by or pertaining to three colors.

trichromatic vision, a normal condition in which the retina perceives all colors.

trichromatism, 1. a trichromatic condition. 2. the use or combination of three colors.

tricrotic, 1. having a threefold beat, as of the arterial pulse. 2. pertaining to such a pulse.

tricuspid, 1. having three cusps or points, as a tooth. 2. pertaining to the tricuspid valve. 3. a tricuspid tooth. 4. the tricuspid valve.

tricuspid valve, a valve of three cusps or folds that prevents the back flow of blood coursing from the right auricle into the right ventricle of the heart.

trifacial, see **trigeminal.**

trigeminal, noting or pertaining to the pair of fifth cranial nerves, each of which divides into three main branches to supply the sensory nerves of the face and head.

trigeminal neuralgia, see **tic douloureux.**

trigonal, of, relating to, or in the shape of a triangle; triangular.

trigone, a triangular space, esp. the one at the base of the bladder.

trilabe, a three-pronged surgical forceps used to remove foreign substances, as stones, from the bladder.

trinitroglycerin, see **nitroglycerin.**

triplet, one of three children born at the same birth.

trismus, a species of tetanus affecting the under jaw with spastic rigidity.

triturable, capable of being pulverized.

triturate, to reduce to fine particles or powder by rubbing, grinding, bruising, or the like.

trituration, any triturated substance, esp. a mixture of a medicinal substance with sugar or milk, triturated to an impalpable powder.

trocar, a perforating surgical instrument, specifically a sharp-tipped rod used to insert a cannula for drawing off fluid from a body cavity.

trochanter, a prominence or process on the upper part of the femur, to which a muscle is attached.

trochanteric, relating to a trochanter.

trochar, see **trocar.**

troche, a small usually medicinal cake or lozenge made of sugar, mucilage, and some drug, to be gradually dissolved in the mouth.

trochlea, a pulleylike structure or arrangement of parts affording a smooth surface upon which another part glides, as the surface of the inner condyle of the humerus, with which the ulna articulates.

trochlear, belonging to or connected with a trochlea; forming a trochlea; pulleylike.

trombidiasis, a state or condition of being overrun with chiggers.

tromomania, see **delirium tremens.**

trophic, 1. of or pertaining to nutrition. 2. concerned in nutritive processes.

trophoblast, a special layer of cells external to the ectoderm of the embryo and having to do with embryonic nutrition.

true rib, one of the seven upper ribs in man directly attached by cartilages to the sternum.

truncal, of or pertaining to the trunk.

trunk, 1. the body of a human being considered apart from the head and limbs; the torso. 2. the main body of an artery, nerve, or the like, as distinct from the branches.

truss, a belt with an affixed pad, used to support a hernia.

truth serum, a drug, as scopolamine or one of certain barbiturates, used to induce a state in which a subject will talk freely when questioned, as about criminal involvement or about repressed memories in psychotherapy.

trypanosoma, see **trypanosome.**

trypanosome, any of the minute flagellate protozoans constituting the genus **Trypanosoma,** parasitic in the blood of man and other vertebrates, and often causing serious diseases, as sleeping sickness, the infection being transmitted by the bite of a tsetse fly.

trypanosomiasis, any disease caused by infection with trypanosomes.

trypsin, the protein-splitting enzyme of the pancreatic juice, capable of converting proteins into peptone, used in medicine and to peptonize milk.

trypsinogen, a pancreatic secretion converted into trypsin by enzyme action.

tryptic, of or pertaining to trypsin.

tryptophan, an essential amino acid in proteins, requisite in the nutrition of humans.

tstetse, a fly of southern Africa, genus **Glossina,** which is the intermediate host or transmitter of the trypanosomes causing sleeping sickness and other diseases in man and domestic animals.

tsutsugamushi disease, an infectious rickettsial disease usually occurring in the Orient, caused by the microorganism **Rickettsia tsutsugamushi,** or **Rickettsia orientalis,** and transmitted by mites.

tubal, of or pertaining to a tube or tubes; tubular.

tubal pregnancy, a pregnancy occurring in one of the fallopian tubes.

tube, any hollow cylindrical vessel or organ.

tubercle, 1. a small, firm, rounded nodule or swelling. 2. the characteristic lesion of tuberculosis.

tubercle bacillus, a short, slender, rodlike, often slightly curved bacterium, **Mycobacterium tuberculosis,** the cause of tuberculosis.

tubercular, 1. of, pertaining to, or of the nature of a tubercle or tubercles; characterized by tubercles. 2. pertaining to or characterized by small rounded nodules or tubercles. 3. pertaining to tuberculosis; tuberculous. 4. a person afflicted with tuberculosis.

tuberculate, having tubercles; tubercled.

tuberculation, 1. the formation of tubercles. 2. the disposition or arrangement of tubercles. 3. a growth or set of tubercles.

tuberculin, a sterile liquid prepared from cultures of the tubercle bacillus, used in the diagnosis and treatment of tuberculosis.

tuberculin test, a test for a hypersensitive reaction to tuberculin indicating present or past tubercular disease.

tuberculoid, resembling tuberculosis or a tubercle.

tuberculosis, (TB), 1. an infectious disease affecting any of various tissues of the body, caused by the tubercle bacillus, and characterized by the production of tubercles. 2. this disease when affecting the lungs.

tuberculous, see **tubercular.**

tuberosity, a rough projection or protuberance of a bone, as for the attachment of a muscle.

tubular, 1. see **tubal.** 2. noting a respiratory sound resembling that produced by a current of air passing through a tube.

tubule, see **tube.**

tubulous, 1. having the form of a tube. 2. containing or composed of tubes.

tularaemia, see **tularemia.**

tularemia, a disease of rabbits, squirrels, and other rodents, caused by a bacterium, **Pasteurella tularensis,** transmitted to man by insects or by the handling of infected animals, and causing prolonged intermittent fever and swelling of the lymph nodes.

tularemic, of or pertaining to tularemia.

tumefaction, 1. the act of tumefying or swelling, or the state of being tumefied. 2. a swollen part; a swelling.

tumefy, to become or to cause to become swollen or tumid.

tumescence, the state of becoming swollen.

tumescent, becoming swollen; swelling; slightly tumid.

tumid, swollen, enlarged, or distended, as a body organ or part.

tumor, an abnormal or morbid swelling in any part of the body; a more or less circumscribed morbid growth of new tissue, not due to inflammation, and differing in structure from the part in which it grows.

tunic, any covering or investing membrane or part, as of an organ.

tunica, see **tunic.**

turbid, foul with extraneous matter; cloudy; not clear.

turbinal, scroll-like; a turbinate bone.

turbinate, pertaining to certain scroll-like spongy bones of the nasal passages.

turbinated, shaped like an inverted bone.

turgescent, growing turgid; in a swelling state.

turgid, swollen; distended beyond its natural state; inflated.

turgor, the state of being swollen or filled out.

tussive, of or relating to a cough.

twelfth cranial nerve, the hypoglossal nerve, one of a pair that gives motor innervation to the tongue.

twilight sleep, a state of semiconsciousness produced by hypodermic injection of scopolamine and morphine usually to effect relatively painless childbirth.

twin, one of two children born at the same birth.

twinge, to affect with sudden, sharp pain or pains, as in body or mind.

twitch, 1. to be suddenly contracted, as a muscle. 2. to move or make motion with a jerk. 3. a brief involuntary contraction of the muscles; a short quick pull; a jerk.

tyloma, a callosity.

tympanal, see **tympanic.**

tympanectomy, the surgical excision of the tympanic membrane.

tympanic, of or pertaining to the tympanum.

tympanic bone, a bone of the skull supporting the tympanic membrane and enclosing part of the tympanum or middle ear.

tympanic membrane, a membrane separating the tympanum or middle ear from the passage of the external ear. Also called **eardrum.**

tympanites, a distention of the abdomen from a collection of air or gas in the intestines or the peritoneum.

tympanitic, of or pertaining to tympanites.

tympanum, 1. the middle ear. 2. the tympanic membrane.

tympany, see **tympanites.**

typhlology, the area of scientific knowledge concerning blindness.

typhoid, 1. an infectious, often fatal, febrile disease, characterized by intestinal inflammation and ulceration, caused by a specific bacillus, **Salmonella typhosa,** which is usually introduced with food or drink. 2. of or pertaining to typhoid fever.

typhoid fever, see **typhoid.**

typhus, an acute infectious disease characterized by great prostration, severe nervous symptoms, and a peculiar eruption of reddish spots on the body, caused by the microorganism **Rickettsia prowazeki,** and transmitted by fleas and lice.

typhus fever, see **typhus.**

tyrocidine, a complex crystalline antibiotic produced by the bacterium **Bacillus brevis,** used in the treatment of bacterial infections.

tyrosinase, a catalytic enzyme containing copper and found in plant and animal tissue, which acts in the oxidation of tyrosine in the natural production of pigments, as melanin.

tyrosine, a common amino acid, isolated by protein hydrolysis.

ula, see **gum.**

ulaemorrhagia, see **ulemorrhagia.**

ulalgia, pain in the gums.

ulatrophia, recession of the gums.

ulcer, a sore open either to the surface of the body or to a natural cavity, and accompanied by the disintegration of tissue and usually the formation of pus.

ulcerate, to make or to become ulcerous.

ulceration, 1. the action or progress of ulcerating, or

the state of being ulcerated. 2. an ulcer or a group of ulcers.

ulcerous, 1. pertaining to or of the nature of an ulcer or ulcers. 2. characterized by the formation of ulcers. 3. affected with an ulcer or ulcers.

ulcus, see **ulcer.**

ulemorrhagia, bleeding from the gums.

ulitis, an inflammation of the gums.

ulna, the long bone of the forearm that is on the side opposite the thumb.

ulnad, in the direction of the ulnar bone..

ulnar, of or relating to the ulnar artery, bone, vein, or nerve.

ulocarcinoma, a carcinoma of the gums; cancer of the gums.

ulorrhagia, see **ulemorrhagia.**

ulosis, scarring; formation of scar tissue.

ulotrichous, 1. pertaining to the crisp- or woolly-haired groups of people. 2. having such hair.

ultramicroscope, an instrument for rendering visible, by means of diffractive effects, objects too small to be seen by the ordinary microscope.

ultramicroscopic, 1. beyond the power of or too small to be seen with a regular microscope. 2. of or pertaining to an ultramicroscope.

ultrared, see **infrared.**

ultrasonic, of or pertaining to frequencies above the range of human audibility, or above 20,000 vibra-

tions per second.

ultrastructure, the submicroscopic, basic arrangement of protoplasm.

ultraviolet, 1. beyond the violet end in the visible spectrum, as of light rays with very short wavelengths, contrasted with **infrared.** 2. producing or pertaining to these rays. 3. ultraviolet radiation.

ultravirus, any filterable, ultramicroscopic virus.

umbilectomy, the surgical excision of the navel.

umbilical, 1. pertaining to the navel or umbilicus. 2. formed or located in the middle, like a navel. 3. central, esp. relating to the abdomen.

umbilical cord, a cordlike structure that passes from the navel of the fetus or embryo to the mother's placenta, carrying nourishment to and wastes from the fetus.

umbilicate, 1. navel-shaped. 2. having a navel or umbilicus.

umbilicus, see **navel.**

unciform, hooklike; having a curved or hooked shape.

unciform bone, a wedge-shaped bone of the wrist having a hooked process.

uncinariasis, see **ancylostomiasis.**

uncinate, hooked; bent at the end like a hook.

uncinus, that which is formed, shaped, or structured like a hook.

unconscious, 1. not conscious or aware of. 2. temporarily devoid of consciousness or not having the mental faculties awake. 3. a general term for the mental processes that are not conscious.

unconsciousness, the condition of being unconscious.

unction, 1. the act of anointing, esp. for medical purposes. 2. an unguent or ointment.

unctuous, 1. of the nature of, resembling, or characteristic of an unguent or ointment. 2. oily; greasy.

uncus, 1. a hooklike structure. 2. a special part of the brain.

underhung, 1. projecting beyond the upper jaw, as applied to the under or lower jaw. 2. having this projection of the jaw.

undersized, of a size or stature less than normal, usual, or average.

undertaker, one whose business it is to prepare the dead for burial and to take charge of funerals.

underweight, 1. weight deficiency. 2. weight below average. 3. having only a weight deficiency.

undinism, a mental state in which the libido is awakened by running water, urination, or the sight of urine.

undulant, wavelike; fluctuating.

undulant fever, see **brucellosis.**

undulate, to have a wavy motion; to rise and fall in waves; to move in curving or bending lines.

undulation, 1. the act of undulating. 2. a waving motion.

undulatory, pertaining to undulation; having an undulating character; moving in the manner of waves.

unfruitful, not producing offspring; barren.

ungual, pertaining to or resembling a fingernail or toenail.

unguent, any soft preparation or salve, either liquid or semiliquid, applied to sores and wounds; an ointment.

unguiculate, having nails or claws, as distinguished from hoofs.

unguinal, see **ungual.**

unguis, a fingernail or toenail.

unhealthy, 1. lacking health; not sound and vigorous of body; habitually weak or indisposed. 2. unfavorable to the preservation of health, as unsanitary living conditions.

uniaxial, having one axis.

unibasal, having one base.

unicellular, consisting of a single cell; exhibiting only a single cell, as a protozoan.

unilateral, pertaining to one side only.

unilocular, having only one cell or chamber.

uniocular, pertaining to or having only one eye.

uniovular, developed from one ovum; see **identical twins.**

unipara, a female who has had only one pregnancy.

uniparous, a female who has given birth to only

one child.

unipolar, pertaining to a nerve cell having a single pole or process, esp. those of the spinal column.

unipotent, said of a cell, having the ability to develop into only one kind of cell or tissue.

unisexual, 1. of or pertaining to only one sex. 2. having only male or female organs in one individual.

unnerve, 1. to deprive of nerve, force, or strength. 2. to deprive of composure, as with shock.

unstable, lacking in emotional control.

urachal, of or pertaining to the urachus.

urachus, an epithelioid cord surrounded by fibrous tissue connecting the urinary bladder with the fetal allantois.

uracil, a crystalline heterocyclic compound, obtained usually by hydrolysis of nucleic acid and used in growth research.

uracrasia, any disordered condition of the urine. See **enuresis.**

uraniscochasma, see **cleft palate.**

uraniscoplasty, plastic surgery to repair a cleft palate.

uraniscus, see **palate.**

urate, a salt of uric acid.

uratic, of or pertaining to urate.

uraturia, an excessive amount of urates in the urine.

urea, the chief nitrogenous constituent of urine and the principal end product of protein metabolism in the body.

ureal, of or pertaining to urea.

ureameter, a device for measuring the amount of urea contained in urine.

urease, an enzyme that decomposes urea with the formation of ammonium carbonate, used in measuring the amount of urea in urine and blood.

uredo, see **urticaria.**

uremia, a toxic condition resulting from the retention in the blood of waste products that should normally be eliminated in the urine.

uremic, of, pertaining to, or characterized by uremia.

ureometer, see **ureameter.**

uresis, see **urination.**

ureter, the duct or tube that conveys the urine from the kidney to the bladder.

ureteral, of or pertaining to the ureter.

ureteralgia, pain in the ureter.

ureterectasis, dilation of the ureter.

ureterectomy, the surgical excision of the ureter.

ureteritis, an inflammation of the ureter.

urethra, a tube extending from the bladder that serves to convey and discharge urine and that, in the male, discharges semen also.

urethratresia, occlusion of the urethra in the newborn, which prevents the passing of urine.

urethrectomy, the surgical removal of the urethra or

part of it.

urethremphraxis, a urethral obstruction.

urethritis, an inflammation of the urethra.

urethroplasty, repair of the urethra by surgery.

urethrorrhagia, hemorrhage from the urethra.

urethroscope, an instrument providing an illuminated view of the urethra for examination.

urethroscopic, of or pertaining to the urethroscope.

urethroscopy, the examination of the urethra by means of a urethroscope.

urge, 1. an involuntary, natural, or instinctive impulse. 2. the act of urging.

uric, pertaining to or obtained from urine.

uric acid, a nitrous, soluble, crystalline acid, found in urine, used in its natural state for agriculture, and extracted or synthesized for both agriculture and industry.

urinal, a vessel used as a receptacle for urine, esp. that of a bedridden person.

urinalysis, the chemical analysis of urine.

urinary, of or pertaining to urine or to the organs connected with its secretion and discharge.

urinary bladder, the distensible membranous organ or sac that receives, holds, and discharges urine.

urinary organs, the organs concerned with the secretion and excretion of urine: the kidneys, the ureters, the urinary bladder, and the urethra.

urinary tract, see **urethra.**

urinate, to discharge or pass urine.

urination, the act of urinating.

urine, the liquid secretion of the kidneys, which is conducted to the bladder by the ureters and discharged through the urethra.

uriniferous, conveying urine.

uriniferous tubule, a tubule of the kidney that carries urine.

urinologist, see **urologist.**

urinometer, an instrument used to determine the specific gravity of urine.

urinoscopy, see **uroscopy.**

urinous, of, pertaining to, or resembling urine or its qualities, as color or odor.

urochrome, the yellow pigment that colors urine.

urocystic, of or relating to the urinary bladder.

urocystitis, see **cystitis.**

urogenital, noting or pertaining to the urinary and genital organs.

urography, X-ray photography of any part of the urinary tract after introduction of radiopaque dyes.

urolith, a urinary calculus.

urologic, of or pertaining to urology.

urologist, a specialist in examining and treating disorders of the urinary organs.

urology, the field of medicine devoted to the study, diagnosis, and treatment of any malfunction or disease of the urinary tract.

urometer, see **urinometer.**

uroncus, a swelling, cyst, or tumor containing urine.

uropyoureter, an infected ureter with an accumulation of urine and pus.

uroschesis, retention of urine with the inability to pass it.

urosepsis, septic poisoning caused by escape of urine into tissue other than the urinary tract.

urticant, inducing itching or stinging.

urticaria, a disorder of the skin characterized by transient eruptions of itching wales, caused by an allergy.

urticarial, of or relating to urticaria.

uteralgia, pain in the uterus.

uterectomy, see **hysterectomy.**

uterine, pertaining to the uterus or womb.

uteritis, an inflammation of the uterus.

uteroplasty, plastic surgery to repair the uterus.

uteroscope, a device used for examining the uterus.

uterotome, a surgical instrument used for uterotomy.

uterotomy, the surgical incision of the uterus.

uterus, the organ in females that serves as a protective place for the ovum while it develops into an embryo or fetus; the womb.

utricle, the larger of two sacs in the membranous labyrinth of the inner ear.

utricular, pertaining to or of the nature of a utricle; baglike; having a utricle or utricles.

utriculitis, an inflammation of the utricle.

utriculus, see **utricle.**

uvea, the vascular or middle layer of the eye, consisting of the ciliary muscle, the choroid, and the iris.

uveal, of or pertaining to the uvea.

uveitis, an inflammation of the uvea.

uvula, 1. a small, conical, fleshy projection suspended from the soft palate over the root of the tongue. 2. any similar structure, esp. at the neck of the bladder.

uvular, relating to the uvula.

uvulatomy, the surgical removal of the uvula.

uvulitis, an inflammation of the uvula.

vaccinal, pertaining or due to vaccine or vaccination.

vaccinate, 1. to inoculate with cowpox vaccine to produce immunity to smallpox or mitigate its attack. 2. to inoculate with microorganisms of any other disease. 3. to practice or perform vaccination as a preventive action.

vaccination, 1. the act of vaccinating. 2. inoculation with vaccine.

vaccine, modified microorganisms used for preventive inoculation.

vaccinia, see **cowpox.**

vaccinial, resembling vaccinia.

vacciniform, see **vaccinial.**

vacciniola, a secondary skin eruption, occasionally following vaccinia.

vaccinogenous, producing vaccine or pertaining to the production of vaccine.

vaccinophobia, a pathological fear of being vaccinated.

vacuolate, containing a vacuole or vacuoles.

vacuolation, 1. the formation of vacuoles. 2. the state of being vacuolate. 3. a system of vacuoles.

vacuole, a space or cavity within the protoplasm of a cell.

vacuous, empty; without contents.

vagal, of or pertaining to the vagus.

vagina, 1. the canal in females leading from the exterior genital orifice to the uterus. 2. an organ or a part having sheathlike characteristics.

vaginal, 1. of or pertaining to a sheath. 2. of or pertaining to the vagina.

vaginalitis, an inflammation of the tunica of the testicles.

vaginate, possessing a sheath; sheathed; enveloped by a sheath.

vaginectomy, 1. the surgical removal of the tunica of a testis. 2. the surgical excision of the vagina or a part of it.

vaginismus, spasms of the vagina from contraction of surrounding muscle fibers.

vaginitis, an inflammation of the vagina.

vaginodynia, pain in the vagina.

vaginoplasty, surgery on the vagina.

vaginoscope, an instrument for examining the vagina.

vaginoscopy, the visual examination of the vagina using a vaginoscope.

vaginotomy, a surgical incision of the vagina.

vagus, either of the tenth pair of cranial nerves extending down through the neck and thorax to the upper part of the abdomen, providing sensory, motor, or secretory impulses through its branches to the larynx, lungs, heart, stomach, and abdominal viscera.

valerian, 1. any of the perennial herbs constituting the genus **Valeriana,** as **Valeriana officinalis,** the root of which yields a drug formerly used as a sedative and an agent to check spasms. 2. the drug obtained from the root of the plant.

valeric, of, obtained from, or relating to valerian.

valeric acid, an acid extracted from the roots of the valerian plant or made synthetically, and used in perfumery and medicines.

valetudinarian, 1. a person of an infirm or sickly constitution. 2. one who is seeking to recover health. 3. one who is overly concerned with poor health.

valetudinarianism, the state of being valetudinarian.

valgus, 1. a condition of turned or twisted leg or foot bones, as knock-knee or bowleg. 2. one so afflicted.

valine, an amino acid, occurring as white, water-soluble crystals derived from the hydrolysis of proteins and used as a dietary supplement in medicine.

vallate, having a surrounding ridge or elevation.

vallecula, a furrow, as on the back of the tongue.

vallecular, of or pertaining to a vallecula.

valval, of or pertaining to a valve.

valvar, see **valvular.**

valvate, 1. furnished with or opening by a valve or valves. 2. serving as or resembling a valve. 3. possessing valves.

valve, a structure within a hollow organ that opens to allow the passage of a fluid in one direction or shuts to prevent its return, as the valves of the heart.

valvotomy, the surgical incision of a valve.

valvular, containing valves; having the character of, pertaining to, or acting as a valve.

valvule, a small valve or a similar structure.

valvulitis, an inflammation of a valve, esp. a valve of the heart.

vaporizer, 1. a person or thing that vaporizes. 2. a mechanism for converting a liquid, esp. a medication for respiratory ailments, into a fine spray or vapor.

varicella, see chicken pox.

variciform, resembling a varix.

varicocele, a varicose enlargement of the spermatic cord veins of the scrotum.

varicocelectomy, the surgical excision of a portion of the scrotum to remove a varicocele.

varicose, 1. abnormally dilated, as a vein. 2. pertaining to or affected with varicose veins. 3. resembling or having the characteristics of a varix.

varicose veins, an enlarged, swollen, and knotted condition of the veins, usually observed in the legs.

varicosity, the state or condition of being varicose.

varicotomy, the surgical removal of a varicose vein.

varicula, a varix in the veins of the conjunctiva of the eye.

variola, see **smallpox.**

variole, a shallow pit or depression like the mark left by a smallpox pustule.

varioloid, 1. resembling smallpox. 2. pertaining to a mild form of smallpox. 3. a mild form of smallpox, esp. as occurring in persons who have been vaccinated or who have previously had smallpox.

varix, an abnormal dilation of a vein or other vessel of the body, usually accompanied by distortion; a varicose vein.

varus, a deformity of a bone or joint, esp. bowleg.

vas, a vessel or duct.

vascular, pertaining to or containing the system of vessels or ducts that convey fluid, as blood.

vascularity, the condition of being vascular.

vasculitis, an inflammation of a blood vessel or other vessel.

vasculum, a small vessel.

vas deferens, the duct that transports sperm from the testis into the urethra for ejaculation.

vasectomy, the surgical excision of the vas deferens or of a portion of it.

Vaseline, a translucent, yellow or whitish, semisolid petroleum product, or a form of petrolatum, used in various preparations for medicinal and other purposes (trademark).

vasifactive, forming new vessels.

vasiform, resembling or having the characteristics of a vas.

vasitis, an inflammation of the vas deferens.

vasoconstriction, a narrowing of the blood vessels.

vasoconstrictive, causing constriction of blood vessels.

vasoconstrictor, 1. serving, when stimulated, to constrict blood vessels, as certain nerves. 2. a drug or other agent causing constriction of blood vessels.

vasodepression, the lowering of blood pressure by dilatation of blood vessels.

vasodilatation, dilatation of, esp. small, arteries.

vasodilator, 1. serving, when stimulated, to dilate or relax blood vessels. 2. a drug, nerve, or other agent that causes relaxation or dilatation of blood vessels.

vasoinhibitor, a drug or other agent that hinders vasomotor nerve action.

vasoinhibitory, tending to depress vasomotor action.

vasoligation, ligation of a vessel; a surgical operation, usually on the vas deferens, which, if done on both sides, causes sterility.

vasomotor nerves, nerves distributed over the muscular coats of the blood vessels, regulating their inner diameter and causing vasoconstriction and vasodilatation.

vasoparesis, a weakness or partial paralysis of the vasomotor nerves.

vasopressor, adrenalin or other substance producing a rise in blood pressure by causing a constriction of artery muscles.

vasosection, 1. the surgical excision of a blood vessel or part of it. 2. see **vasectomy.**

vasospasm, spasm of a blood vessel.

vasostimulant, exciting vasomotor action.

vasotomy, a surgical incision of the vas deferens.

vasotrophic, pertaining to or concerned with the nutrition of the blood vessels.

vector, a carrier of a disease-producing microorganism, as certain insects.

vegetate, to grow or increase by abnormal growth, as an excrescence.

vegetation, an abnormal growth or excrescence, such as seen on the heart valves in endocarditis.

vehicle, an innocuous substance used as a medium for medical ingredients; an excipient.

vein, one of the branching vessels or tubes of the circulatory system conveying blood from various parts of the body to the heart; loosely, any blood vessel.

veined, having or showing veins; characterized by venation; streaked.

veining, an arrangement of veins or veinlike markings.

veinlet, a small vein branching off from a large vein.

velamen, a membranous covering; a velum.

velar, of or pertaining to a velum, or veil, esp. of the palate.

vellication, a twitching or spasm of muscular fibers.

velosynthesis, see **staphylorrhaphy.**

velum, see **velamen.**

vena, see **vein.**

vena cava, either of two large veins discharging

into the right atrium of the heart.

venenous, poisonous.

venereal, 1. of or pertaining to venery. 2. arising from or connected with sexual intercourse with an infected person, as, venereal diseases. 3. adapted to the cure of such diseases, as, a venereal remedy. 4. infected with or suffering from venereal disease.

venereal disease, (VD) any disease contracted from an infected person by means of sexual intercourse.

venereologist, a physician specializing in the treatment of venereal diseases.

venereology, the area of medical science concerned with the study and treatment of venereal disease.

venereophobia, pathological fear of contracting venereal disease.

venesection, see **phlebotomy.**

venin, any one of the poisonous constituents of snake venom.

venine, see **venin.**

veniplex, a network of veins.

venipuncture, the puncturing of a vein, either for intravenous medication or feeding, or for drawing a blood sample for analysis.

venom, the poisonous fluid secreted by certain animals and introduced into the bodies of other animals or man by biting, as in the case of snakes, and stinging, as in the case of scorpions, wasps, or bees.

venomous, 1. having a venom-producing gland or glands, as a venomous insect. 2. capable of causing a poisonous bite or sting.

venous, 1. of or pertaining to the blood that is transported back to the heart through veins, characterized by the absence of oxygen and the presence of carbon dioxide, and of a darker color than arterial blood.

venous hum, the hum heard when listening at a larger vein, esp. of the neck, with a stethoscope.

vent, 1. the external excretory opening, as the anus. 2. any outlet.

venter, 1. the abdomen or belly. 2. a bellylike cavity or concavity, as of bones. 3. a bellylike protuberance, as of muscles.

ventral, belonging or pertaining to the belly or the abdomen, or to the surface of the body opposite to the dorsal or back side.

ventricle, 1. any of various hollow organs or parts in the body, esp. one of the two cavities of the heart that receive the blood from the auricles and propel it into the arteries. 2. one of a series of connecting cavities of the brain, continuous with the central cavity of the spinal cord.

ventricose, 1. swelled out,

esp. unequally on one side. 2. possessing a protruding abdomen.

ventriculus, 1. see ventricle. 2. a hollow organ for digestion; the stomach.

venula, a small vein.

venular, of or relating to a venula.

venule, see **venula.**

vergence, movement of one eye with reference to the other.

vermicide, an agent or drug used to destroy intestinal worms, esp. parasitic worms.

vermicular, 1. pertaining to worms. 2. resembling a worm, esp. in shape or movement. 3. having wormlike, wavy tracks.

vermiform, see **vermicular.**

vermiform appendix, a fingerlike vestigial appendage projecting from the end of the cecum, varying in length from three to six inches, and present in man and some other mammals. See also **appendix.**

vermifuge, a medicine or agent that expels parasitic intestinal worms.

vermin, 1. any of certain undesirable noxious small animals. 2. animal parasites collectively.

verminous, infested with, pertaining to, caused by, or characteristic of vermin.

vermis, see **worm.**

verruca, 1. any wart. 2. any wartlike prominence or projection.

verrucose, 1. warty. 2. having little knobs or warts on

the surface.

verrucous, see **verrucose.**

version, 1. the spontaneous or manual turning of a fetus in the uterus, to facilitate delivery. 2. a condition in which the uterus is turned from its normal position.

vertebra, any of the 33 bones or segments composing the spinal column, consisting typically of a more or less cylindrical body and an arch with various processes, forming a foramen through which the spinal cord passes.

vertebral, 1. of or pertaining to a vertebra or the vertebrae. 2. spinal. 3. composed of vertebrae, as the spinal column.

vertebral column, see **spinal column.**

vertebrate, 1. having vertebrae, a backbone, a spinal column, or, in the embryo, a notochord. 2. belonging to the Vertebrata, a division of animals comprising fishes, amphibians, reptiles, birds, and mammals.

vertebration, a vertebrate development; a segmented backbone.

vertebrectomy, the surgical excision of a vertebra or part of one.

vertex, the crown or top of the head.

vertical, pertaining or related to the top of the head.

vertiginous, affected with vertigo; tending to cause vertigo.

vertigo, a disordered condition in which a person feels that he or his immediate environment is whirling about; dizziness.

vesica, a bladder, esp. the urinary bladder.

vesica fellea, see **gallbladder.**

vesical, of or pertaining to the bladder.

vesicant, 1. a blistering substance or agent. 2. producing blisters.

vesicate, to raise vesicles or blisters on; to blister.

vesication, the formation of blisters.

vesica urinaria, see **urinary bladder.**

vesicle, 1. a small bladder-like structure or cavity. 2. a small sac or cyst. 3. a small bladder or bladder-like air cavity. 4. a circumscribed elevation of the epidermis containing serous fluid.

vesicocele, see **cystocele.**

vesicotomy, see **cystotomy.**

vesicular, 1. of or pertaining to vesicles. 2. having the form of a vesicle. 3. characterized by or consisting of vesicles.

vesiculate, 1. characterized or covered with vesicles. 2. of the nature of a vesicle.

vesiculation, the condition of forming or having vesicles.

vesiculectomy, the surgical excision of the whole or part of a vesicle, esp. the seminal vesicle.

vesiculitis, an inflammation of a vesicle.

vessel, a tube or duct, as an artery, vein, or the like, containing or conveying blood or some other bodily fluid.

vestibular, of or pertaining to a vestibule.

vestibule, 1. any of various cavities or channels regarded as forming an approach or entrance to another cavity or space, as, the vestibule of the ear. 2. to provide with a vestibule or vestibules.

vestige, a degenerate or imperfectly developed organ or structure having little or no utility, but which in an earlier stage of the individual or in ancestral forms performed a useful function.

viable, capable of sustaining independent life, as a normal newborn child; possessing the ability to grow and develop.

vibrate, to move to and fro; to oscillate.

vibratile, capable of vibrating or being vibrated.

vibration, the act or state of vibrating or being vibrated; a quiver or tremor.

vibrator, an electrical device that vibrates and is used for massage.

vibratory, concerned with vibration; marked by vibrations.

vibrissae, long bristlelike hairs located around the mouth and nostrils.

vicarious, pertaining to a body organ assuming a function that it does not normally perform.

view, 1. the power of seeing or perception. 2. sight. 3. the range of vision.

villi, minute, wormlike vascular processes on certain membranes. (Plural of villus.)

villiform, having the form of villi.

villosity, 1. the condition of being villous. 2. a villous surface or coating.

villous, 1. abounding in villi. 2. covered with fine hairs or a woolly substance.

villus, one of the minute hairlike vascular processes on certain membranes.

Vincent's angina, an acute inflammation of the tonsils, the floor of the mouth, and esp. the gums, characterized by ulceration, swelling, fever, and other fever symptoms, often resulting in deterioration of the gums and loss of teeth. Also called **trench mouth.**

vinculum, see **ligament.**

viosterol, a vitamin D preparation used in medicine, made of irradiated ergosterol dissolved in oil.

viral, of, relating to, or as a result of a virus.

viremia, a condition in which viruses are present in the blood.

virile, of, pertaining to, or characteristic of a man; masculine or manly.

virilia, the male sex organs.

virilism, a disorder in which male secondary sexual characteristics, as facial hair, develop in a female.

virologist, a scientist who deals in virology.

virology, the science that deals with viruses and the diseases they cause.

virosis, an infection or disease caused by a virus.

virucidal, of or pertaining to a virucide.

virucide, an agent capable of stopping the activity of or destroying viruses.

virulence, 1. an actively poisonous or malignant quality. 2. the ability of a microorganism to produce disease. 3. venomous hostility.

virulent, 1. malignant; actively or highly poisonous or infectious. 2. having the ability to produce disease, as a bacterium.

viruliferous, conveying or producing a virus.

virus, 1. any of a class of submicroscopic filterable pathogens that cause disease in all life forms and depend upon the host's living cells for their growth and reproduction, considered to be either living organisms or borderline nucleoprotein units that can generally penetrate a fine filter. 2. a virus disease.

viscera, 1. the soft interior organs contained in the cavities of the body, esp. those of the abdomen and thorax, including the lungs, heart, stomach, and intestines. 2. in popular usage, the intestines or bowels.

visceral, 1. of or pertaining to the viscera. 2. affecting or situated within the viscera. 3. having the character of viscera.

viscid, sticking or adhering, and of a glutinous consistency.

viscometer, an instrument for ascertaining the viscosity of fluids.

viscosimeter, see **viscometer.**

viscosity, the state or quality of being viscous.

viscous, 1. sticky, adhesive, thick, or glutinous. 2. of a glutinous character or consistency.

viscus, any internal organ in one of the body cavities; the singular of viscera.

vision, 1. the act, power, or faculty of seeing. 2. sight. 3. the ability to imagine and prepare for the future.

visual, of or pertaining to vision.

visual acuity, sharpness of vision as formulated from a comparison of the distance (usually 20 feet) from a chart at which the patient sees the smallest letters possible for him with the distance at which a normal eye would see those letters.

visual adaptation, the aptitude of the eyes to adjust themselves to changed conditions of light.

visual field, the area within which objects are visible to the fixed eye.

visual purple, see **rhodopsin.**

vital, 1. of or pertaining to life, as, vital functions or processes. 2. being the seat or source of life, as, the vital parts or organs.

3. necessary to life.

vitals, internal parts or organs of the body essential to life.

vital signs, respiration, pulse, and temperature.

vital statistics, facts or figures relating to significant aspects of human existence, as births, deaths, and incidence of disease.

vitamin, one of several organic substances occurring in minute quantities in natural foods and necessary for metabolism, the lack of which causes various diseases.

vitamin A, a terpene, fat-soluble alcohol, obtained from egg yolk and certain other animal products, prescribed for night blindness and for protecting epithelial tissue.

vitamin B$_c$, folic acid.

vitamin B complex, an important group of vitamins including vitamin B$_1$, vitamin B$_2$, and others that are water-soluble.

vitamin B$_1$, thiamine.

vitamin B$_2$, riboflavin.

vitamin B$_6$, pyridoxine.

vitamin B$_{12}$, a water-soluble, crystalline vitamin, obtained from milk, eggs, liver, fish, and meat, which treats pernicious and other anemias and is used as nutriment.

vitamin C, ascorbic acid.

vitamin D, any of a group of fat-soluble vitamins often prescribed for treatment of rickets, whose common sources are fish-liver oils, milk products, eggs, and ultraviolet irradiation of ergosterol.

vitamin E, a vitamin found in wheat germ and other grains.

vitamin G, riboflavin; vitamin B$_2$.

vitamin H, biotin.

vitamin K, a vitamin found in many green vegetables, necessary for normal blood clotting.

vitamin P, a vitamin found in paprika and citrus fruits, which helps to maintain capillary and cell wall permeability.

vitellin, a protein in the yolk of eggs.

vitiligo, a disease in which smooth white patches form on various parts of the body because of the loss of natural pigment.

vitreous, of or pertaining to the vitreous humor of the eye.

vitreous body, see **vitreous humor.**

vitreous chamber, the part of the cavity of the eyeball behind the lens.

vitreous humor, the transparent gelatinous substance filling the body of the eyeball behind the crystalline lens.

vivisect, to dissect the living body of, as an animal. 2. to practice vivisection.

vivisection, the dissection of, or otherwise experimentation on, a living animal, esp. for the purpose of ascertaining or demonstrating some fact in physiology or pathology.

vocal cords, either of two pairs of membranous ligaments projecting into the cavity of the larynx, the edges of which can be drawn together and made to vibrate by the passage of air from the lungs, thus producing vocal sound.

voice, the sound or sounds uttered by living creatures, esp. by human beings in speaking, shouting, or singing.

voice box, see **larynx.**

voiceprint, a spectographic record of modulation, amplitude, and duration of human speech sounds, used chiefly in criminological identification.

volar, relating to the palm of the hand or the sole of the foot.

volsella, a surgical forceps with a sharp pointed hook at the end of each blade.

voluntary, subject to or controlled by the will, as voluntary muscles.

volvulus, a torsion or twisting of the intestine causing intestinal obstruction.

vomer, a bone of the skull in most vertebrates, forming a large part of the nasal septum.

vomerine, of or pertaining to the vomer.

vomit, 1. to eject the contents of the stomach through the mouth; to throw up. 2. the act of vomiting. 3. the matter ejected in vomiting.

vomitory, 1. inducing vomiting. 2. emetic. 3. pertaining to vomiting.

vomiturition, ineffectual efforts to vomit; the vomiting of but little matter.

vomitus, the matter ejected in vomiting.

vulnerability, susceptibility to injury, infection, or illness.

vulnerable, capable of being wounded; liable to injury; subject to being affected injuriously or attacked.

vulnerary, used in healing or curing wounds.

vulnus, an injury or a wound.

vulsella, see **volsella.**

vulva, the female external genital organs.

vulval, of or relating to the vulva.

vulvar, see **vulval.**

vulvitis, an inflammation of the vulva.

wad, a soft mass of fibrous material, as cotton, used for surgical dressing.

waist, the part of the human body between the ribs and the hips.

waiting room, an area provided for the use of persons waiting, as in a physician's office.

wakeful, indisposed or unable to sleep.

wale, a stripe or ridge produced on the skin, as by the stroke of a whip.

walker, a framework designed to support and aid an invalid or elderly person in walking.

walleye, see **strabismus, leukoma.**

walleyed, 1. having one or both eyes with little or no color, as the result of a light-colored or white iris or of white opacity of the cornea. 2. having eyes in which an abnormal amount of the white shows, because of divergent strabismus.

wan, having a pale or sickly color; pallid; indicative of or showing fatigue, emotional distress, illness, or the like.

wart, a small, dry, hard, nonmalignant lesion of the skin.

Wassermann test, a test used for the detection of syphilis.

waste, 1. to wear down or reduce in bodily substance, health, or strength. 2. to emaciate or enfeeble. 3. excrement.

wasting, sapping the bodily strength, as a wasting disease.

water blister, a blister containing a fluid that is clear, watery and devoid of blood or pus.

water brash, see **heartburn.**

waters, see **amniotic fluid.**

water-soluble, having the property of dissolving in water, as many organic compounds.

wax, see **ear wax.**

waxen, pallid or pale, as the complexion.

waxy, pertaining to the degeneration of body tissue resulting from a buildup of waxlike, insoluble protein deposits in some organs; characteristic of amyloid.

weal, see **wale.**

wean, to accustom to do without the mother's milk as food, as a young child.

weanling, a child; a newly weaned child.

welt, see **wale.**

Weltschmerz, a state of melancholy brought about by belief in inevitable disappointment; world-weariness; romantic pessimism.

wen, a nonmalignant tumor, esp. of the scalp, without inflammation and caused by blockage of a sebaceous gland.

wet nurse, a woman who suckles and nurses a child not her own.

wheal, see **wale.**

wheat germ, the embryo or germ of a grain of wheat, used particularly as a vitamin source.

wheeze, to breathe with difficulty and with a whistling sound.

wheezy, affected with or characterized by wheezing.

whelk, a pustule or pimple.

whiplash, an injury to the neck, caused by a sudden jerking of the head.

whipworm, any of certain parasitic nematode worms, of the genus **Trichuris,** having a long body tapered to a whiplike front end.

white blood cell, see **leukocyte.**

white corpuscle, see **leukocyte.**

white matter, nerve tissue, esp. of the brain and spinal cord, containing mostly myelinic nerve fibers, and nearly white in color, distinguished from **gray matter.**

white plague, tuberculosis, esp. pulmonary tuberculosis.

whitlow, see **felon.**

whooping cough, an infectious disease of the respiratory mucous membrane, esp. of children, characterized by a series of short, convulsive coughs followed by a deep inspiration accompanied by a whooping sound.

widow's peak, a point formed on the hairline of the forehead, usually in the middle, by the hair's growth.

will, the faculty or power of conscious and esp. of deliberate action.

willpower, strength of mind; determination; resoluteness.

windburn, discoloration or inflammation of the skin caused by excessive exposure to wind.

windpipe, see **trachea.**

wisdom tooth, a large back molar, so named because it usually appears when a person is nearing or has reached adulthood.

witch hazel, an alcoholic solution of an extract obtained from the bark of a North American shrub, used to treat bruises and sprains and as an astringent.

Wolffian body, see **mesonephros.**

womb, see **uterus.**

woolsorter's disease, pulmonary anthrax acquired by inhaling the spores of the bacterium **Bacillus anthracis,** contained in contaminated hair, esp. wool.

woozy, out of sorts physically, as from nausea.

word-blind, unable to understand written or printed words, even though able to see, write, speak, and understand spoken words.

word-blindness, see **alexia.**

word-deaf, unable to comprehend heard speech, because of cortical lesions.

word salad, the use of jumbled words without apparent meaning, usually occurring in people suffering from a psychosis.

worm, 1. any of various small invertebrates with more or less slender elongated bodies and without limbs, including the platyhelminths, nemahelminths, and annelids. 2. (pl.) a disease or disorder from the presence of parasitic worms in the intestines.

wound, a cut, breach, or rupture in the skin and flesh.

wrinkle, a small crease or fold in the skin.

wrist, the joint by which the hand is united to the arm, and by means of which the hand moves on the forearm; the **carpus.**

writer's cramp, a spasmodic muscle contraction affecting the fingers or hand of a person who has been writing excessively.

wryneck, see **torticollis.**

xanthemia, a yellow pigment in the blood.

xanthine, a crystalline nitrogenous compound, closely related to uric acid, found in urine, blood, and certain body tissues.

xanthinuria, excretion of xanthine in large amounts with the urine.

xanthochromia, a yellow discoloration of patches of the skin or of the spinal fluid.

xanthocyanopia, a form of color blindness in which the person can distinguish between yellow and blue but not between red and green.

xanthocyte, a cell containing yellow pigment.

xanthoderma, yellow skin.

xanthodont, yellow teeth.

xanthoma, a skin condition marked by small, yellow, raised plates or nodules, esp. in the eyelids.

xanthopsia, yellow-colored vision.

xanthuria, see **xanthinuria.**

X chromosome, the sex chromosome carrying or associated with female characteristics, which occurs in a paired state in the female cell and zygote, and with one Y chromosome in the male cell and zygote.

xenodiagnosis, a means of detecting a parasitic disease, as in humans, by feeding an uninfected insect or other host on material believed to be infected and later checking it for the disease or infection.

xenodiagnostic, of or pertaining to xenodiagnosis.

xenogenesis, the supposed production of offspring entirely unlike the parents.

xenogenetic, of or relating to xenogenesis.

xenophobia, a pathological fear of unfamiliar persons.

xeransis, a loss of moisture in the tissues; a gradual drying up.

xeroderma, see **ichthyosis.**

xeroma, see **xerophthalmia.**

xerophthalmia, a dry, red soreness or itching of the eyes, caused by an insufficiency of vitamin A.

xerophthalmic, of or pertaining to xerophthalmia.

xerostoma, excessive dryness of the mouth due to insufficient secretion of the salivary glands.

xiphisternum, the lowermost portion of the sternum.

xiphoid, related or referring to the xiphisternum.

xiphoiditis, an inflammation of the cartilage of the xiphisternum.

X-ray, to examine or treat, as a person, with X rays; to photograph with X rays.

X-ray photograph, a picture produced by X rays, esp. one used for medical diagnosis.

X rays, high-frequency electromagnetic rays of short wavelength, generated by the impact of high-speed electrons on a metal target, capable of penetrating solid masses, destroying living tissue, and affecting a photographic plate.

X-ray therapy, the treatment of certain diseases, as cancer, by the use of X rays.

yawn, to open the mouth involuntarily with a long inhalation of air, through drowsiness or dullness.

yawning, 1. wide open; gaping. 2. expressing boredom or fatigue by a yawn.

yaws, an infectious tropical disease caused by the spirochete **Treponema pertenue,** characterized by skin eruptions resembling raspberries.

Y chromosome, the sex chromosome carrying or associated with male characteristics, occurring with one X chromosome in males.

yeast, a yellowish, somewhat viscid semifluid substance consisting of the aggregated cells of certain minute fungi, used medicinally as a source of B-complex vitamins.

yellow fever, an acute, dangerous, often fatal, infectious disease of warm climates, transmitted by the bite of a mosquito of the genus **Aedes,** characterized by jaundice, vomiting, hemorrhages, and fever.

yoke bone, see **cheekbone.**

yolk, 1. the yellow part of an egg suspended in the

white. 2. food material in the form of protein and fat granules in the ovum of animals.

zein, a protein obtained from corn.

zelotypia, pathologically exaggerated zeal in supporting a cause.

zestocausis, cauterization by the use of steam.

zinc ointment, a preparation consisting of 20% zinc oxide in a base of white petroleum and paraffin, used to treat skin disorders.

zinc oxide, an amorphous white powder, primarily used in paint pigments and cosmetics, and as an antiseptic or astringent in medicine.

zinc white, see **zinc oxide.**

zincold, of, relating to, or resembling zinc.

zoanthropy, a mental illness in which the patient has the delusion that he is an animal.

zoetic, see **vital.**

zonesthesia, the feeling as if a cord constricted the waist; also called girdle pain.

zoonosis, a disease communicable from animals to man.

zoophagous, feeding on animals; carnivorous.

zoophobia, pathological fear of animals.

zooplasty, the surgical transplantation to the human body of tissue from a lower animal.

zoorastia, sexual relations of humans with animals. animals.

zoosperm, see **spermato-**

zoon.

zoster, see **herpes zoster.**

zosteriform, resembling herpes zoster.

zygapophysis, one of the articular processes upon the neural arch of a vertebra, usually occurring in two pairs, anterior and posterior, and serving to interlock each vertebra with the ones above and below.

zygoma, the prominence of the cheekbone, or the part that joins it to the cranium.

zygomatic arch, the arch in the bone beneath the orbit of the skull extending along its front or side.

zygomatic bone, a bone on each side of the face that forms a section of the zygomatic arch and its orbit.

zygomatic process, one of the bony processes that are joined to the zygomatic bone.

zygote, a cell formed by the union of two gametes, as an egg and a sperm; the fertilized ovum.

zymase, an enzyme in yeast that causes the decomposition of sugar into alcohol and carbon dioxide, and that may be obtained in the form of an extract.

zymogen, any of various substances that, by internal change, give rise to an enzyme.

zymology, the branch of science that deals with ferments and fermentation.

zymolysis, 1. the fermentative action of enzymes. 2. the resulting fermentation.

zymolytic, of or pertaining to zymolysis.

zymoplastic, producing an enzyme or enzymes.

zymosis, 1. fermentation. 2. a zymotic disease; the infective process by which certain diseases were once believed to evolve.

zymosthenic, tending to intensify the functional activity of enzymes.

zymotic, 1. of, pertaining to, or relating to fermentation. 2. denoting an infectious disease.